616.8 B R

D1076476

M

Mobilisation of the Nervous System

To Carol and Juliet

The cover artwork is based on a figure showing plexus formation in the brachial plexus. Adapted from Kerr A. T., 1918, *The Brachial Plexus of Nerves in Man — the Variations in its Formations and its Branches*. American Journal of Anatomy 23: 285

Mobilisation of the Nervous System

David S. Butler B. Phty, Grad Dip
Adv Manip Ther, M.A.P.A, M.P.A.A.

Lecturer, School of Physiotherapy, University of South
Australia, Adelaide

with a contribution by
Mark A. Jones B. S (Psych), R. P. T., Grad Dip
Adv Manip Ther, M. App. Sc. (Manipulative Therapy)

Lecturer, School of Physiotherapy, University of South
Australia, Adelaide

artwork by
Richard Gore Dip. Art

CHURCHILL LIVINGSTONE
MELBOURNE EDINBURGH LONDON TOKYO AND NEW YORK 1991

CHURCHILL LIVINGSTONE
Medical Division of Longman Group UK Limited

Distributed in Australia by Longman Cheshire Pty
Limited, Longman House, Kings Gardens, 95 Coventry
Street, South Melbourne 3205, and by associated
companies, branches and representatives throughout the
world.

First published 1991

ISBN 0-443-04400-7

National Library of Australia
Cataloguing in Publication data
Butler, David S. (David Sheridan), 1956–
  Mobilisation of the nervous system.

  Includes index.
  ISBN 0 443 04400 7.

  1. Nervous system. I. Jones, Mark A.
612.8

Library of Congress Cataloging-in-Publication Data

Butler, David S. (David Sheridan), 1956–
    Mobilisation of the nervous system/David S. Butler;
  with a contribution by Mark A. Jones; artwork by
  Richard Gore.
      p.   cm.
    Includes bibliographical references and index.
    ISBN 0-443-04400-7
    1. Nerves, Peripheral — Wounds and injuries.
  2. Stress (Physiology) 3. Manipulation (Therapeutics)
  4. Physical therapy. I. Jones, Mark A. II. Title.
    [DNLM: 1. Manipulation, Orthopedic. 2. Neurologic
  Examination — methods. 3. Peripheral Nerves —
  injuries. 4. Physical Therapy. 5. Stress, Mechanical. WL
  500 B985m]
  RD595.B88   1991
  615.8′2 — dc20
  DNLM/DLC
  for Library of Congress   91–385
                                                     CIP

Produced by Longman Singapore Publishers (Pte) Ltd

Printed in Singapore

Acknowledgments

Many people over a number of years have helped put this book together, some of whom may not be aware that they have helped.

Don Griffith, Ivor Cribb, Gwen Jull, Robyn Cupit, Marion Grover, Margaret Bullock, Geoff Maitland, Ruth Grant, Pat Trott, Mary Magarey, Sir Sydney Sunderland, Peter Wells, Megan Dalton, Robbie Blake, Paul Ryan, Paul Lew, Liellie McLaughlin, Bern and Ellen Guth, Libby Brooke, Ted Huber, Shirley Gore, Libby Gore, course members on the graduate diploma in advanced manipulative therapy in Adelaide over the last five years, the physiotherapy staff at the West Hill Hospital in Dartford, Kent. There are many others.

Thanks to photographers Itzik Yossef and Peter Cox from the South Australian Institute of Technology.

Thanks to librarians at the South Australian Institute of Technology, University of Adelaide, British Medical Library, West Hill Hospital and at the Institute of Neurology, London.

Special thanks to Helen Slater and Michael Shacklock for editing chapters and for constructive advice and support.

Special thanks to Louis Gifford and Philippa Tindle for stimulating my initial thoughts and for sharing ideas over the last 5 years.

Special thanks to Mark Jones for his superb contribution on clinical reasoning processes in manipulative physiotherapy.

A grateful acknowlegement to the music of Leonard Cohen, Bob Marley, Rembetico and Paco Peña.

My very special admiration and thanks go to Richard Gore for his devoted and diligent artwork.

Many thanks also to Judy Waters and John Macdonald from Churchill Livingstone. The mistakes are mine.

Despite all this dispensation of gratitude, by far the most is reserved for Juliet who has contended with more than anyone.

Preface

It seems remarkable that only 30 years have passed since Phalen's description of 'carpal tunnel syndrome' made it an easily recognisable clinical entity. Equally remarkable is that only 20 years have passed since the realisation that there are specific pathways for pain. Research from the last three decades has provided a mass of information about the nervous system; much of this information is still waiting to be sifted and analysed by those who have patient contact.

In the last ten years, some physiotherapists have not been idle either. In the search for better results and answers for symptom and sign mechanisms and treatment responses, many orthopaedically orientated physiotherapists have turned to the nervous system. A nervous system mobilisation treatment, based on clinical observations and research, is evolving. The examination carried out by many present day physiotherapists could well be called neuro-orthopaedic.

In retrospect, these changes seem logical. Why is manual therapy dominated by joint approaches? Surely not all the answers lie with the joint. It must take its place as just one of the innervated structures we deal with. Is it because the joint provides a convenient lever to hold on to? Are we at a stage in evolution that still sees manual therapy under the orthopaedic umbrella? I feel that many physiotherapists treat a joint, muscle or fascia yet forget it is connected to the nervous system. All structures are connected in some way to the nervous system and the nervous system has complex biomechanics just like the structures it innervates.

Some people have been instrumental in these developments. In physiotherapy, Geoff Maitland stands out. It was his open ended 'signs and symptoms' concept that inevitably drew his attention to what he called 'the pain sensitive structures in the spinal canal' and ultimately the development of the Slump Test as an assessment and treatment tool. It is the clinical reasoning processes inherent in Maitland's concept that have facilitated the development of material presented in this book. Maitland's texts are necessary companion texts to this book. Robert Elvey deserves credit for introducing the Upper Limb Tension Test into clinical use. This and the Slump Test have become more than just techniques. They created an awareness in a number of physiotherapists, myself included, that tension testing was not merely a diagnostic tool to test structures such as the disc. They had a far greater role because they tested the normal mechanics and physiology of the nervous system during body movements. This allowed greater recognition of the fact that if the nervous system's movement and elasticity were impaired, then very frequently symptoms could arise from its own tissues. Ultimately there could be repercussions for impulse traffic to and from non-neural tissues. The next step was to turn examination procedures into treatment techniques. The nervous system must have optimal mechanical functions just like the other structures in the body.

In medicine, some clinicians and researchers stand out, perhaps unwittingly. Although without an experimental basis, but by paying careful attention to his patients, Cyriax was able to develop the notion of 'dural pain'. In retrospect, and judging by the number of recent citations, Breig was ahead of his time with his work on the biomechanics of the central nervous system and with his insistence that we are only just beginning to realise the neurophysiological sequelae to adverse tension in the nervous system. Sunderland's work on the internal structure of peripheral nerve and the role of ischaemia in entrapment lesions stands out. His classic text, *Nerves and Nerve Injuries*, is as relevant for physiotherapists as it is for surgeons. The recent work on the role of vascular factors and axoplasmic transport in nerve injuries by Lundborg, Rydevik, Dahlin and their colleagues has afforded explanations to much which physiotherapists encounter clinically. Mackinnon & Dellon have furthered study on nerve compression and its treatment and are challenging the pathological bases of many syndromes such as de Quervain's tenosynovitis. Like Breig with the central nervous system, Mackinnon & Dellon are putting forward evidence that, in the peripheral nervous system, the clinical consequences of nerve injuries are greatly underestimated. In Australia, Bogduk has been of great assistance with anatomical studies clarifying spinal innervation. His writings demystify neuroanatomy for physiotherapists and doctors. These are among many others. Most would not realise that their work is of great significance to manual therapy. From a physiotherapist's perspective, there is an obvious link between these men and women in that they all realise the nervous system structure is related to function and one of those functions is movement.

Modern physiotherapists are in an awkward situation. Not only do they require knowledge of gross anatomy of the entire body, they also need to go to a microscopic level and understand the relevant microanatomy. It is at the microscopic level where answers to the existence of symptoms and responses to treatment exist. In this book I have presented information which I consider is relevant and necessary for a physiotherapist to mobilise and to understand some of the reasoning for the mobilisation of the nervous system. Some is rather basic knowledge, but unfortunately not taught in the physiotherapy schools — the emphasis was on orthopaedics. If it was taught, it was quickly forgotten because it was never practised clinically.

There is still much research to be done in order to unravel the problems of the nervous system. However, there is already much that is now accepted fact and can be integrated and used in assessment, treatment and prognosis. The blood/nerve diffusion barriers are an example. It would be gratifying if some of the information in this text could be used as a lever into research. There is no shortage of studies to be undertaken. It must be admitted that clear proof of the existence of neuropathy as outlined is not always available. Much of the assessment and treatment of the more minor nerve injury, where there is no proof of neural involvement, is at this stage, speculative and dependent on inference from clinical reasoning experiences. Still, recent research from the physiotherapy world is encouraging and I have great hope for the establishment of experimental validity of the structural differentiation procedures discussed throughout this book.

Clinical reasoning processes in manual therapy are discussed in some depth in this book. Because a 'recipe' treatment is not followed and each patient's treatment is dependent on the subjective and physical assessment findings and previous clinical reasoning experiences, this may mean that we are in some ways ahead of the literature. Already there is an enormous gap between the neuroscientists and those at the 'battlefront'; it is hoped that all realise the battlefront is not necessarily surgery. The link between physiotherapist and scientist is weak, in many areas missing, and in need of development.

Much of this work is directed at the peripheral nervous system (PNS), probably mirroring the available research work and present understanding of the central nervous system (CNS). More is known about the PNS. It is more accessible, has far better regenerative powers and is more amenable to movement than the more protected CNS. However, despite recent attention to the peripheral nervous system, due respect must be given to the CNS as a contributing factor to symptoms, signs and treatment responses. It is a sobering thought that, for every axon in the peripheral nervous system, there are 1000 in the central nervous system.

Physiotherapists have always had a role in the

treatment of severe nerve injury. However, what is emerging is an important role in the minor, but sometimes equally incapacitating, injury at the other end of the nerve injury spectrum — the neuropraxias, irritative lesions and injuries that may not even rate the label of neuropraxia. Hopefully this role will not only be in treatment but one of a contribution to scientific knowledge regarding these injuries.

Finally, this book has been written by a physiotherapist who is primarily a clinician and who has dabbled in the areas of biomechanics and pathology looking for answers to the clinical problems he encounters daily. I sometimes feel that I have only just scratched the surface.

Adelaide, 1991   D. B.

Contents

Introduction — towards a multifactorial
approach   xiii

PART I

The basis for adverse neural tension

1. Functional anatomy and physiology of the
   nervous system   3

   Introduction   3
   The peripheral nervous system   5
   The central nervous system   10
   Nervous system relations — spaces and
      attachments   16
   The basis of symptoms   19
   Circulation   19
   Axonal transport systems   25
   Innervation of the nervous system   26
   Summary   30

2. Clinical neurobiomechanics   35

   Introduction   35
   The spinal canal, neuraxis and meninges   37
   The Straight Leg Raise   41
   Upper limb adaptive mechanisms   43
   Autonomic nervous system adaptive
      mechanisms   44
   The concept of tension points   46
   Further biomechanical considerations   49

3. Pathological processes   55

   Injury to the nervous system   55
   Pathological processes   58
   Further consequences of nerve injury   64
   Minor nerve injury   69
   Other factors in adverse tension processes   69

4. The clinical consequences of injury to the
   nervous system   75

   Where can the pain come from?   75
   Signs and symptoms following neural
      injury   79
   Area of symptoms   80
   Kinds of symptom   82
   History   83
   Postural and movement patterns   84

PART II

Examination

5. Clinical reasoning   91
   Mark Jones and David Butler

   Introduction   91
   The clinical reasoning process   92
   Characteristics of expertise   95
   Analysing structures and contributing
      factors   96
   Inquiry strategies   98
   Structural differentiation   102
   Precautions and contraindications   104

6. Examination of nerve conduction   107

   General points   107
   Subjective neurological examination   108
   Physical examination of sensation   109
   Examination of motor function   115
   Further testing and analysis   122
   Tests of cord function   122
   Electrodiagnosis   123

7. Tension testing — the lower limbs and
   trunk   127

The concept of base tension tests   127
Passive Neck Flexion   128
Straight Leg Raise   130
Prone Knee Bend   136
The Slump Test   139

8. Tension testing — the upper limbs   147

Upper Limb Tension Test 1   147
Upper Limb Tension Test 2   153
Upper Limb Tension Test 3   156
Other upper limb tension tests   159

9. Application, analysis and further testing   161

Essentials of testing   161
The relevance of examination findings   161
Essential features of tension test analysis   163
Establishing sites of adverse tension   165
Taking tension testing further   167
Recording   171
Palpation of the nervous system   172
Classifications of nerve injury   175

PART III
Treatment and treatment potential

10. Treatment   185

History   185
General treatment points   185
Basic principles of mobilisation   187
The irritable disorder (pathophysiological dominance)   188
The non-irritable disorder (pathomechanical dominance)   190
Treatment of the interfacing structures   193
Commonly asked questions about treatment   194
Prognosis making   198
Communication   199

11. Self Treatment   203

Introduction   203
Self mobilisation   203

Some useful techniques   205
Posture   209
Prophylaxis   210

PART IV
Selected disorders and case studies

12. Adverse neural tension disorders centred in the limbs   213

Introduction   213
The extremities   213
The foot and ankle   214
The hand and wrist   218
Thoracic outlet syndrome   222
Meralgia paraesthetica   222
The nerve lesion in lower limb muscle tears   223
Peripheral nerve surgery   224
Repetition strain injury (RSI)   226

13. Adverse neural tension disorders based on the spinal canal   231

Nerve root injuries   231
Loss of spinal extension   235
Whiplash   236
Epidural haematomas   238
Coccydynia and spondylolisthesis   238
Post lumbar spine surgery   239
Headache   241
T4 syndrome   242
Trauma and inflammation of the neuraxis   243

14. Selected case studies   247

An unusual and vague foot pain   247
An example of extraneural pathology   251
The 'pain everywhere' kind — where to start?   253
A typical tennis elbow?   255
A passing mention of fingertip pain   258

Courses   259

Index   261

Introduction — towards a multifactorial approach

Joint-specific thinking is dominant in the systems of manual therapy in use in the world today. There are, however, other schools of thought which favour treatment via muscle or fascia. The obvious implications are that the best approach will be 'structure selective'. I believe that optimum open-mindedness in manual therapy must lead to a questioning of a one-structure approach in the treatment of so-called 'musculoskeletal' disorders.

In any neuro-orthopaedic disorder, it is impossible to have just one structure involved. For example, in the kind of pure nerve injury that might happen from a misplaced injection, there will probably be manifestations in non-neural structures related via impulse conduction and axoplasmic transport. The patient who turns and locks his or her neck is likely to have reflex spasm in associated neck musculature. The longer the neck stays locked, the greater the likelihood of there being changes in the associated muscles, in other structures and in affective responses. Still, at a certain stage of a disorder it is likely that a problem could be cured with treatment directed at one structure. However, in terms of speed of recovery and preventive management, it is doubtful that a one-structure approach will be optimal.

With a model using joint structure as the focus, acknowledgement of the role of the nervous system and its control of symptom presentation can be diminished, even belittled. The nervous system is certainly involved, directly or indirectly, in all patient problems. It could be injured and be a source of symptoms. Even if uninjured, it still carries the afferent impulses from non-neural structures and efferent signals for responses such as muscle spasm. Symptoms are an expression of the status of the tissues involved (e.g. joint, muscle, fascia, dura mater etc.), as conducted through the nervous system and modified by the environment. They provide the physiotherapist with invaluable clues to understand the patient's problem and discover the most effective management. Thus, attention to all potential factors influencing a patient's symptoms is essential and requires a model which is not dominated by any single structure, but rather, where all structures and contributing factors (e.g., environment and culture) are taken into account. Classic structural or direct approaches in manual therapy focus on one structure such as joint (e.g., Cyriax, McKenzie, Kaltenborn, early Maitland, chiropractics and osteopathy), or muscle (e.g., Janda and Lewit). Their survival is testimony to measures of success. However, other approaches without a structural focus which might be called 'facilitative' or 'indirect' (e.g., Proprioceptive Neuromuscular Faciliation, Feldenkrais, Alexander, psychological), are also successful in their results. These approaches could be said to attend more to the quality of movement rather than to specific structures or biomechanics. The point of this discussion is to encourage the use of a multifactorial approach to patient examination and management.

While one cannot hope to achieve expertise in all approaches, awareness and understanding of what is available will facilitate utilisation and consultation for the benefit of the patient and the physiotherapist. It is tempting to suggest the nervous system is the central system linking both the structural/direct and facilitative/indirect approaches as they both must communicate their effects via the nervous system. However, this could inhibit open-minded thinking, as it would if any other structure or system were considered 'central'. Present day scientific understanding of the processes involved in neuro-orthopaedic disorders are an unknown distance along the path to their total understanding. If we prematurely adopt what appears to be logical or obvious as absolute fact, it discourages our further search for knowledge and understanding. The intervertebral disc had long been considered a structure that is not innervated and hence not a direct source of symptoms. This has since been refuted (Bogduk et al 1981) and I am certain the story is still not finished. Historically, it has been the rigid and, at times, blind acceptance of a theory which has held up and misdirected the advancement of knowledge in science. Bergland (1985) has argued that, to the detriment of science, the nervous system has been wrongly seen as an electrical organ rather than a gland. Physiotherapists too, must have an open mind and consider the role of hormones in the function/dysfunction of our body and its subsequent expression in behaviour. They should, in this regard, consider whether they have the means of influencing hormone distribution by mobilising the nervous system and effecting the quality and quantity of the axoplasmic flow. It is essential that continued research explores all avenues.

Thus, we must take care to consider all possible structures and utilise both 'structural/direct' and 'facilitative/indirect' approaches. This book aims to present science, theory, concepts, hypotheses and techniques related to examination and treatment of the nervous system in neuro-orthopaedic disorders, but with full acknowledgement of and open-mindedness towards other structures and approaches.

REFERENCES

Bergland R 1985 The fabric of mind. Penguin, Melbourne
Bogduk N, Tynan W, Wilson A S 1981 The nerve supply to the human lumbar intervertebral discs. Journal of Anatomy 132: 39–56

PART I

The basis for adverse neural tension

1. Functional anatomy and physiology of the nervous system

INTRODUCTION

To interpret the signs and symptoms of injury to the nervous system accurately, a physiotherapist requires an understanding of its static and dynamic anatomy; and this understanding is also fundamental to safe and effective mobilisation.

This chapter is a study of the anatomy and physiology associated with movement of the nervous system. In the context, the study of movement of the nervous system is no different from that of joint or muscle. The nervous system is built primarily for impulse conduction. The main aim of the chapter is to show that the impulse conducting function is supported by anatomy that allows conduction while accomodating body movements.

Because this chapter has a bias toward the functional anatomy of the nervous system related to the function of its own movement, the all important function of impulse conduction may seem neglected. There are many worthwhile texts on this subject. Recent and recommended ones, among others, are Walton (1982), Mathers (1985) and Bowsher (1988).

The concept of the continuous tissue tract

The peripheral and central nervous systems need to be considered as one since they form a continuous tissue tract. For the majority of functions, any division into peripheral and central components can only be artificial.

The system is a continuum in three ways. Firstly, the connective tissues are continuous, although in different formats, such as epineurium and dura mater. A single axon can be associated with a number of these connective tissues. Secondly, neurones are interconnected electrically so that, for example, an impulse generated at the foot may be received at the brain. Lastly, the nervous system may be regarded as continuous chemically. The same neurotransmitters exist peripherally as centrally and there is a flow of cytoplasm inside axons.

Arguably, there is no other structure in the body with such connectedness. Stresses imposed upon the peripheral nervous system during movement are transmitted to the central nervous system. Conversely, tension can be conveyed from the central nervous system to the peripheral nervous system.

If the nervous system were to be considered as an organ rather than the multisegmented structure it is commonly thought to be, it would lead to a far better understanding of the system and of the pathomechanical and pathophysiological consequences of altering its mechanics. One of the greatest implications of 'organ thinking' is that, if there is some change in part of the system, then it will have repercussions for the whole system. The continuous tissue tract makes this inevitable.

The need for specialised anatomy

There is one outstanding difference between the mechanical features of the nervous system and the mechanical features of other body structures. That is, the nervous system carries impulses to and from those other structures. This feature underlines the importance of the normal mechanics of neural tissue and its associated connective tissues.

3

Humans are capable of highly skilled movements with the nervous system stretched or slack, stationary or mobile. Observation of dancers, or sportsmen and women, for example, makes this obvious. The nervous system not only has to conduct impulses during a remarkable range and variety of movements, it has to adapt mechanically during the movements. Some biomechanical facts help to emphasise this. The spinal canal is from 5 cm to 9 cm longer in flexion than extension (Inman & Saunders 1942, Breig 1978, Louis 1981). It may be even longer in hypermobile individuals. This rather remarkable variation in the length of the spinal canal and its repercussions on the tissues contained within is of great clinical importance.

Because of the continuous tissue tract, any limb movement must have mechanical consequences for nerve trunks and the neuraxis. (Neuraxis is a term used when the CNS is considered along its length irrespective of its bends and folds (Bowsher 1988)). Consider also what happens at the elbow and hip. Here, major nerves are on opposite sides of the axes of movement. So, in elbow flexion, while the ulnar nerve stretches, its counterparts, the median and radial nerves, must adaptively shorten. The same tissues, while still conducting impulses, undergo very different mechanical deformations. The reverse will obviously happen during elbow extension.

Peripheral nerves have to adapt to marked changes in the length of the nerve bed. For example, Millesi (1986) calculated that, from wrist and elbow flexion to wrist and elbow extension, the bed of the median nerve is approximately 20% longer. Somehow, the median nerve has to adapt to this and conduct impulses at the same time. Nerve trunks also need a protective mechanism from compressive forces. This is especially so where the trunks lie close to the exterior, such as cutaneous nerves, or where nerves run over bone, such as the common peroneal nerve at the head of the fibula.

It appears that nervous system mechanics go further than adapting to movement and protection from compression. The continuous tissue tract also has the ability to limit certain combinations of movement. A review of the anatomy

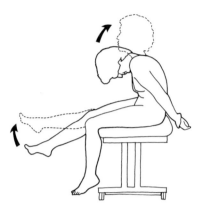

Fig. 1.1 In the Slump position the range of movement of knee extension will be dictated by the head position. With the neck extended, the subject can extend her knee further

and biomechanics in following chapters will show that it has a functional anatomy easily capable of such a purpose. A combination of movements, such as the Slump Test position (Fig. 1.1), is an example. This test is discussed in detail in Chapter 7.

Thus, to cater for this dual role of impulse conduction and a variety of related movements, complex anatomical adaptations which protect neurones and allow conduction in any desired posture or movement are inbuilt in the system. Such varying roles for a structure demands a complex functional anatomy.

Gross shape and features

There are two main kinds of tissue making up the nervous system: those associated with impulse conduction and those associated with support and protection of the impulse conducting tissues. Examples of the former are axons, myelin and Schwann cells, examples of the latter are the connective tissues such as neuroglia, the meninges and perineurium. These two kinds of tissues have an intimate relationship to allow for uninterrupted impulse conduction while the body moves.

Some gross features of neuroanatomy are relevant for a study of its mechanics. The peripheral nervous system requires more adaptive mechanisms than the central nervous system.

Much of the neuraxis and the meninges is protected by the cranium and, to a lesser degree, the spinal column. A noted problem area is where peripheral nerves join on to the less mobile neuraxis. Most peripheral nerves and trunks run deep and are on the flexor aspect of limbs. This keeps them close to the axes of movement as well as affording protection. The ulnar nerve at the elbow is a notable example of a nerve on the extensor aspect and is consequently vulnerable to injury.

Overall, and rather simply, the entire nervous system forms an 'H' on its side. Being a continuous tissue tract, this means that any tension placed at any part of the 'H' can be dissipated in two directions. Such thinking will be helpful in the examination of the mechanics of areas that contribute to adverse tension.

The peripheral nervous system forms many subdivisions and plexuses, both internal and external. The main purpose of this is to assemble the necessary sensory, motor and autonomic components to a nerve trunk. However, with a little 'mechanical thinking', the gross shape of the subdivisions and plexuses could also be seen as a convenient force distributor. Take the interconnections of the brachial plexus for example (Fig. 1.2). During movement, the mesh of nervous system keeps excessive forces away from a single branch. An even more complex branching of nerve fibres occurs inside the nerve trunks. This is discussed and illustrated later in this chapter.

In its course through the body, the nervous system comes in contact with many different structures: firm and unyielding, such as the radial nerve in the spiral groove of the humerus, or soft, such as the tibial nerve surrounded by posterior thigh muscles. The system also courses through tunnels that may be osseous, fibro-osseus or solely soft tissue. With injury, the nature of the surrounding structure will be consequential for the type and extent of injury.

THE PERIPHERAL NERVOUS SYSTEM

In this section, for convenience's sake, the nervous system is discussed under the traditional headings of the peripheral and central nervous systems. The peripheral nervous system is traditionally defined in anatomical terms as the cranial nerves (except the optic nerve), the spinal nerves with their roots and rami, the peripheral nerves and the peripheral components of the autonomic nervous system (Gardner & Bunge 1984). The peripheral nervous system is associated with Schwann cells; these are replaced by glial structures in the central nervous system.

The neurone

A neurone comprises a cell body (perikaryon), some dendrites and usually one axon. Axons are either myelinated or unmyelinated and are grouped together into bundles, or fascicles. Axons are usually referred to as 'nerve fibres'. The cytoplasm of the neurone, known as axoplasm, is contained, and flows within and around a system of microtubules and neurofilaments, within the axon. Each axon is surrounded by Schwann cells, which, in the case of the myelinated fibres, produce myelin and ensheath the axon. In non-myelinated fibres, one Schwann cell is associated with a number of axons whereas, in the myelinated fibres, the ratio is one Schwann cell per axon. Nodes of Ranvier interrupt the continuity of the sheath (refer to Fig. 1.3). This discontinuity in the myelin sheath allows rapid impulse conduction as the action potential leaps from one node to the next. An individual axon can extend the length of a limb, for example, from the cell body in a lumbar dorsal root ganglion to a synaptic terminal in the foot. Yet, even

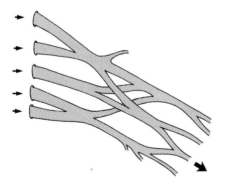

Fig. 1.2 The brachial plexus as a force distributor. Tension on one trunk will be distributed throughout the whole plexus

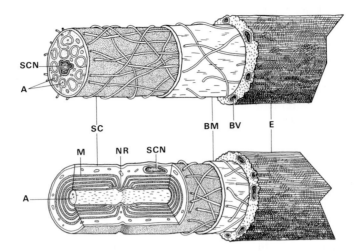

Fig. 1.3 Diagrammatic myelinated and unmyelinated neurones. A axons, BM basement membrane, BV blood vessel, E endoneurium, M myelin, NR node of Ranvier, SC Schwann cell, SCN Schwann cell nucleus

though the blood supply of the distal axon may be different from the cell body and the connective tissues differ, there is a special connectedness about the neurone — it is still the one cell. An abnormality in one part of the neurone will have consequences for the whole neurone. Surrounding the Schwann cells, or the Schwann/myelin complex in myelinated fibres, is a collagenous basement membrane, which, in turn, is surrounded by the endoneurium, the innermost of three connective tissue layers (Fig. 1.3).

Although the connective tissues combine their physical attributes and provide the nerve fibres with protection, these nerve fibres are also equipped to handle tensile and compressive forces. Axons run an undulatory course in the endoneurial tubules as do the fascicles in the epineurium. The slight undulatory course run by axons in the endoneurial tubules allows some stretch. These undulations cause an optical phenomenon known as the 'spiral bands of Fontana' — these bands disappear in areas of nerve compression (Mackinnon & Dellon 1988).

It seems as though the myelin sheath possesses features which serve a biomechanical purpose. When a nerve fibre is stretched, the internodal distance in the myelinated fibres expands, thus safeguarding the less protected node of Ranvier (De Renyi 1929, Landon & Williams 1963). With stretch, the lamellae of the myelin sheath

slide on each other. Clefts or incisures (incisures of Schmidt-Lantermann) in the myelin sheath run oblique to the axon, and part during nerve stretch; the axon cylinder being more elastic than the myelin (De Renyi 1929, Glees 1943, Robertson 1958, Singer & Bryant 1969) (Fig. 1.4). It is reasonable to assume that, if the axon is elongated, then its diameter will lessen. Friede & Samorajski (1969) calculated that the clefts would allow considerable elongation and changes in axon volume. Other than these mainly aged references, little attention has been directed to the biomechanical properties of the myelin sheath. However, there must be adaptive mechanisms. Those who treat by movement must

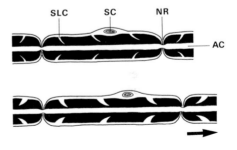

Fig. 1.4 Diagrammatic representation of the biomechanics of the myelin sheath. With stretch of a nerve fibre, the lamellae of myelin slide on each other and the Schmidt Lantermann Clefts (SLC) open up. AC axon cylinder, SC Schwann cell, NR node of Ranvier

also consider movement at this microscopic level. Given that minor demyelination is a possible source of ectopic impulse generation (Calvin et al 1982), abnormal biomechanics of the myelin sheath may also contribute.

Three kinds of nerve fibres are carried in peripheral nerve — motor, sensory and autonomic fibres. Motor fibres originate from cell bodies in the ventral horn of the spinal cord and terminate at the neuromuscular junction. Cell bodies of presynaptic sympathetic nerve fibres also lie in the ventral horn from cord segments T1 to T3. Postganglionic fibres arise from the sympathetic trunk. Sensory fibres originate from cell bodies in the dorsal root ganglia and terminate at receptors such as Meissner's corpuscles, Pacinian corpuscles or as free nerve endings. The proportion of fibres in each nerve depends on the function of the nerve. The median nerve and sciatic nerve, both destined primarily for the extremities, have the greatest proportion of autonomic fibres. Some nerves, such as the lateral femoral cutaneous nerve, are purely sensory, whereas there are no pure motor nerves. All nerves carry at least a few afferent fibres, perhaps from joint structures if not from muscle.

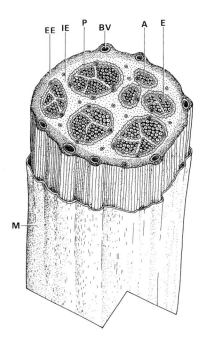

Fig. 1.5 The connective tissue sheath of a multifascicular segment of peripheral nerve. A axon, BV blood vessel, E endoneurium, EE external epineurium, IE internal epineurium, M mesoneurium, P perineurium

Endoneurium

Surrounding the basement membrane is the endoneurial tube: a distensible, elastic structure made up of a matrix of closely packed collagenous tissue (see Fig. 1.3). Note the endoneurium and the two outer connective tissue layers in Figure 1.5. The matrix contains fibroblasts, capillaries, Mast cells and Schwann cells. There is no evidence of any lymphatic channels (Sunderland 1978, Lundborg 1988).

Endoneurium plays an important role in the maintenance of the endoneurial space and fluid pressure, hence a constant nerve fibre environment. A slightly positive pressure is maintained in the space. Without lymphatics, any alteration in the pressure, as may occur with oedema (Ch. 3), could interfere with conduction and movement of the axoplasm (axoplasmic flow). According to some researchers (Granit & Skoglund 1945, Sunderland 1978), if the tubes become severely damaged, neural disorganisa-

tion, including neuroma formation and artificial synapses between neighbouring fibres, is possible.

The collagen fibril orientation in the endoneurium is essentially longitudinal — evidence that the endoneurium has a role in protecting the axons from tensile force. The three connective tissue sheaths, the endoneurium, perineurium and epineurium, all have collagen fibres arranged longitudinally, although with some cross fibres forming a lattice. Cutaneous nerves have a greater percentage of endoneurium, probably due to the extra cushioning a nerve requires when it is close to the surface (Gamble & Eames 1964).

Perineurium

Each fascicle is surrounded by a thin lamellated sheath known as the perineurium (see Fig. 1.5). Up to 15 layers may be present in mammalian nerve trunks (Thomas & Olsson 1984). There is no basal lamina between perineurial cells, and the cells overlap. Thus they form 'tight junctions'

(Thomas & Olsson (1984). Lundborg (1988) outlines the roles of the perineurium as:–

- Protecting the contents of the endoneurial tubes
- Acting as a mechanical barrier to external forces
- Serving as a diffusion barrier, keeping certain substances out of the intrafascicular environment.

With lamellae composed of collagen and a small amount of elastin, the perineurium is thought to be the structure most resistant to tensile force (Sunderland 1978). Much of the collagen fibres run parallel to the direction of the nerve fibre, although there are circular and oblique bundles which may protect the nerve from kinking when it has to go around an acute angle, as does the ulnar nerve at the elbow (Thomas 1963). The perineurium is the last peripheral nerve connective tissue sheath to rupture in tensile testing (Sunderland 1978). Although, recently, Kwan et al (1988) found that the perineurium of rabbit tibial nerve ruptured first under tensile testing while leaving the nerve grossly intact. Intrafascicular pressure has to be raised to approximately 300–750 mmHg before the perineurium will rupture (Selander & Sjostrand 1978). It is a tough, strong tissue. Its important role as a diffusion barrier is discussed later in this chapter.

Epineurium

This outermost connective tissue investment surrounds, protects and cushions the fascicles. Collagen bundles are arranged primarily in the longitudinal axis of the nerve trunk (Thomas & Olsson 1984). Longitudinally orientated elastic fibres close to the perineurium have been identified (Thomas 1963). Note in Figure 1.5 that epineurium keeps fascicles apart (internal epineurium) as well as forming a definite sheath around the fascicles (external epineurium). The internal epineurium facilitates gliding between fascicles — a necessary adaption to movement, especially when a peripheral nerve has to bend to an acute angle during a limb movement (Millesi 1986). The relative content of epineurium differs between

nerves and individuals (Sunderland & Bradley 1949). For example, there is more epineurium where nerve trunks cross joints, or in tunnel areas such as the carpal tunnel. Epineurium forms a distinct sheath, well differentiated from surrounding fascia. Considerable range of motion of the nerve trunk in relation to neighbouring fascia, as in the nerve bed, is allowed (McLellan & Swash 1976, Sunderland 1978, Wilgis & Murphy 1986). The amount of movement varies depending on the area of nerve trunk. At various positions along the trunk, the epineurium is anchored to the surrounding tissue.

The supporting connective tissues of peripheral nerve are highly reactive, far more than tendon, for example (Daniel & Terzis 1977). Cells within the connective tissues can react to injury by multiplying and synthesising collagen. Connective tissue can flourish and proliferate, supported by the well developed intrinsic circulation. A lymphatic capillary network exists in the epineurium, drained by channels accompanying the arteries of the nerve trunk (Sunderland 1978).

Quantities of fat exist in peripheral nerves and probably have a cushioning role. There is more fat in the sciatic nerve in the buttocks than elsewhere (Sunderland 1978). This fat disappears with wasting and may predispose the nerve to compression neuropathy.

All connective tissues of peripheral nerve are highly innervated (see page 29).

Mesoneurium

Mesoneurium is a loose areolar tissue around peripheral nerve trunks, so called because it resembled the mesentery of the small intestine (Smith 1966) (see Fig. 1.5). Van Beek & Kleinert (1977) suggested the tissue be called the 'adventitia' because nerve does not have a true mesentry as does the gut. In many areas, blood vessels enter the nerve via the mesoneurium. This tissue allows the peripheral nerve to glide alongside the adjacent tissue, plus, it can contract in an 'accordion like arrangement' (Smith 1966). In 1989, Sunderland acknowledged that a non-specialised fascial connective tissue exists around peripheral nerve and that this tissue provides a loose framework so the nerve can slide. Lundborg

(1988) referred to this as a 'loose conjunctiva like connective tissue'. Nerve movement will not always be the sliding type. As Sunderland (1989) pointed out, those familiar with injection techniques know the cord-like nerve can slip sideways away from the point of pressure. The mesoneurium is an important structure if the nervous system is thought of in mechanical terms. Its role is not yet completely understood. While the nerve probably slides through the mesoneurium to some degree, there are likely to be attachments both inside the mesoneurium and from mesoneurium to adjacent structures.

Fascicular arrangement in the epineurium

Nerves are not uniform structures. Fascicles run in a wavy course throughout the nerve trunk and form constantly changing plexuses within the trunk. Figure 1.6 shows this in a segment of musculocutaneous nerve. The position within the trunk differs as does the number and size of fascicles. An inverse relation exists between the number and size of the fascicles (Sunderland 1978). It does appear, however, that the fascicular mesh as described by Sunderland (1978) is more complex in the proximal portion of the nerve trunk and less so distally (Jabalay et al 1980). Together with assembling the required afferent and efferent constituents of a nerve branch, the constantly changing position within the trunk offers protection from compression and tensile forces, more so than if the fascicles ran in a straight line.

When a greater number of fascicles are present, a nerve is better protected from compressive forces (Fig. 1.7). The common peroneal nerve at the knee provides a nice example. At the knee

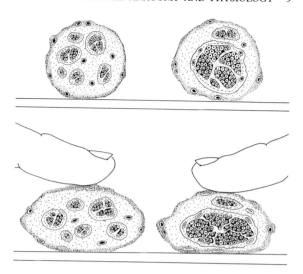

Fig. 1.7 Compression of the fascicles. Where a peripheral nerve is multifascicular, a greater pressure will be required to affect nerve fibres than where there is a small number of fascicles

crease the nerve is composed of approximately eight fascicles, yet a few centimetres further distally, at the head of the fibula, approximately 16 fascicles are present (Sunderland & Bradley 1949). At the head of the fibula the common peroneal nerve is subject to compressive forces; for example, it is rather inconveniently placed at bumper bar height. Also, the nerve is attached quite firmly to the head of the fibula, making it difficult to slip away from any external forces. There is also a greater amount of connective tissue in the common peroneal nerve at the head of the fibula (68%), compared to 51% in the popliteal fossa (Sunderland & Bradley (1949). In general, at least half of a peripheral nerve is connective tissue. The range is from 21% to 81%, with greater percentages present where a nerve is located near a joint (Sunderland 1978).

The significance of the fascicular arrangement is obvious for nerve surgery — some knowledge will be vital to get the best fascicular match during nerve suture. The significance is less so for physiotherapists. If the nervous system is palpated (Ch. 9) it will be easier to get a neural response in areas where there are few fascicles (see Fig. 1.7). In segments where there are a greater number of fascicles, it will require firmer palpation and the connective tissue may be symp-

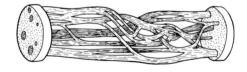

Fig. 1.6 The fascicular branching in the musculocutaneous nerve. From: Sunderland S 1978 Nerves and nerve injuries, 2nd edn. Churchill Livingstone, Edinburgh. With kind permission from the publishers and author

tomatic before the neural tissue. This may also assist in the interpretation of Tinel's sign (Ch. 6). If a nerve is tapped in an area where there are few fascicles, response from nerve fibres is more likely. I have used the interpretation of the fascicular arrangement as part of a hypothesis regarding the biomechanics of the nervous system. Simply, where the nervous system moves significantly in relation to interfacing tissues, such as in the mid humeral area, there is a smaller number of fascicles and less connective tissue than where the nervous system has better attachments, such as at the head of the fibula. With this ever changing intraneural plexus, the presentation of signs and symptoms may well be the 'luck of the draw' depending on which fascicles are injured. An injury of one part of a peripheral nerve trunk may have greatly differing clinical repercussions from a similar injury a centimetre or so further along the trunk.

The autonomic nervous system

The autonomic nervous system (ANS) is often the forgotten nervous system. Its division from the somatic nervous system must be regarded as artificial. It consists of two succeeding neurones. The axons of the first are known as 'preganglionic' fibres. They originate in the brain or spinal cord, lie in the lateral grey columns of the spinal cord and exit over some cranial nerves and ventral roots, synapsing in autonomic ganglia. The axons of cell bodies originating in the autonomic ganglia are referred to as 'post-ganglionic' and are distributed to glands and smooth muscle. Both preganglionic and post-ganglionic fibres are arranged into complementary sympathetic and parasympathetic divisions. Each preganglionic neurone may synapse with approximately 20 postganglionic neurones — surely an important factor in the diffuse dissemination of sympathetic activity (Williams & Warwick 1980). The autonomic nervous system to the limbs is a system of efferent nerve fibres. There is no evidence of any afferent fibres.

The sympathetic trunk and ganglia

The sympathetic trunk comprises two chains of preganglionic fibres, one on either side of the vertebral column, extending from the base of the skull to the coccyx. Some 21–25 ganglia are contained in the chain. A number of postganglionic fibres (rami communicantes) emerge from the ganglia and connect to the corresponding spinal nerve or to other fibres in the chain (Gardner & Bunge 1984).

The sympathetic ganglia are capsulated, the capsules being a continuation of the epineurium of attached branches. In the cervical spine, the chain is anterior to the transverse processes of the cervical vertebrae. In the thorax, it is anterior and attached to the head of the ribs, close to the costotransverse joints. Finally, in the abdomen, it is anterolateral to the bodies of the vertebrae. The chains are anterior to the sacrum and join together anterior to the coccyx (Williams & Warwick 1980). The location of the chain to axes of movement and its connection with adjacent structures will be important in body movement. These issues are discussed and illustrated in the section on biomechanics of the autonomic nervous system in Chapter 2.

The preganglionic fibres for the head and neck arise from segments C8 to T5. Those for the upper limb arise from T2 to T10 and those for the lower limb from T10 to L2. However, with the continuum of the chain, mechanical influences may be from further afield.

THE CENTRAL NERVOUS SYSTEM

Nerve roots

Nerve roots are considered to be more a part of the central than the peripheral nervous system. They involve the meninges, lack Schwann cells and receive at least half of their nutrition from the cerebrospinal fluid.

The connective tissues of nerve trunks are very different to those in the nerve roots, even though the same axon may be present as in the ventral roots. Many authors have drawn attention to the fact that the connective tissue coverings in nerve roots are much weaker, or not present at all. Thus, the suggestion arises, also based on clinical findings, that nerve roots are more susceptible to injury (Murphy 1977). Morphologically and physiologically, the connective tissues are different and no purpose is served by comparison. Nerve roots lack the connective tissues that are so much a part of a peripheral nerve. Gamble (1964) conducted an electron microscopy study and found that connective tissues of the nerve roots were more like the leptomeninges (arachnoid and pia mater) than that of the peripheral nerve trunk. In agreement, Park & Watanabe (1985), using a scanning electron microscope, observed that each rootlet, as it emerged, was ensheathed by a pial layer, the outermost of which formed a covering around individual fascicles. When examined under the microscope this resembled a 'wispy sheet of gauze'. Park & Watanabe (1985) have called these layers the 'radicular pia' and noted, under microscopy, that the open meshed nature of the sheath allowed free percolation of the cerebrospinal fluid (CSF).

This decrease in content and strength of the connective tissue structures does not mean that fibres in the nerve roots are left without protection. Otherwise it would seem that nerve root avulsion from the cord and severe injury to the nerve roots would be commonplace. For the most part, this does not happen. Injuries to nerve roots are commonly not from traction, but rather, indirectly from the neighbouring structures such as discs and zygapophyseal joints. It is extremely difficult to avulse nerve roots from the cord by applying tension onto nerve trunks and plexuses (Barnes 1949, Frykolm 1951). Observations of birth paralysis, where the injuries are in the brachial plexus and not at nerve root level, point to considerable safety mechanisms at root level. Tension and movement, which can be easily absorbed in peripheral nerve, is transmitted elsewhere at nerve root level. There are a number of features at nerve root level allowing this transmission.

1. The fourth, fifth and sixth cervical spinal nerves have a strong attachment to the gutter of their respective transverse process. Sunderland (1974) examined cadaver material from the lower cervical spine and found that, 'the neural structures and their coverings were not attached to the foramen'. The vertebral artery presses the spinal nerves back onto the gutters. Sunderland (1974), in his study of the cervical and upper thoracic spine, noted that such attachments were not evident elsewhere.

Extrathecal attachments of lumbosacral nerve roots have been well described (Spencer et al 1983, Tencer et al 1985) and are reviewed below. No comparison has been made between these attachments in the various regions of the body.

Although the nerve root complex is allowed movement in the intervertebral foramen, there are other areas of attachment, such as the midline dural attachments to the spinal canal (see page 17).

2. At segmental levels, dural and epidural tissues form a connective tissue sheath. The epidural tissues must include the epidural sheath described by Dommisse (1975) and Hasue et al (1983). Beyond the dorsal root ganglion, this sheath forms the epineurium and perineurium. The three peripheral nerve connective tissue sheaths do not join up exactly with the three meninges as is often taught. Functionally this arrangement would not be the best. The strong perineurium has no mechanical equivalent in the nerve roots, and if there were some means of tension transmission, it would be far too strong for the delicate arachnoid. The epidural tissues and the dura combine to form the epineurium and the outer layers of the perineurium. The endoneurium is a continuation of the pia (Shantaveerappa & Bourne, 1963; Sunderland, 1974). Haller et al (1971) noted the 'open endedness' of the perineurium in that its outer layers are continuous with the dura/arachnoid and the inner layers form the pial sheath (Fig. 1.8). This arrangement is best for force distribution together with preserving a constant environment around the nerve fibre. The perineurium can continue its diffusion barrier mechanisms with the dura and its contained CSF, and the blood nerve barrier of the endoneurial vessels is continued in some way with the pia mater. This junctional area is often misunderstood. Most descriptions of the area are of animals, especially rats.

3. The dural sleeve forms a plugging

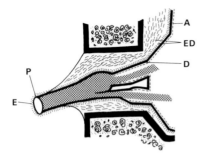

Fig. 1.8 The junctional zone between peripheral and central nervous systems. A arachnoid, D dura, ED epidural tissue, P perineurium, E epineurium. Not to scale. From: Sunderland S 1978 Nerves and nerve injuries, 2nd edn. Churchill Livingstone, Edinburgh. With kind permission from the publishers and author

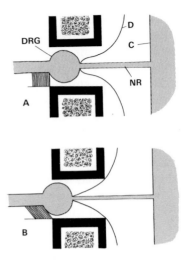

Fig. 1.9 Plugging of the intervertebral foramen. C cord, D dura mater, NR nerve root, DRG dorsal root ganglion. From: Sunderland S 1978 Nerves and nerve injuries, 2nd edn. Churchill Livingstone, Edinburgh. With kind permission from the publishers and author

mechanism. This not only stops the nerve roots being pulled out of the intervertebral foramen, it is also a convenient force distributor (Fig. 1.9). Plugging of the foramen occurs as the dural sleeve is pulled into the intervertebral foramen (Sunderland, 1974). Sunderland (1974) also noted that traction was finally transmitted to the cord via the denticulate ligaments and this partially eased the tension on the nerve roots.

4. Nerve roots also have their own inbuilt mechanisms in that they lie in undulations and are able to unfold. Cerebrospinal fluid (CSF) supplies approximately half of the nerve root's metabolic needs (Park & Watanabe, 1985). CSF also cushions and protects the roots (Louis, 1981; Rydevik et al, 1984). Individual fascicles within the nerve root have the ability to slide on each other as they do in peripheral nerve. The kinking and 'pig-tailing' in the blood vessels supplying the fascicles, further expanded upon and illustrated later in this chapter, provides plenty of evidence (Parke & Watanabe, 1985).

Some forces will ultimately be transmitted centrally. It is important to realise that both the connective tissues and the neural tissues will absorb the force.

It seems that nerve roots do not always have a straightforward exit from the spinal canal in the lower cervical and upper thoracic regions. There

are persistent reports in the literature of angulated nerve roots between C3 and T9 (Baldwin, 1908; Frykolm, 1951; Reid, 1958, 1960; Nathan & Feuerstein, 1970). Angulated or 'ascending' nerve roots mean the roots descend in the dural theca and then ascend to emerge from their respective intervertebral foramina (Fig. 1.10). Reid (1960) dissected 80 cadavers, 5 years old and over, and found that 71% had nerve roots running in an 'anomalous' direction. Nathan & Feuerstein (1970) reported an incidence of angulated nerve roots in 38 out of 50 cases. Reid (1960) noticed also that, by changing the flexion/extension position of the head, the roots could be made to run rostrally or caudally. This was more evident in younger cadavers. His results were derived from positioning the head in a representation of 'normal erect posture'. Extension increased the number of ascending roots. This occurrence is likely to place the roots and dural sleeves at risk during movement. An observation of Figure 1.10 shows that these angulated nerve roots will be at risk from movement in all directions. Angulated nerve roots may be, at least in part, a result from some pathology such as degenerative shrinkage of the spinal column or the dura being tethered below with the rest of the

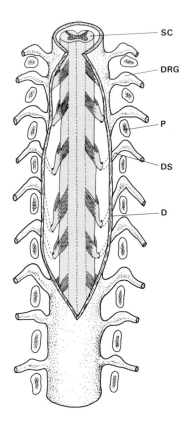

Fig. 1.10 Angulated course of nerve roots. D dura, DS dural sleeve, P pedicle, DRG dorsal root ganglion, SC spinal cord. Adapted from Nathan & Feuerstein (1970)

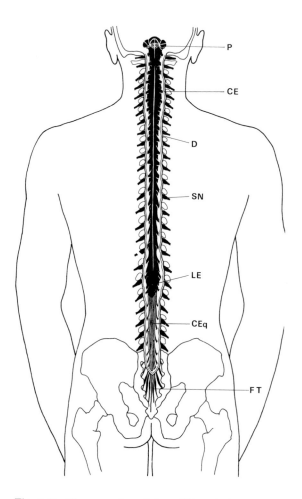

Fig. 1.11 The neuraxis and dura. CE cervical enlargement, CEq cauda equina, D dura, cut and reflected, FT filum terminale, P pons, SN spinal nerve LE lumbar enlargement. Adapted from Mathers (1985)

meninges and neuraxis adapting by angulating. In both studies, such changes were rarely noted in cadavers under the age of 25 years. It should be noted that Dommisee (1986) debated their existence.

The neuraxis

The neuraxis (spinal cord) is a continuation of the medulla oblongata. At approximately the L2 vertebral segment, it tapers to a point, forming the conus medullaris (Fig. 1.11). Roughly, the neuraxis occupies half of the space in each direction in the spinal canal (Hollinshead & Jenkins 1981). The ascending tracts are located in the periphery of the cord. This not only makes them more susceptible to compressive forces from herniated disc material or blood, for example, but also means they will have to contend

with greater amounts of movement. In spinal flexion, the posterior columns will need to move more than tracts on the anterior side of the neuraxis (Breig 1978), the axis of flexion/extension being well forward of the neuraxis. It seems likely that the opposite will happen during spinal extension. In spinal lateral flexion movements, tracts on the convex side will be stretched more than those on the concave side (Fig. 1.12).

Axons in the central nervous system are well protected by a variety of connective tissue structures, but, like peripheral nerve, the nerve fibres are not without their own intrinsic protection. In normal physiological movements the fibres have

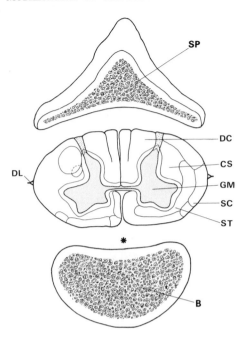

Fig. 1.12 Tracts of the cord — with the approximate location of the axis of flexion and extension. The dorsal columns will need to move further than the other tracts during flexion and extension. * approximate centre of rotation, B body, CS corticospinal tract, DC dorsal columns, GM gray matter, SC spinocerebellar tract, SP spinous process, ST spinothalamic tract, DL denticulate ligament

no problem keeping up with the body movements they control via conduction. Axons are not straight, as countless textbooks would have it, but are arranged in folds and spirals which straighten as the spinal cord elongates (Fig. 1.13). The posterior columns are more folded and twisted than the anterior columns since they are further away from the instantaneous axis of rotation than the other tracts (White & Panjabi, 1978).

Breig (1978) notes two methods of neuraxial adaptation to stretch:

- Unfolding and untwisting as axons straighten
- Movement in relation to neighbouring vertebral segments.

The cut end of fresh spinal cord will actually flow like a mucoid gel if devoid of connective tissue attachments (Breig 1978). Transfeldt & Simmons (1982) reported similar movement adaptive mechanisms present in the spinal cords of cats.

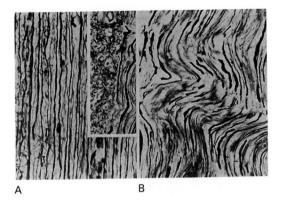

Fig. 1.13 The effect of elongation on a segment of human spinal cord taken from the area of the anterior median fissure and the anterior white commissure (× 525) A The effect of elongation as in spinal flexion. B The effect of shortening. Note separation of nerve fibres, in some areas increased thickness and because of the folding of the fibres, they cannot be followed throughout their length. From: Breig A 1978 Adverse mechanical tension in the central nervous system. Almqvist & Wiksell, Stockholm, with permission

The meninges

Three connective tissue membranes, known as meninges, surround the spinal cord. The inner two, the arachnoid and pia mater, are known as the leptomeninges. The much thicker outer layer is the dura mater (Figs. 1.14, 1.15).

Pia mater and arachnoid mater

These are very delicate membranes, far more so than the dura mater. A mesh, or lattice, of collagen fibres make up the pia and arachnoid maters. This allows stretch and some compression without kinking (Breig 1978) (Fig. 1.16). It thus offers protection to the neural elements while, at the same time, allowing a movement mechanism. This latticing is also present in the neuroglia of both grey and white matter and in lymph ducts within the neuraxis (Breig 1978). Pia mater is a continuous tissue, separating the CSF fluid of the subarachnoid space from the spinal extracellular fluid spaces. Arachnoid trabeculae cross from pia to the arachnoid. Nicholas & Weller (1988) documented the existence of an intermediate leptomeningeal layer between arachnoid and pia (see Fig. 1.14). They suggested that

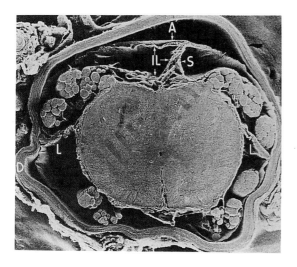

Fig. 1.14 Scanning electron micrograph of the lumbar spinal cord of a 15 month old child. L denticulate ligaments, D dura (note the layers) A arachnoid, S dorsal septum, IL intermediate leptomeningeal layer. From: Nicholas D S, Weller R O 1988 The fine anatomy of the human spinal meninges. Journal of Neurosurgery 69: 276–282, with kind permission from the publishers and authors

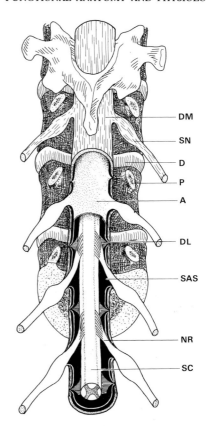

Fig. 1.15 Diagrammatic cutaway section of the spinal canal, meninges and spinal cord. A arachnoid, D disc, DL denticulate ligament, DM dura mater, NR nerve root, P pedicle (cut), SAS subarachnoid space, SC spinal cord, SN spinal nerve

this layer, along with the arachnoid trabeculae, may serve to dampen pressure waves in the CSF during body movements. The arachnoid must contain the CSF and it appears well adapted to do this, consisting of multiple layers with some of the membranes fused (Waggener & Beggs 1967).

CSF, subarachnoid and subdural spaces

The subarachnoid space (see Fig. 1.14, 1.15) contains CSF. CSF has a primarily nutritive role, but also assists with cord biomechanics. It is thought to act as a hydraulic cushion, surrounding the cord and nerve roots with fluid and thus offering protection during body movement (Louis 1981). The significance of the mechanical role is evident by the complications that may follow dural puncture or durotomy, either accidental or intentional. The CSF cushion is lost with CSF leakage through the resulting dural defect. The consequent traction on cranial dura and blood vessels (all innervated) is likely to cause symptoms (Spielman 1982). The dural theca is able to change its capacity and shape rapidly in re-

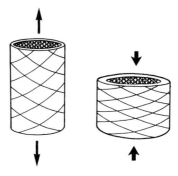

Fig. 1.16 The collagen arrangement of the arachnoid and pia allows some stretch and compression

sponse to changes in intracranial, intra-abdominal and intrathoracic pressure (Martins et al 1972). This indicates that CSF has considerable dynamics in response to movement. Due to the relatively incompressible shape of the spinal canal, the shape of the dural theca must change as the pressure in the epidural venous plexus does. The inclusion of pathology inside the spinal canal could easily interfere with these mechanisms.

The subdural space (see Fig. 1.14) is a potential space, containing a little serous fluid, which probably allows sliding of the arachnoid on the dura.

Dura mater

Dura mater is the outermost meningeal layer and by far the toughest and strongest (see Figs 1.14 & 1.15). It consists primarily of collagen fibres and some elastin fibres aligned in the longitudinal axis and in layers (Tunturi 1977). This gives the dural theca great axial strength, although it is considerably weaker in the transverse direction (Haupt & Stofft 1978). Surgeons have often commented that, if the dura tears, it tears in an axial direction. Dura mater is a remarkable tissue, it does not deteriorate with age and is suitable as a material for heart valve replacement (van Noort et al 1981). This suggests a toughness, combined with good vascularisation and innervation. Dural innervation and its consequences are discussed later in this chapter and in Chapter 4.

The spinal dural theca is a continuous enclosed tube running from the foramen magnum to the filum terminale at the coccyx. At segmental levels there are prolongations — the nerve root sleeves. Spinal dura mater is continuous with the cranial dura.

Other spinal canal contents

The epidural space contains the internal vertebral venous plexus, discussed in more detail later in this chapter. There are also fat deposits. Fat deposits are localised in the intervertebral foramina and in the posterior recess between the ligamenta flava (Parkin & Harrison 1985). The fat appears to be regulated by the space available. In spinal stenosis the amount of fat in the spinal canal diminishes.

NERVOUS SYSTEM RELATIONS — SPACES AND ATTACHMENTS

A relationship between component parts exists in any moving structure. In the nervous system, this is defined by the space around the component parts and the connections between component parts. Adequate space is needed around the neural and connective tissue and there must be enough space at rest and during physiological movements of the spine. Within the spinal canal, the CSF-filled subarachnoid space, the potential subdural space and the epidural space are the main considerations. The integrity of these spaces is essential for movement.

The nervous system is attached to surrounding tissues and structures. These attachments differ in different areas of the body, but are repeatable anatomical features and are essential for normal range of movement of the nervous system. This is an important concept for physiotherapists. Just as the knee, for example, has collateral and cruciate ligaments to guide and limit the movement of the knee, a similar role is played by the connections of the nervous system. Alterations in the structure and nature of the spaces and attachments are likely to be of clinical significance in adverse tension syndromes. Attachments need consideration in terms of those attaching neural tissue onto connective tissue, such as the denticulate ligaments, and those attaching connective tissue (and thus the neural tissue) onto other structures, such as the dural ligaments.

Hasue et al (1983) have shown that the space around neural tissue, both in the spinal canal and the intervertebral foramen, is less in males than in females. These authors also point out that developmental and degenerative stenosis is more common in the male.

The external connections of the dura

Inside the cranium, the dura mater is loosely adhered to the central portions of the cranial bones and tightly adhered at the suture levels (Murzin & Goriunov 1979). The spinal dura mater is continuous with the cranial dura mater. There is a firm attachment at the foramen magnum and, at the caudal end, to the coccyx by the external filum terminale. This is a thin elastic tube, more elastic than the spinal cord, and a likely buffer to cord overstretch (Tani et al 1987). It is a regular occurrence for physiotherapists investigating coccydynia (Ch. 13) to find that patients with this common disorder present with altered nervous system mechanics.

A network of dural ligaments (Hoffman ligaments) attaches the anterior theca to the anterior and anterolateral aspect of the spinal canal (Figs 1.17 & 1.18). Early anatomists were well aware of these tethering ligaments. A revival of interest has spurred a resurgence of study into these ligaments as a part of neuraxial and meningeal biomechanics (Spencer et al 1983, Tencer et al 1986). In the lumbar spine, the ligaments are particularly well developed and not only do they tether the dura centrally, they also tether it in the lateral recess. Blikna (1969) noted that the dural

ligaments around L4 were stronger and more numerous than elsewhere — so strong that they could not be displaced with a probe. Thoracic dural ligaments tend to be filmier and longer, and in the cervical spine, they are shorter and thicker (Romanes 1981). The studies of Tencer et al (1985) have revealed that, in the lumbar spine, dural ligaments, nerve roots and trunks are of equal importance in the distribution of forces. Yet, Tencer et al (1985) also found that these ligaments provided minimal restraint to dural movement in the longitudinal axis. Nevertheless, the peripheral nervous system provides the neuraxis and its membranes with a very strong physical attachment to the rest of the body.

Dorsally, a plica or septum (dorsomedial septum) has been shown to be a consistent feature in the posterior aspect of the spinal canal between the flaval ligament and the posterior dura mater. (Parkin & Harrison 1985, Blomberg 1986, Savolaine et al 1988) (see Fig. 1.17). These attachments are longer than the anterior

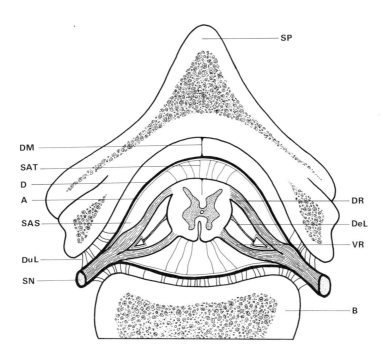

Fig. 1.17 Diagrammatic transverse section of the spinal canal and the attachments of the neuraxis and meninges. A arachnoid, B body, D dura, DuL dural ligament, DeL denticulate ligament, DMS dorsomedian septum, DR dorsal root, SAS subarachnoid space, SAT subarachnoid trabeculae, SN spinal nerve, SP spinous process, VR ventral root.

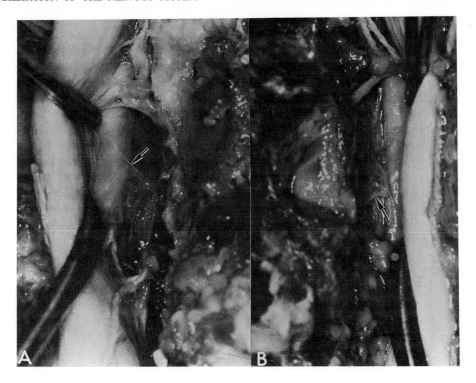

Fig. 1.18 Dural ligaments. A thoracic, B lumbar. The dural theca is held back with a probe. From: Tencer A F, Allen B L, Ferguson R L 1985 A biochemical study of thoracolumbar spine fractures with bine in the canal. Part III. Mechanical properties of the dura and its tethering ligaments. Spine 10: 741–747, with kind permission from the publishers and authors

attachments (Parkin & Harrison 1985). They are anatomically complex, strong, and it seems inevitable that they will be involved in the biomechanics of neuromeningeal tissues, particularly in the considerable antero-posterior movements noted by Penning & Wilmink (1981). This posterior dural attachment could also be a reason why some epidural injections may not have the desired effect. If the plica is a continuous tissue, all the dura may not be bathed in the injection material.

Internal dural attachments

Inside the dural sac there are 21 pairs of denticulate ligaments (see Figs 1.14, 1.15 & 1.17). These run from the pia mater to the dura and are orientated to keep the cord central in the dural theca. With the cord 'slung' in the theca, any tension or movement is far greater in the theca than in the cord (Epstein 1966, White &

Panjabi 1978) (Fig. 1.19). Tani et al (1987) have shown that the denticulate ligaments, as well as the filum terminale, prevent excessive elongation of the cord during flexion. Thickened denticulate ligaments associated with cervical spondylosis have been implicated in cord degeneration (Bedford et al 1952).

The subarachnoid trabeculae run from the arachnoid to the pia. They form large channels for the CSF, and probably dampen pressure waves in the CSF (Nicholas & Weller 1988).

Attachments of the peripheral nervous system

The peripheral nerves are also attached to surrounding tissue. However, they are allowed movement in their nerve beds, less in some areas than in others, such as where blood vessels enter or where nerves branch. This is an understudied area, probably mirroring the importance given to

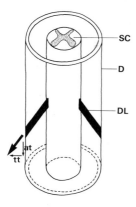

Fig. 1.19 The denticulate ligaments sling the cord in the dural theca. These ligaments stabilise the cord centrally in the dural theca and provide stability against axial and transverse forces. D dura, DL denticulate ligaments, SC spinal cord. at axial tension, tt transverse tension. Adapted from White & Panjabi (1978)

nerve biomechanics at present. The mesoneurial tissues, the nerve itself and the structure to which it attaches, clearly possess quite complex anatomy for movement purposes. What is unmistakable is that, along the course of a peripheral nerve, there are some areas where the nerve is more attached than others, for example, the common peroneal nerve at the head of the fibula, and the radial nerve to the head of the radius. Yet in other areas, a remarkable amount of movement of over 1.5 cm occurs (McLellan & Swash 1976). In an earlier section I discussed the mesoneurium. Where a peripheral nerve is attached to an adjacent structure it must attach in some way through the mesoneurium, if the mesoneurium is a continuous structure. This connection needs histological analysis.

THE BASIS OF SYMPTOMS

Knowledge of three processes is important to an

understanding of symptom reproduction related to the nervous system:

- The supply of blood to the nervous system
- The axonal transport systems
- The innervation of the connective tissues of the nervous system.

All of these processes will be influenced by mechanical deformation.

CIRCULATION

The nervous system consumes 20% of the available oxygen in the circulating blood yet consists of 2% of body mass (Dommisse 1986). Among cells, neurones are especially sensitive to alterations in blood flow. An uninterrupted vascular supply is imperative for the metabolic demands of normal neural function. The blood supply to the nervous system (vasa nervorum) is well equipped to ensure that blood flow to neurones is unimpeded in all dynamic and static postures. Blood supplies the necessary energy for impulse conduction and also for the intracellular movement of the cytoplasm of the neurone.

A general pattern of blood supply to neurones exists. There are extrinsic vessels supplying feeder arteries to the nerve. Once inside the nervous system, there is a well developed intrinsic system (Fig. 1.20). In many parts of the body, blood supply is so assured that if some feeder vessels are compromised, the intrinsic system can provide enough blood for normal neural function. With such an assured supply, it may seem that the nervous system can be relatively independent of its blood supply. Stripping of feeder vessels, as occurs in peripheral nerve surgery, may not give rise to a defect. However, if after stripping,

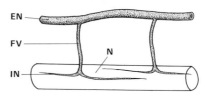

Fig. 1.20 The extraneural and intraneural design of the circulatory system. EN extraneural vessel, IN intraneural vessel, FV feeder vessel, N nervous system

a vital feeder artery is blocked, the nerve will fail rapidly (Porter & Wharton 1949).

Vasculature of the spinal canal and neuraxis

These structures have a multiple supply. The vertebral artery, the deep cervical, the posterior intercostal and the lumbar arteries supply the vertebral column. They also supply, via segmental subdivisions, the spinal canal and contents. At certain vertebral levels, medullary feeder branches arise and join the longitudinally running anterior and two small posterior spinal arteries. At every level, the segmental spinal arteries give rise to radicular arteries which supply the distal half of the nerve roots. The anterior spinal artery supplies about 75% of the cord. It is more a longitudinal system of functionally independent vascular entities with a related feeder vessel.

There are usually around eight medullary feeder arteries (Lazorthes et al 1971, Dommissee 1974). These arteries are more common in the lumbar and cervical spines, although great variation between cadavers has been noted (Dommisse 1986). Some cadavers have been noted with only two anterior medullary feeders, while others may have up to 17 (Dommisse 1986). It is clear that the person with only two such arteries is more at risk and may present different signs and symptoms from the same injury than a patient with many medullary feeder arteries. Most of the arteries enter the cord in the low cervical spine and the lumbar spine. This is a sensible design, for, not only are there neurones of the brachial and lumbosacral plexuses to supply, but during spinal movements these plexus areas have limited movement in relation to the spinal canal (Louis 1981) (Fig. 1.21). These issues of cord and spinal canal movements are taken up in the next chapter.

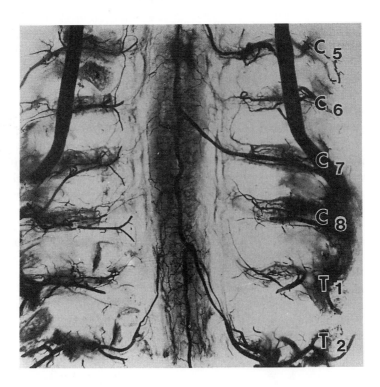

Fig. 1.21 Photograph of an injected and cleared cervicothoracic section of a neonatal spinal cord. This shows the arterial medullary vascularisation at the C5–7 level of the cervical spinal canal. At this level of the spinal canal the lumen is at its narrowest. From: Parke W W 1988 Correlative anatomy of cervical spondylotic myelopathy. Spine 13: 831–837, with kind permission from the publishers and author

Clefts in the cord allow blood vessel access to neurones. These perivascular spaces are also lymph ducts draining the cord. A similar latticed collagen arrangement to the leptomeninges exists in these clefts or ducts whereby the lattice of collagen fibres protects the blood vessels in stretch and compression (Breig 1978). With this mechanism, plus a multiple segmental supply to all areas of the system, blood supply is normally assured. Also, the system of segmental feeder vessels running transversely, together with intraneural vessels running longitudinally, will assist. When the cord is elongated the vessels running longitudinally are stretched while those running transversely are folded. The opposite effect occurs on shortening of the cord (Fig. 1.22). Another protective mechanism may come from the strong pulse in the cord continually 'bumping' it away from possible impinging structures (Jockich et al 1984).

A multi-use venous system exists in the spinal canal. Intramedullary veins drain into a series of longitudinal veins in the epidural space — the vertebral venous plexus. These veins in the spinal canal are valveless and under little pressure (Penning & Wilmink 1981). This allows flow reversibility, and an accommodating mechanism to sudden in-rushes of blood, as may occur from coughing and straining. Together with the CSF pressure, via the alterations in the venous system, a balance of intraspinal canal pressure is maintained. The venous plexuses take up much of the remaining non-neural space in the spinal canal. This also offers the cord some protection. These veins consequently have a function as 'pressure stabilisers', according to Penning and Wilmink (1981).

A critical vascular zone exists from the T4 to T9 vertebral levels. The spinal canal is at its narrowest and the blood supply is less rich in this area (Dommisse 1974). This may be relevant in syndromes such as the 'T4 syndrome' (Ch. 13).

Vasculature of the nerve roots

Blood is supplied to each root from two distinct afferent vessels. In the proximal radicular artery, blood arises from a longitudinal spinal artery and flows distally. The distal radicular artery arises segmentally and blood flow is proximal. (Parke et al 1981) (Fig. 1.23). At the meeting of the two systems there is an area of relative hypovascularity. Within the root itself, the intraneural supply is very complex. Parke & Watanabe (1985) produced a detailed study examining the compensatory adaptations that the vascular supply of the nerve roots have for movement. In Figure 1.24, the full range of adaptations to movement are evident in order to allow the fascicles to slide on each other during movement. These features are more evident in the lumbar nerve roots than cervical (Parke & Watanabe 1985). Parke & Watanabe (1985) refer to the adaptations as 'coils, T-Bars and pig tails'. The coils and pig tails allow stretch while the T-Bar branches allow rapid shunting of blood if

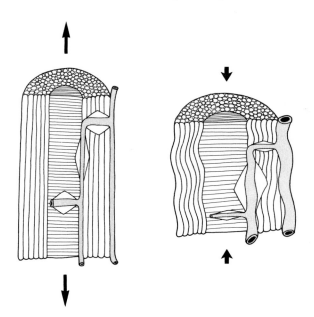

Fig. 1.22 The blood supply during stretch and compression of the spinal cord. Adapted from Breig (1978)

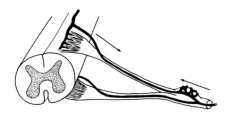

Fig. 1.23 Extraneural blood flow to the nerve roots. Adapted from Bogduk & Twomey (1987)

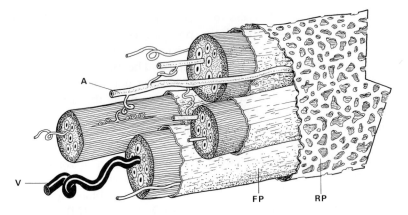

Fig. 1.24 The intrinsic blood supply to a nerve root. A arteriole, FP fasicular pia, RP radicular pia, V venule. Adapted from Parke & Watanabe (1988)

a branch is blocked. Watanabe & Parke (1986) noted that, in a cadaver with spinal stenosis, the 'pig tails' were accentuated to the sides of the constriction but absent under the constriction. The overall arrangement permits lateral and axial movement between fascicles. These are necessary adaptations for movement given the 'piston-like' movement of the nerve roots that occurs in the foramina during spinal movements (Sunderland 1978).

The radicular veins are few in number, and to some extent mimic the arterial supply, although obviously with a reversed flow of blood (Parke & Watanabe 1985).

Vasculature of the peripheral nervous system

The peripheral nervous system has a vascular supply as good as, if not better than, the central nervous system (Fig. 1.25). Perhaps this vasculature has developed due to the greater ranges of movements required of the peripheral nervous system. The vulnerability of axons of the peripheral nervous system to vascular changes is well known (Sunderland 1976, Rydevik et al 1981 Gelberman et al 1983, Powell & Myers 1986). The vascular arrangement is, once again, designed for uninterrupted flow, regardless of the position of the nerve in relation to the surrounding tissue. The extrinsic supply of the peripheral nerves is such that it allows leeway for movement;

that is, there is slack in the feeder vessels so that a nerve can glide without alteration in the blood supply. Note in Figure 1.26, where a nerve has bent, how the adaptations of the circulatory system have ensured adequate blood supply. In general, major feeder vessels enter nerves at areas where there is minimal or no nerve movement in relation to surrounding tissue. Examples of this are at the elbow for the median and radial nerves. These issues are discussed in detail in the next chapter. However, if part of the extrinsic supply is occluded, the intrinsic supply is also sufficient for the needs of the nerve fibres (Lundborg 1970, 1975).

The intrinsic vascular system is extensive, linking endoneurium, perineurium and epineurium. Only capillaries cross the perineurium and thus into the endoneurial environment. These vessels run in an oblique direction across the perineurium and this may allow a valve mechanism, squeezing the vessels closed if the intrafascicular pressure rises. Note the inset in Figure 1.25 (Lundborg 1988).

Under normal conditions, only part of the intraneural vascular system is used. However, if traumatised, many more vessels come into use (Lundborg 1970). Intraneural blood flow is reversible and collateral systems exist. Note the arterial loops in Figure 1.25. Such anatomy emphasises the need for uninterrupted blood supply to nerve fibres and the importance of maintaining a constant endoneurial environment. (Lundborg

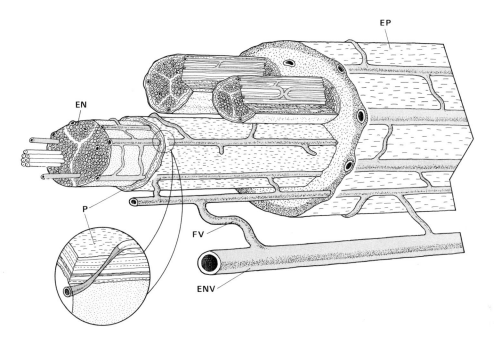

Fig. 1.25 The blood supply of a multifascicular segment of peripheral nerve. EN endoneurium, ENV extraneural vessel, EP epineurium, FV feeder vessel, P perineurium. The inset shows the oblique direction of a blood vessel entering the fascicle. Adapted from Lundborg (1988)

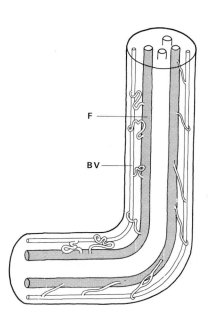

Fig. 1.26 Diagrammatic illustration of the adaptations in feeder vessels to allow intrafascicular movement. F fascicle, BV blood vessel

1975, Bell & Weddell 1984). Intraneural blood vessels are sympathetically innervated (Hromada 1963, Lundborg 1970, Appenzeller et al 1984). According to Appenzeller et al (1984), the nerve supply to a particular blood vessel arises from the nerve trunk that the blood vessel supplies. This probably allows an adjustable blood supply for functional demands on the nerve.

Stretch and compression will surely alter the circulation, although, the mechanisms are not fully understood. Stretch will lessen the diameter of the longitudinally running vessels, plus raise intrafascicular pressure and perhaps result in squeezing closed the vessels crossing the perineurium. Arrest of blood flow will begin at approximately 8% elongation (rabbit sciatic tract) and complete arrest will occur at approximately 15% elongation (Lundborg & Rydevik 1973, Ogata & Naito 1986). The clinical consequences of this are discussed in Chapter 3.

The blood nerve-barriers

A slightly positive pressure exists in the intrafascicular environment. This tissue pressure is referred to as the endoneurial fluid pressure (EFP) and is probably maintained by the elasticity of the perineurium. Lundborg (1988) has shown how the endoneurial contents will 'mushroom' through the perineurium, if cut. Alterations in the ionic composition or pressures within this environment may interfere with blood flow and, consequently, conduction and the flow of axoplasm. There are two barriers which maintain the endoneurial environment — the perineurial diffusion barrier and the blood-nerve barrier at endoneurial microvessels. The perineurium is the more resistant barrier (Lundborg 1981). Perineurial lamellae are part of the diffusion barrier mechanism. The junctions form 'tight cells' and, by control of substance flow, can regulate the intrafascicular environment (Lundborg 1988). Only small capillaries and venules pass through the lamellae and these travel in an oblique direction (Myers et al 1986) (see Fig. 1.25). The barrier function is bi-directional. As well as protection from the exterior, this mechanism means that if the intrafascicular pressure increases, such as from an oedematous reaction (Lundborg & Rydevik 1973), the barrier may close. A good example of the protective function of the diffusion barrier is where peripheral nerves travel through infected areas without nerve conduction being altered. The perineurial barrier is resistant to trauma, and, even after surgery to epineurium, the resultant epineurial oedema will not breach the perineurium (Rydevik et al 1976). Nor will an ischaemic induced epineurial oedema affect the barrier, at least initially (Lundborg et al 1973, Lundborg 1988). In Chapter 3, the consequences of a prolonged oedematous reaction in and around the nervous system are discussed.

The endoneurial capillary bed can be considered a peripheral example of the blood-brain barrier, known as the 'blood-nerve' barrier (Waksman 1961). Substances such as radioactive tracers and dyed proteins will cross through epineurial blood vessels but not through the tight endothelial cells of the endoneurial microvessels (Olsson & Reese 1971, Olsson et al 1971). One notable exception to this, and relevant to diabetes, is that simple sugars can cross the barrier

(Mackinnon & Dellon 1988). Both these barriers will break down after acute or chronic compression (Rydevik & Lundborg 1977, McKinnon et al 1984).

The perineurial barrier function is illustrated in Figure 1.27. Simply, a reaction outside the perineurium will not gain access to the endoneurial environment. Yet, a reaction such as ischaemic damage to microvessels, leading to oedema, will increase the endoneurial fluid pressure from within and consequently close the barrier (Sunderland 1976, Lundborg 1988, Mackinnon & Dellon 1988). The perineurium of the peripheral ganglia has a barrier function similar to that of

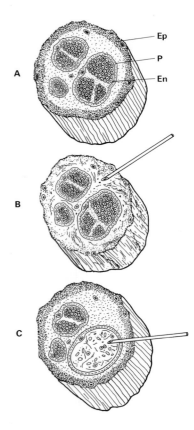

Fig. 1.27 The perineurial diffusion barrier. E endoneurium, Ep epineurium, P perineurium.
A Normal segment of peripheral nerve. B If a reaction is introduced around the nerve and into the epineurium, the perineurial diffusion barrier, via substance control protects the intrafascicular environment. C If a reaction begins inside the perineurium (e.g., virus, oedema) and intrafascicular pressure increases, the barrier closes and the reaction is kept within the perineurium. Destruction of neural tissue may follow

peripheral nerve. McKinnon & Dellon (1988) have postulated that breakdown of the blood nerve barrier may mean a breakdown of an immunological barrier, similar to the blood-brain barrier, which can be broken with inflammation or injury.

Physiotherapists need knowledge of the properties of the perineurium and the diffusion barriers. Many answers in disorder interpretation and prognosis lie within its structure. Techniques of mobilisation and prognosis will differ depending on whether a pathology is inside the perineurium or outside of it. In Chapter 3 the pathological processes that follow impairment of the function of the diffusion barriers are discussed.

AXONAL TRANSPORT SYSTEMS

Within the cytoplasm of all cells, there is movement of materials and substances. The cytoplasm of the neurone (axoplasm) is no different. However, due to the length of the axon and its function, specialised intracellular movement mechanisms occur. Axons of cell bodies can be over one metre long, such as a motor axon from a muscle in the foot to its cell body in the ventral horn. If the cell body of a neurone were 100 cm in diameter, it would have an axon diameter of 10 cm and a length of around 10 kilometres (Rydevik et al 1984). The volume of material in an axon and terminals may be thousands of times

as great as in the cell body (Lundborg 1988). Mammalian axoplasm is quite viscous, about five times that of water (Haak et al 1976). Of necessity, the intracellular transport mechanisms are complex. These mechanisms are referred to as axonal transport systems and are a major direction for research in present day neurological science. The axon contains smooth endoplasmic reticulum, ribosomes, microtubules and neurofilaments comprised of actin like material — all structures likely to be part of the axoplasmic transport mechanisms. Perhaps human movement plays a role in this intracellular motility.

Within the axon, the flow of substances is constant and controlled. Remarkably, there are many different axonal transport systems within a single axon, of which three main flows have been identified. From the cell body to the target tissues (antegrade flow) there is a fast and a slow transport system. From the target tissues to the cell body there is a retrograde flow of axoplasm (Fig. 1.28). This bi-directional flow is evident because a nerve will swell both distally and proximally from circumferential pressure (Mackinnon & Dellon 1988).

Antegrade transport

Materials produced in the cell body are transported along the axon at various velocities. Two groups based on the speed of transport, can be identified. The fast transport moves at approxi-

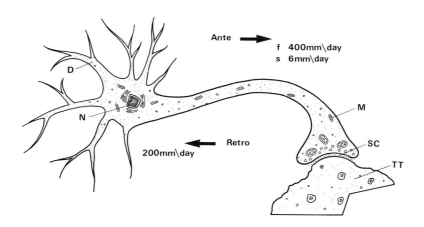

Fig. 1.28 Axoplasmic transport systems within a single neurone. D dendrite, N nucleus, M mitochondria, SC synaptic cleft, TT target tissue

mately 400 mm per day and the substances carried, such as neurotransmitters and transmitter vesicles, are for use in transmission of impulses at the synapse (Droz et al 1975). This transport depends on an uninterrupted supply of energy from the blood. Various toxic substances and deprivation of blood will slow or block the transport (Ochs 1974).

In the slow antegrade transport (1–6 mm per day), cytoskeletal material such as microtubules and neurofilaments are carried (Levine & Willard 1980, McLean et al 1983) Essentially, the slow transport exists for maintenance of the structure of the axon.

The exact mechanisms of transport are unknown. Various hypotheses, including force generating enzymes and transport filaments, have been summarised by Lundborg (1988).

Retrograde transport

Retrograde transport from target tissues to the cell body moves rapidly (approx 200 mm per day). The system carries recycled transmitter vesicles and extracellular materials such as neurite growth promoting factors from the nerve terminal or from damaged segments of nerve.

It also seems very likely that the retrograde flow carries 'trophic messages' about the status of the axon, the synapse and the general environment around the synapse, including the target tissues (Kristensson & Olsson 1977, Varon & Adler 1980, Bisby 1982). If the retrograde flow is altered by physical constriction or from loss of blood flow, nerve cell body reactions are induced (Ochs 1984, Dahlin & McLean 1986, Dahlin et al 1987). Viruses, such as herpes simplex, can be transported via the retrograde transport to the cell body (Kristensson 1982). In Chapter 3, the circumstances leading to, and the effects of, depletion of the axoplasmic flow are discussed in more detail.

An understanding of the concepts of axonal transport is important for physiotherapists employing mobilisation of the nervous system as a treatment. As Korr has suggested for some years (1978, 1985) many of the disorders we treat and the responses from treatment may be related to the axonal transport systems. In this regard, Korr

is referring to treatment via joint structures. The effects of mobilising the nervous system as well as joint structures will logically have a greater effect on the flow of axoplasm. Knowledge of these systems is also important in order to understand the development of symptoms along the nervous system (ie, double crush, multiple crush syndromes) and the need to treat often more than the local area for optimum results.

INNERVATION OF THE NERVOUS SYSTEM

The title of this section is somewhat paradoxical. However, the connective tissues of the nervous system are innervated. They are, thus, able to be a source of symptoms. Already in this chapter, the design of the nervous system for a movement function has been outlined. By the innervation of the supporting structures, some protection to the primary neurones is given. This innervation also means that the connective tissues of the nervous system can contribute to altered sensory input in the same way that muscle, joint and other tissues can.

Documentation about the innervation of the nervous system is far from complete, and the clinical consequences not fully understood. Many major textbooks on the subjects of neurology and orthopaedics neglect it. Of importance also with 'mechanical thinking' are the connections of the nervous system to other tissues. These attachments and the structures they attach to are likely to be innervated.

The meninges

Dura mater is innervated by segmental, bilateral, sinuvertebral nerves, first described by Luschka (1850). These are tiny nerves, hardly, if at all, visible to the unaided eye. Each sinuvertebral nerve emerges distal to the dorsal root ganglion, from the union of a somatic root arising from the ventral rami and an autonomic root from the grey rami communicantes or a sympathetic ganglion (Fig. 1.29). The nerve is sometimes known as the recurrent meningeal nerve. Each sinuvertebral nerve pursues a perivascular course back into the spinal canal through the intervertebral foramen.

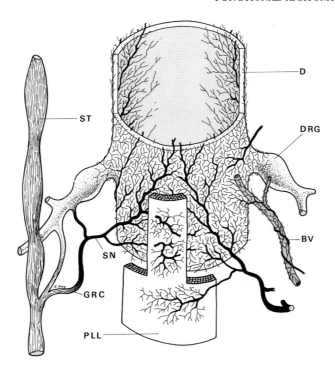

Fig. 1.29 Diagrammatic representation of the sinuvertebral nerve innervating the dura mater, from the ventral aspect. BV blood vessel, D dura, DRG dorsal root ganglion, GRC gray rami communicantes, PLL posterior longitudinal ligament, SN sinuvertebral nerve, ST sympathetic trunk. Note that the dura is innervated directly by the sinuvertebral nerve and that some fibres go via the posterior longitudinal ligament. Nerve fibres from blood vessels also supply the dura

(Hovelacque 1927, Bridge 1959, Kimmel 1961, Edgar & Nundy 1966, Edgar & Ghadially 1976, Bogduk 1983, Groen et al 1988, Cuatico et al 1988).

As well as supply to the dura, branches of the sinuvertebral nerve innervate the posterior longitudinal ligament, periosteum, blood vessels and the annulus fibrosis (Edgar & Ghadially 1975, Bogduk 1983). Hovelacque (1927) found that, from the initial part of the nerve, there were branches supplying the neck of the rib and the periosteum of the vertebral arch.

Dural innervation is intrinsic as well as extrinsic. A dural plexus is formed once each nerve pierces the dura (Groen et al 1988) and the result is a mesh of nerve (Fig. 1.30). Some branches of the sinuvertebral nerve may travel for some distance along the dura before piercing it. Ectopic impulses via a sinuvertebral nerve could come from the extrinsic part, say from a microneuroma in the nerve (neurogenic pain) or from irritation

of the nerve endings in the dura mater (nociceptive pain). Branches of the sinuvertebral nerve spread to the opposite side and up and down a number of segments. Edgar & Nundy (1966) measured the extent of axial spread of innervation as a total of four segments, while Groen et al (1988) measured a maximum of eight segments, four rostral and four caudal.

The sinuvertebral nerves may go directly to the dura or go via the posterior longitudinal ligament. Groen et al (1988) noted two previously unrecorded features of the sinuvertebral nerve. Firstly, the nerve travelled as 'curled bundles' representing an adaptation to dural movements (see Fig. 1.30). Secondly, an additional supply to the ventral dura came from the perivascular nerve plexus of the radicular ramus of a segmental artery.

The innervation density varies depending on the spinal segment. It is richer in the superficial dural layers than in those deeper. Root sleeves at cervical and lumbar levels have a richer nerve

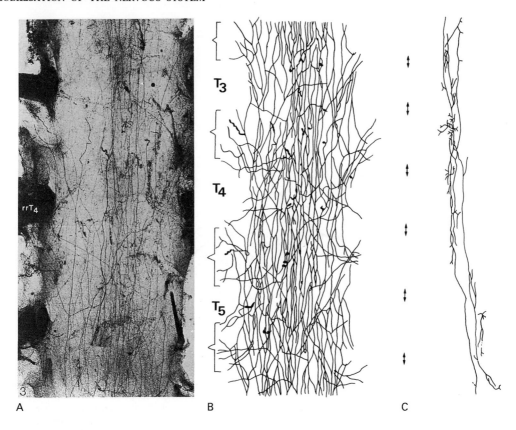

Fig. 1.30 The multisegmental meshwork of dural innervation. A Dorsal view of ventral dura mater (T2–T5). The plexus is primarily longitudinally arranged and in the 'intersleeve' parts the nerves run dorsally. B Tracing of the photograph. Note the cut and curled segments of nerves. C Drawing of major dural nerve and the extent of semental innervation
From: Groen G J, Baljet B, Drukker J 1988 The innervation of the spinal dura mater: Anatomy and clinical implications. Acta Neurochirurgica 92: 42, with kind permission from the publisher and the authors

supply than the thoracic root sleeves (Cuatico et al 1988).

All recent authors on the subject agree that the ventral aspect of the dura mater has a far denser innervation than the dorsal aspect. Cyriax (1982) uses painless needle entry from lumbar puncture into the posterior dura as an example of this dorsal insensitivity. Towards the midline, the dorsal dura may be completely insensitive (Groen et al 1988).

Branches of the sinuvertebral nerve also supply the dura mater and blood vessels of the posterior cranial fossa (Kimmel 1961). The greater proportion of the rest of the cranial dura is supplied by the trigeminal nerve (Bogduk 1989). The likelihood of some headaches originating from cranial dura has been long suggested (Penfield & McNaughton 1940). These headaches are discussed in Chapter 13.

An inferior branch of the sinuvertebral nerves passes through the dural ligaments (Parke & Watanabe 1990) and probably innervates them. Dural ligaments span two highly innervated tissues, the posterior longitudinal ligament and the ventral dura mater and may well be a bridge for branches of the sinuvertebral nerve. This very plausible suggestion was made by Groen et al (1988) who also thought that some anatomists may have confused sinuvertebral nerves for dural ligaments. In the absence of literature, Sunderland (pers. comm. 1989) feels they are likely to be innervated. Certainly, the scar formation involved in pathological tethering will have a nerve supply and it may also entrap the nerve itself.

The innervation of the arachnoid and pia maters has had far less experimental attention. Bridge (1959) noted nerves running longitudinally in the pia mater, though not in the arachnoid mater. In recent years arachnoiditis has become a more frequent diagnosis, yet the nerve supply to the arachnoid is far from clear and needs further study. There appear to be no studies supporting an innervation of the denticulate ligaments. Edgar & Nundy (1966) searched for such a nerve supply but were unsuccessful.

The connective tissues of nerve roots

Dural sleeve nerve supply is similar to the dura mater. The innervation of the radicular pia (nerve root representatives of endoneurium and perineurium) is slightly different to their counterparts in peripheral nerve. The ventral nerve root connective tissues receive their innervation from fibres originating in the dorsal root ganglion. Connective tissues of the anterior nerve roots are innervated by fine branches from the sinuvertebral nerve (Hromada 1963).

The peripheral nervous system

The distribution and type of nerve fibres in the connective tissues of peripheral nerve has received scant examination. This is a remarkably understudied area of neurology.

The connective tissues of peripheral nerves, nerve roots and the autonomic nervous system have an intrinsic innervation: the 'nervi nervorum' from local axonal branching. There is also an extrinsic vasomotor innervation from fibres entering the nerve from the perivascular plexuses (Hromada 1963, Thomas & Olsson 1984). Free nerve endings have been observed in the perineurium, epineurium and endoneurium (Fig. 1.31). Encapsulated endings, such as Pacinian corpuscles, have been observed in the epineurium and perineurium (Fig. 1.32). In the literature on peripheral nerve, very few authors have been aware of this innervation or have associated clinical consequences to it. Thomas (1982) believes that the nervi nervorum must be considered a source of symptoms in diabetic neuropathy and in inflammatory polyneuropathies.

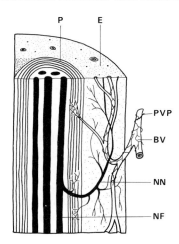

Fig. 1.31 The innervation of the connective tissues of peripheral nerve — the nervi nervorum. E epineurium, BV blood vessel, NN nervi nervorum, NF nerve fibre, P perineurium, PVP perivascular plexus. Adapted from Hromada (1963)

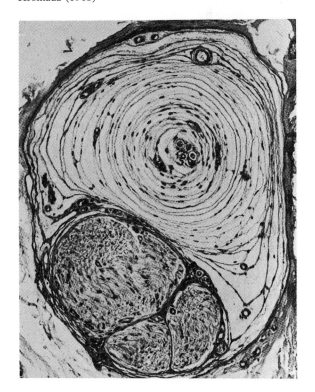

Fig. 1.32 Photograph of a Pacinian corpuscle in peripheral nerve perineurium. From: Thomas P K & Olsson Y 1975 Microscopic anatomy and function of the connective tissue components of peripheral nerve. In: Dyck P J, Thomas P K, Lambert E H (eds) Peripheral Neuropathy. W B Saunders, Philadelphia Vol 1, with kind permission from the authors and publishers

Sunderland (1978) considers the pain from local pressure on a nerve to be due to the nervi nervorum but also acknowledges (1979) that there is a lack of information regarding the status of the nervi nervorum in pain states. It seems logical that stretch, rather than compression, of a segment of peripheral nerve would involve more nociceptive endings. Perhaps there is some special relationship between the nervi nervorum and the primary neurones. Perhaps nociception from the connective tissues could 'close down' when ectopic impulses of a particular nature are generated along the primary neurones.

More study on the physiology of the nervi nervorum and its role in pain states is necessary. The most recent reference to this innervation is Hromada in 1963. Newer staining and examination techniques may reveal more information about the nerve endings of the nervi nervorum. We can still only presume that the nerve endings are nociceptive. The blood vessels of the perineurium and epineurium are sympathetically innervated (Hromada 1963, Lundborg 1970, Appenzeller et al 1984 Thomas & Olssen 1985). This no doubt helps to maintain a constant intrafascicular environment.

Hromada (1963) also noted that the connective tissues of the dorsal root and sympathetic ganglia receive innervation from fibres whose cell bodies are located in the ganglia themselves. A second source of innervation arises from fibres entering the ganglion from associated perivascular plexuses.

The innervation of the nervous system cannot be neglected — it seems very likely that it plays a part in adverse tension syndromes. Perhaps innervation could be regarded as a protective mechanism for the nervous system, symptom production being a warning that the impulse conducting mechanisms may be in danger from mechanical or chemical compromise.

SUMMARY

If the nervous system is examined in terms of the features required to maintain normal impulse conduction and axonal transport systems, it becomes clear that many of these relate to body movements. Each component of the nervous system from peripheral nerve axon cylinder to the dural theca possess features which protect it, and other related structures, during normal physiological movement. As such, it is no different from joint or muscle. With such wonderful adaptations, it is tempting to ask 'Why should anything go wrong?' Indeed one of the main messages I would like to deliver in this book is that things can very easily go wrong with these movement mechanics. I believe these mechanisms which allow normal movement are impaired more easily and far more frequently than may have previously been recognised. Reasons for this predisposition to injury can be generalised as the complexity of structure, intimate connectedness throughout the body, and multi-tissue components which react differently to injury, yet ultimately influence all neural and perhaps non-neural structures. This also must be analysed in terms of what humans do to their bodies.

REFERENCES

Appenzeller O, Dithal K K, Cowan T, Burnstock, G 1984 The nerves to blood vessels supplying blood nerves: the innervation of vasa nervorum. Brain Research 304: 383–386
Baldwin W M 1908 The topography of spinal nerve roots. Anatomical Record 2: 155–156
Barnes R 1949 Traction injuries of the brachial plexus in adults. Journal of Bone and Joint Surgery 31B: 10–16
Bedford P D, Bosanquet F D, Russel W R 1952 Degeneration of the spinal cord associated with cervical spondylosis. Lancet July 12: 55–59
Bell M A, Weddell A G M 1984 A morphometric study of intrafascicular vessels of mammalian sciatic nerve. Muscle & Nerve 7: 524–534

Bisby M A 1982 Functions of retrograde axonal transport. Federation Proceedings 41: 2307–2311
Blikna G 1969 Intradural herniated lumbar disc. Journal of Neurosurgery 31: 676–679
Blomberg R 1986 The dorsomedian connective tissue band in the lumbar epidural space of humans. Anesthesia and Analgesia 65: 747–752
Bogduk N 1983 The innervation of the lumbar spine. Spine 8: 286–293
Bogduk N 1989 The anatomy of headache. In: Dalton M (ed) Proceedings of headache and face pain symposium, Manipulative Physiotherapists Association of Australia, Brisbane
Bowsher D 1988 Introduction to the anatomy and physiology of the nervous system, 5th edn. Blackwell, Oxford

Breig A 1978 Adverse mechanical tension in the central nervous system. Almqvist & Wiksell, Stockholm

Bridge C J 1959 Innervation of spinal meninges and epidural structures. Anatomical Record 133: 533–561

Cuatico W, Parker J C, Pappert E, Pilsl S 1988 An anatomical and clinical investigation of spinal meningeal nerves. Acta Neurochirurgica 90: 139–143

Cyriax J 1982 Textbook of Orthopaedic Medicine 8th edn. Baillierre Tindall, London, Vol 1

Dahlin L B, McLean W G 1986 Effects of graded experimental compression on slow and fast axonal transport in rabbit vagus nerve. Journal of the Neurological Sciences 72: 19–30

Dahlin L B, Nordborg C, Lundborg G 1987 Morphological changes in nerve cell bodies induced by experimental graded nerve compression. Experimental Neurology 95: 611–621

Daniel R K, Terzis J K 1977 Reconstructive microsurgery. Little Brown, Boston

De Renyi G St 1929 The structure of cells in tissues as revealed by microdisection. Journal of Comparative Neurology 47: 405–425

Dommisse G F 1974 The blood supply of the spinal cord. Journal of Bone and Joint Surgery 56B: 225–235

Dommisse G F 1975 Morphological aspects of the lumbar spine and lumbosacral region. Orthopaedic Clinics of North America 6: 163–175

Dommisse G F 1986 The blood supply of the spinal cord. In: Grieve G P (ed) Modern manual therapy of the vertebral column. Churchill Livingstone, Edinburgh

Droz B, Rambourg A, Koenig H L 1975 The smooth endoplasmic reticulum: structure and role in the renewal of axonal membrane and synaptic vesicles by fast axonal transport. Brain Research 93: 1–13

Edgar M A, Nundy S 1966 Innervation of the spinal dura mater. Journal of Neurology, Neurosurgery and Psychiatry 29: 530–534

Edgar M A, Ghadially J A 1976 Innervation of the lumbar spine. Clinical Orthopaedics and Related Research 115: 35–41

Epstein B S 1966 An anatomical, myelographic and cinematographic study of the dentate ligaments. American Journal of Roentgenography 98: 704–712

Friede R L, Samorajski T 1969 The clefts of Schmidt-Lantermann: a quantitative electron microscopic study of their study in developing and adult sciatic nerves of the rat. Anatomical Record 165: 89–92

Frykolm R 1951 Lower cervical nerve roots and their investments. Acta Chirurgica Scandinavica 101: 457–471

Gamble H J, Eames R A 1964 An electron microscope study of the connective tissues of human peripheral nerve. Journal of Anatomy 98: 655–663

Gamble H J 1964 Comparative electron microscopic observations on the connective tissues of a peripheral nerve and a spinal nerve root in the rat. Journal of Anatomy 98: 17–25

Gardner E, Bunge R P 1984 Gross anatomy of the peripheral nervous system. In: Dyck P J, Thomas P K, Lambert E H, Bunge R (eds) Peripheral neuropathy, 2nd edn. Saunders, Philadelphia, Vol 1

Gelberman R H, Szabo R M, Williamson R V 1983 Tissue pressure threshold for peripheral nerve viability. Clinical Orthopaedics and Related Research 178: 285–291

Glees P 1943 Observations on the connective tissue sheaths of nerves. Journal of Anatomy 77: 153–159

Groen G J, Balget B, Drukker J 1988 The innervation of the spinal dura mater: anatomy and clinical considerations. Acta Neurochirurgica 92: 39–46

Haak R A, Kleinhaus F W, Ochs S 1976 The viscosity of mammalian nerve axoplasm measured by electron spin resonance. Journal of Physiology 263: 115–137

Haller F R, Haller A C, Low F N 1971 The fine structure of cellular layers and connective tissue space at spinal nerve root attachments in the rat. Americal Journal of Anatomy 133: 109–124

Hasue M, Kikuchi S, Sakuyama Y, Ito T 1983 Anatomic study of the interrelation between lumbosacral nerve roots and their surrounding tissues. Spine 8: 50–58

Haupt W, Stofft E 1978 Uber die denbarkeit und Reissfestkeit der dura mate spinalis des menchen. Verhandlungen der Anatomischen Gesellschaft 72: 139–142

Hollinshead W H, Jenkins D J 1981 Functional anatomy of the limbs and back, 5th edn. Saunders, Philadelphia

Hovelacque A 1927 Anatomie des nerfs craniens et rachidiens et du sisteme grand sympathique chez l'homme. Gaston Doin et Cie, Paris

Howe J F, Calvin W H, Loeser J D 1976 Impulses reflected from dorsal root ganglia and from focal nerve injuries. Brain Research 116: 1390–144

Howe J F, Loeser J D, Calvin W H 1977 Mechanosensitivity of dorsal root ganglia and chronically injured axons: a physiological basis for the radicular pain of nerve root compression. Pain 3: 25–41

Hromada J 1963 On the nerve supply of the connective tissue of some peripheral nervous system components. Acta Anatomica 55: 343–351

Inman V T, Saunders J B 1942 The clinico-anatomical aspects of the lumbosacral region. Radiology 38: 669–678

Jabaley M E, Wallace W H, Heckler F R 1980 Internal topography of major nerves of the forearm and hand. A current view. Journal of Hand Surgery 5: 1–18

Jokick P M, Rubin J M, Doirman G B 1984 Intra-operative ultrasonic evaluations of spinal cord motions. Journal of Neurosurgery 60: 707–717

Kimmel D L 1961 Innervation of the spinal dura mater and dura mater of the posterior cranial fossa. Neurology 10: 800–805

Korr I M (ed) 1978 The neurobiologic mechanisms in manipulative therapy. Plenum, New York

Korr I M 1985 Neurochemical and neurotrophic consequences of nerve deformation. In: Glasgow E F, Twomey L T, Scull E R, Kleynhans A M (eds) Aspects of manipulative therapy, 2nd edn. Churchill Livingstone, Edinburgh.

Kristensson K, Olsson Y 1977 Retrograde transport of horseradish peroxidase in transected axons. 3. Entry into injured axons and subsequent localisation in perikaryon. Brain Research 126: 154–159

Kwan M K, Rydevik B L, Myers R R et al 1988 Stretch injury of rabbit peripheral nerve: a biomechanical and histological study. In: Proceedings 34th annual meeting, Orthopaedic Research Society, February 1–4, Atlanta Georgia

Kristensson K 1982 Implications of axoplasmic transport for the spread of virus infections in the nervous system. In: Weiss D G, Gorio A (eds.) Axoplasmic transport in physiology and pathology. Springer-Verlag, Berlin

Landon D N, Williams P L 1963 The ultrastructure of the node of Ranvier. Nature 199: 575–577

Levine J, Willard M 1980 The composition and organisation of axonally transported proteins in the retinal ganglion cells of the guinea pig. Brain Research 194: 137–154

Louis R 1981 Vertebroradicular and vertebromedullar dynamics. Anatomica Clinica 3: 1–11

Lundborg G 1970 Ischaemic nerve injury: experimental studies on intraneural microvascular pathophysiology and nerve function in a limb, subjected to temporary circulatory arrest. Scandinavian Journal of Plastic and Reconstructive Surgery (Suppl) 6: 1–113

Lundborg G 1975 Structure and function of the intraneural microvessels as related to trauma, edema formation and nerve function. Journal of Bone and Joint Surgery 57A: 938–948

Lundborg G 1981 Mechanical effects on circulation and nerve function. In: Gorio A, Millesi H, Mingero S (eds.) Post-traumatic nerve regeneration. Raven Press, New York

Lundborg G 1988 Nerve injury and repair. Churchill Livingstone, Edinburgh

Lundborg G, Rydevik B 1973 Effects of stretching the tibial nerve of the rabbit: a preliminary study of the intraneural circulation and the barrier function of the perineurium. Journal of Bone and Joint Surgery 55B: 390–401

Lazorthes G, Gauaze A, Zadeh J O 1971 Arterial vascularisation of the spinal cord. Journal of Neurosurgery 35: 253–261

Luschka H von 1850 Die nerven des menschlichen eirbelkanales. Tubingen, Laupp

MacKinnon S E, Dellon A L 1988 Surgery of the peripheral nerve. Thieme, New York

Martins A M, Wiley J K, Myers P W 1972 Dynamics of the cerebrospinal fluid and the spinal dura mater. Journal of Neurology, Neurosurgery and Psychiatry 35: 468–473

Mathers L H 1985 The peripheral nervous system. Butterworths, Boston

MacKinnon S E, Dellon A L, Hudson A R et al 1984 Chronic nerve compression – an experimental model in the rat. Annals of Plastic Surgery 13: 112–120

McLellan D C, Swash M 1976 Longitudinal sliding of the median nerve during movements of the upper limb. Journal of Neurology, Neurosurgery and Psychiatry 39: 566–570

Millesi H 1986 The nerve gap: theory and clinical practice. Hand Clinics 4: 651–663

Murphy R W 1977 Nerve roots and spinal nerves in degenerative disc disease. Clinical Orthopaedics and Related Research 129: 46–60

Murzin V E, Goriunov V N 1979 Study of strength of fixation of dura mater to the cranial bones. Zh Vopr Neirokhir 4: 43–47

Myers R M, Murakami H, Powell H C 1986 Reduced nerve blood flow in edematous neuropathies: a biomechanical mechanism. Microvascular Research 32: 145–151

Nathan H, Feuerstein M 1970 Angulated course of spinal nerve roots. Journal of Neurosurgery 32: 349–352

Nicholas D S, Weller R O 1988 The fine anatomy of the human spinal meninges. Journal of Neurosurgery 69: 276–282

Ochs S 1974 Energy metabolism and supply of ^p to the fast axoplasmic transport mechanism in nerve. Federation Proceedings 33: 1049–1058

Ochs S 1984 Basic properties of axonplasmic transport. In: Dyck P J, Thomas P K, Lambert E H, Bunge R (eds) Peripheral neuropathy, 2nd edn. Saunders, Philadelphia

Ogata K, Naito M 1986 Blood flow of peripheral nerve. Effects of dissection, stretching and compression. Journal of Hand Surgery 11B: 10–14

Olsson Y, Reese T 1971 Permeability of vasa nervorum and perineurium in mouse sciatic nerve studies by fluorescence and electron microscopy. Journal of Neuropathology and Experimental Neurology 30: 105–119

Olsson Y, Kristensson, K, Klatzo J 1971 Permeability of blood vessels in connective tissue sheaths in the peripheral nervous system to exogenous proteins. Acta Neuropathologica Berlin (Suppl) 5: 61–69

Parke W W, Gammell K, Rothman R H 1981 Arterial vascularization of the cauda equina. Journal of Bone and Joint Surgery 63A: 53–62

Parke W W, Watanabe R 1985 The intrinsic vasculature of the lumbosacral spinal nerve roots. Spine 10: 508–515

Parke W W, Watanabe R 1990 Adhesions of the ventral dura mater. Spine 15: 300–303

Parkin I G, Harrison G R 1985 The topographical anatomy of the lumbar epidural space. Journal of Anatomy 141: 211–217

Penfield W & McNaughton F 1940 Dural headache and the innervation of the dura mater. Archives of Neurology and Psychiatry 44: 43–75

Penning L & Wilmink J T 1981 Biomechanics of the lumbosacral dural sac: a study of flexion-extension myelography. Spine 6: 398–408

Powell H C, Myers R R 1986 Pathology of experimental nerve compression. Laboratory Investigation 55: 91–100

Porter E L, Wharton P S 1949 Irritability of mammalian nerve following ischaemia. Journal of Neurophysiology 12: 109–116

Reid J D 1958 Ascending nerve roots and tightness of dura mater. New Zealand Medical Journal 57: 16–26

Reid J D 1960 Ascending nerve roots. Journal of Neurology, Neurosurgery and Psychiatry 23: 214–221

Robertson J D 1958 The ultrastructure of the Schmidt-Lantermann clefts and shearing defects of the myelin sheath. Journal of Biophysics, Biochemistry and Cytology 4: 39

Romanes G L 1981 Cunningham's manual of practical anatomy, 14th edn. Oxford, London

Rydevik B, Lundborg G 1977 Permeability of intraneural microvessels and perineurium following acute graded experimental nerve compression. Scandinavian Journal of Plastic and Reconstructive Surgery 11: 179–187

Rydevik B, Lundborg G, Nordborg C 1976 Intraneural tissue reactions induced by internal neurolysis. Scandinavian Journal of Plastic and Reconstructive Surgery 10: 3–8

Rydevik B, Lundborg G, Bagge U 1981 Effects of graded compression on intraneural blood flow. Journal of Hand Surgery 6: 3–12

Rydevik B, Brown M D, Lundborg G 1984 Pathoanatomy and pathophysiology of nerve root compression. Spine 9: 7–15

Savolaine E R, Pandja J B, Greenblatt E H et al 1988 Anatomy of the lumbar epidural space: new insights using CT-epidurography. Anesthiology 68: 217

Selander D, Sjostrand J 1978 Longitudinal spread of intraneurally injected local anesthetics. Acta Anaesthologica Scandinavica 22: 622–634

Shanthaveerappa T R, Bourne G H 1963 The perineural epithelium: nature and significance. Nature 199: 577–579

Singer M, Byrant S V 1969 Movements in the myelin schwann sheath of the vertebrate axon. Nature 221: 1148–1150

Smith J W 1966 Factors influencing nerve repair 1. Blood supply of peripheral nerves. Archives of Surgery 93: 335–341

Spielman F J 1982 Post lumbar puncture headache. Headache 22: 280–283

Spencer D J, Irwin G S, Miller J A A 1983 Anatomy and significance of function of the lumbosacral nerve roots in sciatica. Spine 8: 672–679

Sunderland S, Bradley K C 1949 The cross sectional area of peripheral nerve trunks devoted to nerve fibres. Brain 72: 428–439

Sunderland S 1974 Meningeal-neural relations in the intervertebral foramen. Journal of Neurosurgery 40: 756–763

Sunderland S 1976 The nerve lesion in carpal tunnel syndrome. Journal of Neurology, Neurosurgery and Psychiatry 39: 615–616

Sunderland S 1978 Nerves and nerve injuries, 2nd edn. Churchill Livingstone, Edinburgh

Sunderland S 1979 The painful nerve lesion: a prologue. In: Bonica J J et al (eds) Advances in Pain Research and Therapy. Raven Press, New York, 3: 36–37

Sunderland S 1989 Features of nerves that protect them during normal daily activities. In: Jones H M, Jones M A, Milde M R (eds) Sixth Biennial Conference Proceedings, Manipulative Therapists Association of Australia, Adelaide

Tani S, Yamada S, Knighton R S 1987 Extensibility of the lumbar and sacral cord: pathophysiology of the tethered spinal cord in cats. Journal of Neurosurgery 66: 116–123

Tencer A F, Allen B L, Ferguson R L 1985 A biomechanical study of thoracolumbar spine fractures with bone in the canal. Part 3 Mechanical properties of the dura mater and its tethering ligaments. Spine 10: 741–747

Thomas P K 1963 The connective tissue of peripheral nerve: an electron microscope study. Journal of Anatomy 97: 35–44

Thomas P K 1982 Pain in peripheral neuropathy : clinical and morphological aspects. In: Culp W J, Ochoa J (eds.) Abnormal nerves and muscles as impulse generators. Oxford, New York

Thomas P K, Olsson Y 1984 Microscopic anatomy and function of the connective tissue components of peripheral nerve. In: Dyck P J, Thomas P K, Lambert E H, Bunge R (eds) Peripheral Neuropathy, 2nd edn. Saunders, Philadelphia

Transfeldt E E, Simmons E H 1982 Functional and pathological biomechanics of the spinal cord: an in-vivo study. International society for the study of the lumbar spine, Toronto.

Tunturi A R 1977 Elasticity of the spinal cord dura in the dog. Journal of Neurosurgery 47: 391–396

Van Beek A, Kleinert H E 1977 Practical microneurorraphy. Orthopaedic Clinics of North America 8: 377–386

Van Noort R, Black M M, Martin T R P, Meanley S 1981 A study of the uniaxial mechanical properties of human dura mater preserved in glycerol. Biomaterials 2: 41–45

Varon S, Adler R 1980 Nerve growth factor and control of nerve growth. Current Topics in Developmental Biology 16: 207–252

Waggener J D, Beggs J 1967 The membranous coverings of neural tissues: an electron microscopy study. Journal of Neuropathology and Experimental Neurology 26: 412–416

Waksman B H 1961 Experimental study of diphtheric polyneuritis in the rabbit and guinea pig. III The blood-nerve barrier in the rabbit. Journal of Neuropathy and Experimental Neurology 21: 35–77

Walton J 1982 Essentials of neurology, 5th edn. Pitman, London

White A A, Panjabi M M 1978 Clinical biomechanics of the spine. Lippincott, Philadelphia

Wilgis S, Murphy R 1986 The significance of longitudinal excursions in peripheral nerves. Hand Clinics 2: 761–768

Williams P L, Warwick R 1980 Gray's anatomy, 36th edn. Churchill Livingstone, Edinburgh

2. Clinical neurobiomechanics

INTRODUCTION

The neurobiomechanics discussed in this chapter have emerged from a number of sources, such as animal and human cadaveric studies, human invivo studies and surgical observations. A combination of this background and my own clinical observations has enabled the formation of a hypothesis linking neurobiomechanics, neuropathology, and ultimately the delivery of mobilisation techniques. This hypothesis appears clinically valid and I hope it will stimulate research in the area of biomechanics of the nervous system. In this area, the literature is somewhat scanty. There is some information about areas of normal nerves, although little is available on the whole nervous system or on damaged nervous systems.

It would be convenient to include the nervous system in an established joint motion segment model, such as that presented by White & Panjabi (1978), a treatment system such as that of McKenzie (1981) or a joint combined movements model such as that of proposed by Edwards (1987, 1988). However, the complexity of movement and tension mechanisms in nervous system biomechanics precludes this. As I have suggested in the introduction, an open-minded, multi-factorial approach to neuro-orthopaedic disorders is required to include the nervous system.

There are two main allied biomechanical concepts related to the nervous system. First is that of the structure adjacent to the nervous system (referred to as the mechanical interface), and the effects of its biomechanics on the system. The second is the neurobiomechanics themselves, where two broad mechanics of movement can be identified; sliding next to the interface, and elongating. These concepts are reviewed prior to their analysis in the trunk and limbs.

The mechanical interface

One of the most outstanding features of the nervous system's biomechanics, relevant to manual therapy, is the mobility of the nervous system. Its mobility is such that it can act dependently or independently of the structures it spans. For example, a Straight Leg Raise (SLR) involves movement and tension of the nervous system in the calf and foot, yet negligible activity in the foot non-neural structures. However, if the SLR was performed including ankle dorsiflexion, the neural structures in the calf and foot will lose their independence from the surrounding structures and be affected by the joint position. Thus, the continuum of the nervous system, secures its ability to move either alone or be influenced by surrounding structures. The considerable avenues for diagnosis and treatment produced by this feature are discussed in later chapters.

The interfacing tissues, or more specifically, the mechanical interfaces, are central to an understanding of adverse tension. The mechanical interface may be defined as 'that tissue or material adjacent to the nervous system that can move independently to the system' (Butler 1989) (Fig. 2.1). The supinator muscle, for example, is an interface to the posterior interosseus branch of the radial nerve as it passes through the radial tunnel (Fig. 2.2). The ligamentum flavum is an interface to the posterior aspect of the spinal dura

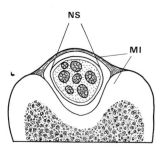

Fig. 2.1 Diagrammatic representation of the mechanical interface. MI mechanical interface NS nervous system

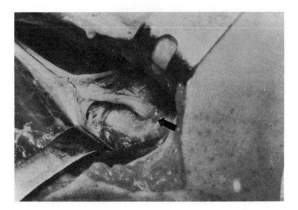

Fig. 2.2 The posterior interosseus nerve passing into a constricted arcade of Frohse (arrow) in the supinator muscle. From: Dawson D M, Hallett M, Millender L H 1983 Entrapment neuropathies. Little, Brown, Boston, with permission

mater. Zygapophyseal joints are yet another important interface. A known sources of pain themselves (Mooney & Robertson 1976), they also have a close topographical relationship with nerve roots and vascular structures which may have less protection from chemical and mechanical deformation than elsewhere in the body. Although the pure mechanical interface may be a fascial sheet or a blood vessel, a more relevant interface such as muscle or ligament may be adjacent to it. Interfaces of a pathological nature certainly exist. Examples of possible pathological interfaces are osteophytes, ligamentous swelling or fascial scarring. A tight plaster or bandage could be considered as a further example. The introduction of a fluid such as oedema or blood around the nervous system could also engender a pathological interface. For the purposes of the concepts presented in this book, interfacing tissues may be regarded as extraneural or extradural structures, that is, 'outside' the nervous system.

In this chapter, the biomechanics of the clinically important and central mechanical interface, the spinal canal, are discussed. Some peripheral interfaces, such as the interfacing structures involved in the carpal tunnel, are discussed in Chapter 12 under individual syndromes. Prior to a discussion of the spinal canal, a review of how the nervous system adapts to movement is warranted.

Nervous system adaptations to movement.

Rather simply, and yet conveniently for physiotherapists, the nervous system adapts to lengthening in two basic ways. This can only be a generalisation of the nervous system as a whole since the individual structural components of the nervous system have different biomechanical properties. The nervous system adapts to lengthening by:

1. The development of tension or increased pressure within the tissues, i.e., increased intraneural pressure, or increased intradural pressure. This pressure develops as a consequence of elongation and occurs in all tissues and fluids enclosed by and including the epineurium and the dura mater.

2. Movement. On closer analysis movement may be considered as (a) gross movement or (b) movement occurring intraneurally between the connective tissues and the neural tissues.

(a) gross movements refer to movement of the system as a whole in relation to interface. A peripheral nerve sliding through a tunnel such as the median nerve in the carpal tunnel or the dural theca sliding in relation to a vertebral segment are clear examples of this gross movement. A pathological situation such as blood in the epidural space, oedema in a nerve bed, or pathological tethering of the dura to the spinal canal would interfere with this movement adaptation.

(b) intraneural movement refers to movement of the neural tissue elements in relation to the connective tissue interfaces. The brain can move in relation to the surrounding cranial dura mater, the spinal cord can move in relation to the dura mater, nerve fibres unfold and move in relation to endoneurium. A fascicle can slide in relation to another fascicle in peripheral nerves and in nerve roots. An intraneural fibrosis or oedema would affect these mechanisms.

Relationship between movement and tension

These adaptive mechanisms are all constituents of normal movement and must occur together. However, certain body and limb movements seem more likely to move the nervous system rather than tension it and vice versa. Shoulder depression and elevation with the arm in a neutral position and the elbow flexed to 90° is an example of the nervous system moving in relation to surrounding interfaces (Fig. 2.3A). More tension could be produced in the nervous system if the same movement was performed with the neck laterally flexed away from the arm and the elbow and wrist extended (Fig. 2.3B). In cadaver studies of the SLR, neural movement commences early in the range. Beyond 70° there is little movement although tension

increases rapidly (Charnley 1951, Fahrni 1966, Goddard & Reid 1965, Breig 1978). In the spinal canal, Breig (1978) noticed the dura could be easily picked up and moved with forceps if the body were in a neutral position. The movement was markedly decreased if the thoracolumbar spine was flexed thus imposing a tension component. As a generalisation, if a body part is moved with the other body parts in a neutral position, there will be less tension and more movement of the nervous system in relation to interfaces. Conversely, if the same movement were performed with body parts in tension, there will be great increases in intraneural tension but little movement of the nervous system.

THE SPINAL CANAL, NEURAXIS AND MENINGES

The spinal canal as a mechanical interface

The typical spinal canal is capacious enough in all directions to allow the development of some intrusion, such as spondylitic changes, without any clinically detectable neural dysfunction. There is also a considerable amount of space for the neuraxis and meninges to move. These canal

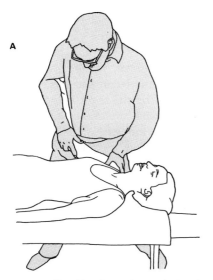
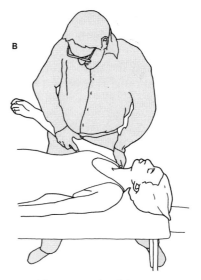

Fig. 2.3 Shoulder depression and elevation with the arm in neutral is an example of the nervous system moving in relation to surrounding interfaces. More tension could be placed upon the nervous system if the neck was laterally flexed away from the arm, and the elbow and wrist, extended as in Figure 2.3B

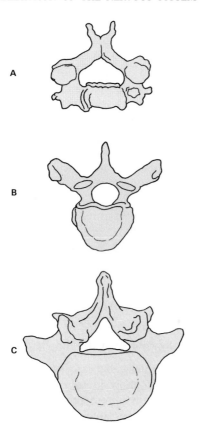

Fig. 2.4 Segmental variations in the shape of the spinal canal A cervical, B mid thoracic, C low lumbar

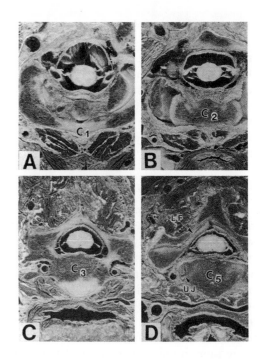

Fig. 2.5 The changing spaces available for the neuraxis and meninges in the cervical spinal canal. LF ligamentum flavum, UJ unco-vertebral joint. From: Parke W W 1988 Correlative anatomy of cervical spondylotic myelopathy. Spine 13: 831–837, with kind permission from the publishers and author

spaces are quite variable, both along the entire spinal canal and within smaller segments such as the cervical and lumbar canals. Note in Figure 2.4 that the cervical canal is large and triangular, particularly in the upper cervical spine. The thoracic spinal canal is smaller and more cylindrical while the lumbar spinal canal is larger than the thoracic canal, rounded in the upper segments, and becoming trefoil caudally. The canal is uniformly wider in its transverse measurement than in its antero-posterior measurement. The shape of the spinal canal varies quite quickly according to the spinal level. At the T6 intervertebral level it is at its narrowest and roundest (Dommisse 1975).

In the cadaver sections illustrated in Figure 2.5, there are quite marked differences in the dimensions of the canal in relation to the contained neuraxis and meninges in the cervical spine. At the C1 vertebral level the cord occupies less than half of the canal whereas, at C5, it occupies about three quarters of the available space. Therefore, any structure invading the canal, pathological or otherwise, will have a greater potential to compromise the neuraxis and/or meninges at the lower level. Similarly, in the thoracic spine, the T6 level would be the most vulnerable.

The spinal canal undergoes substantial length changes during movement. From spinal extension to spinal flexion, it elongates by between 5–9 cm with most of the movement occurring in the cervical and lumbar regions (Inman & Saunders 1942, Breig 1978, Louis 1981) (Figs 2.6 & 2.7). During the early ranges of flexion, the cross-sectional area of the spinal canal increases, largely due to an increase in the antero-posterior diameter. In extension, the cross-sectional area lessens (Penning & Wilmink 1981, Liyang et al 1988). Clinically, this is evident when patients with lumbar disc lesions, apparently crowding the spinal canal, get some relief by adopting a posture with a few degrees of lumbar flexion. Dyck

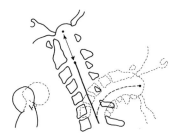

Fig. 2.6 Change in length of the cervical spinal canal during flexion and extension. Tracing from a radiograph. From: Troup J D G 1986 Back and neck injuries. In: Reilly T (ed) Sports fitness and sports injuries. Faber & Faber, London, with permission from the publishers and author

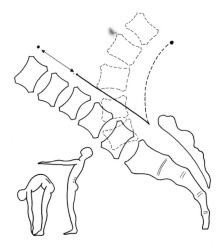

Fig. 2.7 Change in length of the lumbar spinal canal during flexion and extension. Tracing from a radiograph. From: Troup J D G 1986 Back and neck injuries. In: Reilly T (ed) Sports fitness and sports injuries. Faber & Faber, London, with permission from the publishers and author

(1979) utilises this for his 'stoop test' whereby progressive spinal flexion is used to minimise the extent that structures may invade the spinal canal.

The walls of the spinal canal do not move as one. Due to the axis of flexion and extension being anterior to the neuraxis, the posterior wall of the canal elongates more than the anterior wall during flexion movements. These movements have been measured radiographically in 35 subjects where it was found that the posterior aspect increased in length by 23%–30% and the anterior wall of the canal increased from 6.5%–13% (Babin & Capesius 1976).

Lateral flexion movements elongate one side

of the canal and shorten the other. It has been estimated that there is a 15% change in length between the two extremes of spinal lateral flexion (Breig 1978).

The effects of rotation on the shape of the spinal canal has not been investigated. Most spinal rotation occurs in the cervical spine and will probably alter the shape of the spinal canal in some way. Changes are less likely in the less mobile thoracic and lumbar spines. Few functional movements are in the pure coronal or sagittal planes and rotation will nearly always be combined with other movements such as flexion and extension which have a greater effect on the nervous system.

Traction elongates the spinal canal and thus, by necessity, alters the contained structures. Breig (1978) used superimposed radiographs and measured a 10 mm length increase in a patient's cervical spine following 5 kg of traction. There are photographs in Cyriax (1978) showing marked distraction of lumbar vertebrae during traction. Patients occasionally complain of headaches after lumbar traction. Perhaps this is due to the elongation of the lumbar spinal canal and the resultant forces on the neuraxis and meninges at that level and higher. In these patients, a finding of a positive Slump Test (Ch. 7) is very common.

Certain limb movements such as the Straight Leg Raise test (SLR) will increase neuraxial and meningeal tension. This is due to the connections of the peripheral nervous system to the central nervous system. A limb movement such as the SLR also elongates the lumbar spinal canal by pelvic rotation (Breig 1978, Bohannon et al 1985).

Effects at the intervertebral foramen

Extension of the spine decreases the cross sectional area of the intervertebral foramen (IVF). Conversely, the cross sectional area is increased by flexion. This effect has been measured in the lumbar spine. Panjabi et al (1983) reported, from cadavers with no degeneration of the spine, that flexion increased the IVF area by 30% from the neutral and extension decreased the space by 20%. Lateral flexion and rotation movements caused minimal (2–4%) alterations in cross sectional area, although in specimens with degenerative joints, these movements influenced the cross-sectional areas far more. These are marked changes in an area containing such structures as nerve roots, dorsal root ganglion, radicular artery and grey ramus communicans (Breig 1978).

Due to the containment of the neuraxis and meninges together with their attachments to the spinal canal, movements of the canal and IVF structures will inevitably have repercussions on these structures.

Neuraxial and meningeal adaptive mechanisms

In this area, Breig's work (1978) is outstanding and his text is recommended reading for anyone attempting to mobilise the nervous system.

With the spinal canal being 5–9 cm longer in flexion than extension, the contained structures must adapt in order to function normally. Since the structures are composed of different tissues (compare neuraxis to dura mater), they will adapt differently. These features are discussed in Chapter 1.

The Slump Test and the Passive Neck Flexion Test are two of the most useful tension tests. Both employ spinal flexion. In flexion, the neuraxis and meninges elongate and move anteriorly in the spinal canal. In extension, they move posteriorly. Extension, as well as allowing relaxation of the neuraxis, also creates transverse folds in the dura mater (Breig 1978). While the dural theca moves posteriorly in the lumbar spine, the tip of the theca moves caudally (Penning & Wilmink 1981). With lateral flexion movements, the nervous system on the concave side shortens and elongates on the convex side, thus mirroring the spinal canal (Breig 1978). In rotation, although it seems the shape of the spinal canal stays reasonably constant, the neuraxis and meninges do not. Farfan (1975) considers that persistent rotation of one vertebrae on another can stretch a nerve root by 0.5–1.0 cm. Logically, spinal rotation to the left should stretch the left dorsal root more than the left ventral root. Breig

(1978) notes that, due to the denticulate ligaments, rotation of the thoracic spine causes deformation of the spinal cord with an accompanying decrease in the spinal cord circumference. Few functional movements are in the pure coronal or sagittal plane and rotation will nearly always be combined with other movements. The thoracic spine is the least mobile segment and the neuraxis in this area is governed by tension and movement alterations in the more mobile lumbar and cervical spines (Jirout 1963, Breig 1978).

If the dural theca and the spinal cord are lengthened, the pressure in these two structures will increase. Changes in tension in the spinal cord during flexion are evident from alterations in the shape of blood vessels and in the shape of the cord (Fig. 2.8). There will be a further increase in pressure if the dural theca is drawn onto a ridge of bone or soft tissue during flexion.

The adaptive mechanisms of tension and movement of the structures within the spinal canal are nicely summed up in Figure 2.8, a photograph taken from Breig's book *Adverse Mechanical Tension in the Central Nervous System* (1978). In this picture, the adaptive mechanisms of both movement and tension are clearly illustrated. Also evident is movement of the cord and nerve roots in relation to the dura and dural sleeves.

The sliding of the nervous system next to the interface can be analysed further into directions of movement. In spinal flexion of 24 cadavers, Louis (1981) could demonstrate a consistent pattern of neuraxial, meningeal and nerve root movement in relation to interfaces, and also areas where the relationship was constant. According to Louis (1981) the C6, T6 and L4 vertebral levels are the approximate areas where no nervous system movement occurs in relation to interfaces. I have referred to such an occurrence in the body as a 'tension point', and have elaborated on this concept later in the chapter. In Figure 2.9 Louis's work has been extrapolated to spinal flexion in the sitting position. Reid (1960) also noted that, with spinal flexion, there was little movement at C5 root level and, at the T12

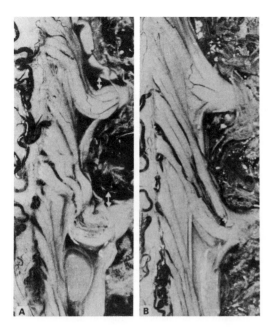

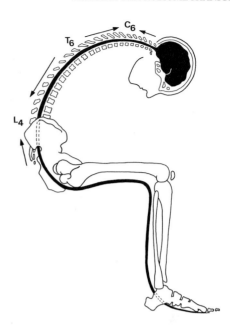

Fig. 2.8 Normal deformation of the dura, cord and nerve roots in the cervical canal in the cadaver due to full extension and flexion of the cervical spine. A total laminectomy has been performed and the dura opened and retracted although still able to transmit tension.
In A the cervical spine is in extension, the nervous system is slack, the root sleeves have lost contact with the pedicles (lower arrows) and the nerve roots with the inner surfaces of the sleeves (upper arrows).
In B the cervical spine has been flexed, the nervous system including the dura mater has been stretched and moved in relation to surrounding structures. Note that the root sleeves have come in contact with the pedicles and the nerve roots with the inner surface of the sleeves. Note also the change in shape of the blood vessels. From: Breig A 1978 Adverse mechanical tension in the central nervous system, Almqvist & Wiksell, Stockholm, with permission

Fig. 2.9 Postulated neurobiomechanics from spinal extension to spinal flexion. The approximate points C6, T6 and L4 are where the neuraxis and meninges do not move in relation to the movements of the spinal canal. Adapted from Louis (1981)

THE STRAIGHT LEG RAISE (SLR)

The SLR is probably the most widely known tension test, although its main use traditionally is to assist in the diagnosis of a low lumbar disc injury. However, the complex neurobiomechanics that occur in and around the sciatic tract during the test suggest a far greater role for the test in the analysis of symptomatology.

Both movement and elongation occur in the sciatic tract during the SLR. Figure 2.10 clearly demonstrates the degree of nerve movement at the intervertebral exit and within the pelvis during a SLR.

It is well known and obviously supported by the photographs that, during a SLR, lumbosacral nerve roots move caudal in relation to their respective intervertebral foramen and in a caudal direction within the pelvis (Goddard & Reid 1965, Breig 1978, Breig & Troup 1979). However, little thought has been given to the dynamics of the remaining sciatic nerve trunk. Nerves have some elastic properties such

root level, there was downward movement. With cervical flexion alone, most movement occurred in a rostral direction from C7 to the T3 vertebrae. Smith (1956) conducted radiographic examinations of cord shift in rhesus monkeys. He found that, from spinal extension to flexion, the cord converged towards the C4,5 disc; moving downwards from above and upwards from below. Where both the neuraxis and the meninges have been studied during movement, it has been noted that their biomechanics are different. They do not move as one, and the neuraxis has a movement relationship with the dural theca (Adams & Logue 1971, Louis 1981).

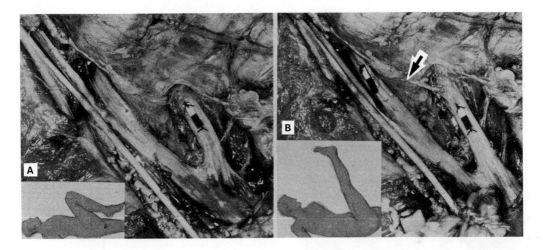

Fig. 2.10 The sacral plexus and the exits of the spinal nerves through the intervertebral foramina. Paper markers have been sutured to the nerves. In A, with the rest of the body in an 'anti-tension' position and the hip in some flexion, the nerve is drawn into the intervertebral foramina. In B, the effect of the Straight Leg Raise on the nerve is evident as the nerve is drawn out of the foramen. Note also the sympathetic trunk (arrow) tightening up during the SLR. From: Breig A 1978 Adverse mechanical tension in the central nervous system, Almqvist & Wiksell, Stockholm, with permission

that, if the entire nerve is tensed, caudal movement in relation to its interface cannot continue throughout the entire leg. There needs to be a reversal of movement somewhere along the trunk. Smith (1956) conducted studies with monkeys and one human cadaver to investigate this process. It was been found that, while the sciatic and tibial nerves superior to the knee move caudal in relation to interfaces, this relationship is reversed inferior to the knee. That is, the tibial nerve below the knee moves cephalad in relation to surrounding tissue. Thus a point exists somewhere posterior to the knee where no movement occurs in relation to the interface (Fig. 2.11). Note that the SLR in this study was performed by extending the knee while the hip was in flexion. The mechanisms of adaptation may be different in the traditional SLR where hip flexion is superimposed on the extended knee. Certainly, patients' responses to the alternative methods of SLR differ.

It may be easier to apply the concept of 'tension points' to the common peroneal trunk. Here the tension point appears to be at the attachment of the nerve to the head of the fibula and presumably, during knee extension in hip flexion, the common peroneal nerve and branches move in opposite directions on

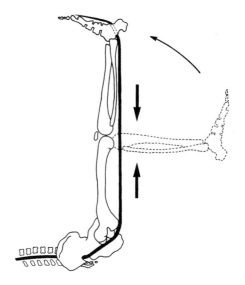

Fig. 2.11 Postulated neurobiomechanics during knee extension in hip flexion. The nervous system proximal to the knee is drawn caudal in relation to the interface and the nervous system distal to the knee moves rostral. At the point of movement, there is no movement of the nervous system in relation to the surrounding interfacing structures. Adapted from Smith (1956)

either side of the attachment. In the traditional SLR (hip flexion with knee extended), the tension point may be posterior to the hip (Smith 1956). The concept of tension points is discussed later in this chapter. These postulated physical

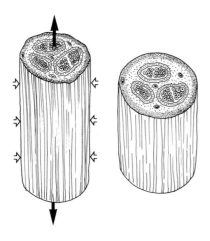

Fig. 2.12 Tension along a nerve will increase the intraneural pressure as the cross-sectional area decreases

properties of nerve may, in some way, explain the distribution of symptoms during tension testing.

When tension is applied to a nerve, the intraneural pressure will increase as the cross-sectional area decreases (Fig. 2.12). This increase in pressure will compromise the amount of blood allowed access to the nerve fibres, probably by stretched extraneural vessels or by closing of the small vessels crossing the perineurium. This blood deprivation may interfere with conduction and also, in combination with the pressure, affect the axonal transport systems (Ch. 3). The exact degree of rise in intraneural pressure during a test such as the SLR is unknown. From extrapolation of data on the ulnar nerve (Pechan & Julis 1975), it is possible to quadruple the pressure within a peripheral nerve by activities that stretch limbs. Thus, it seems that normal activities, perhaps even moving from sitting to standing, could greatly increase the intraneural pressure in the sciatic nerve. This study by Pechan & Julis (1975) is examined in detail in the next section on upper limb adaptive mechanisms. It is known that, in association with such deformation of nerve, the blood supply to nerve fibres will begin to diminish at around 8% elongation of the nerve and stop at around 15% elongation (Lundborg & Rydevik 1973, Rydevik et al 1981, Ogata & Naito 1986). How this relates to the elongation of nerves during a tension test is unknown.

Clinically, the SLR will rarely be used alone. The biomechanics of additional movements which further sensitise the test, such as ankle dorsiflexion, hip adduction, hip medial rotation and cervical flexion are discussed in Chapter 7. So too is the Prone Knee Bend test.

UPPER LIMB ADAPTIVE MECHANISMS

The mechanical function of the nervous system in the upper limb is also impressive. In a classic study, McLellan & Swash (1976) placed needles in the median nerves of 15 volunteers and measured the movement of these needles during various arm and neck movements. This rather ingenious study meant that in vivo movement could be measured. The amount of movement of a segment of nerve was ascertained by measuring the excursion of the head of the needle and the depth of the needle in the limb. The rest was simple geometry. In this study, active and passive movements were of equal effect. With the needles positioned in the median nerve, midway in the upper arm, wrist and finger extension pulled the nerve down an average of 7.4 mm. Flexion of the elbow allowed 4.3 mm of movement upwards. In one volunteer, the median nerve could be displaced by 2–3 cm in some arm movement combinations (unfortunately unrecorded). Similar amounts of movement have been recorded in cadaver studies (Shaw Wilgis & Murphy 1986). One unfortunate drawback for physiotherapists seeking information from these two studies is that the position of the whole arm and trunk during the experiments was not recorded. Nevertheless, the ranges and directions of movement recorded give a valuable insight into upper limb biomechanics.

When Macnicol (1980) studied ulnar nerve biomechanics at the elbow in 40 fresh cadaveric arms, he noted the ulnar nerve migrated proximally during flexion. He also measured the pressure of the ulnar nerve against interfacing tissues, including bone, at the elbow in 10 specimens. Elbow flexion to 90° did not significantly alter the pressure. However, full flexion caused marked increases at the postcondylar groove and within the cubital tunnel. These pressures were increased by concomitant abduction of the arm.

The position of the rest of the body was not stated.

The other adaptive mechanism to movement is the development of pressure or tension in the system. Pechan & Julis's study (1975) has already been mentioned and is worthy of elaboration. They measured the intraneural pressure in the ulnar nerves of fresh cadavers with the elbow in various positions. A pressure transducer was connected to a needle placed in the ulnar nerve at the elbow. With the elbow position constant they could change the intraneural pressure considerably by wrist and shoulder movements. In a position similar to the Upper Limb Tension Test 3 (Ch. 8), intraneural pressure within the ulnar nerve was quadrupled.

It is very likely that tension points occur in the vicinity of the elbow and shoulder during arm movements and that their behaviour would be dependent on the kind of arm movement. Rubenach (1987) noted very little movement of the median nerve at the elbow during upper limb tension manoeuvres in a cadaver, and Sunderland (1978) has suggested that, where nerves branch or enter a muscle at an abrupt angle, the movement is likely to be far less than elsewhere along the nerve.

These two adaptive mechanisms of tension and movement must occur simultaneously, although in certain situations one mechanism will predominate. Pathological processes or injury may effect one or both of these adaptive mechanisms. In later chapters, an explanation of how treatment can be directed accordingly is offered.

Physiotherapists involved in the treatment of joints will be well aware of the importance of accessory ('joint play') and physiological movements. In the examination and treatment of the nervous system, adaptive mechanisms of movement and tension should be accorded the same importance.

AUTONOMIC NERVOUS SYSTEM ADAPTIVE MECHANISMS

Often overlooked is the fact that the autonomic nervous system (ANS) must also adapt to body movements if it is to function correctly. Autonomic fibres in the peripheral nervous system and the neuraxis must adapt in a similar fashion to neighbouring motor and sensory fibres. However, equally important biomechanics exist where the ANS is physically separate from the rest of the nervous system, i.e., in the trunks, rami and ganglia. Where the ANS forms chains, the likelihood of mechanical involvement is greater. Of particular interest is the sympathetic trunk. The location of the trunk, just anterior to the ever-moving costo-transverse joints, should provide ample initial evidence. In Figures 2.13 and 2.14 the location of the sympathetic chain in relation to the vertebral column and ribs is shown. The anterior view (Fig. 2.13) shows that lateral flexion movements, particularly of the thoracic spine, must move and tighten the sympathetic chain. The side view is probably more revealing. Flexion is likely to stretch the thoracic and lumbar chains, since the trunk is posterior to the axis of flexion and extension.

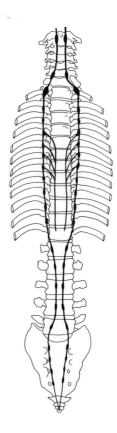

Fig. 2.13 Anterior view of the sympathetic trunk and its bony relations

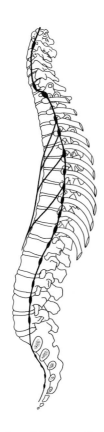

Fig. 2.14 Lateral view of the sympathetic trunk and its bony relations

Conversely, cervical extension could stretch the cervical sympathetic trunk and ganglia. In the cervical spine, damage to the cervical sympathetic plexus has been observed by Macnab (1971) in simulated whiplash incidents in monkeys. Most damage occurred during the extension phase. People who sit with a kyphotic thoracic spine combined with lumbar spine flexion and upper cervical spine extension as the chin 'pokes' could quite conceivably be placing undue tension on the sympathetic trunk. Cervical flexion could tense the sympathetic plexuses around the carotid and vertebral arteries (Schneider & Schemm 1961).

As well as movement and tension created in the thoracic sympathetic trunk by thoracic spine and rib movements, given the continuum of the system, movements such as a SLR will have mechanical effects on the sympathetic trunk. Breig (1978) realised there could be considerable clinical repercussions from altered biomechanics of

the lumbar sympathetic trunk. In the photograph (Fig. 2.15) the large excursion of the lumbar sympathetic trunk during a SLR is evident. Excitation and deficit symptoms from the ANS may presumably be provoked by chemical irritation or mechanical stimulus such as stretching or compression.

Clear documentation of widespread patho-anatomical changes in and around the sympathetic trunk and ganglia in 1000 cadavers has been detailed by Nathan (1986). Further details of this study and the changes in this part of the nervous system are presented in Chapter 3. It should be noted that no normative studies of the attachments of the sympathetic structures have been carried out. Perhaps there is a series of normal attachments similar to the dural ligaments. This possibility has never been investigated in the terms we are now considering.

The effect of adverse tension on preganglionic neurones of the autonomic nervous system also requires consideration. These neurones are located in close proximity to the centre of the cord and are thus somewhat protected. Yet, the possibility of symptoms from irritation or inhibition or a neuropraxic type of injury of these neurones exists. This is particularly so in the thoracic spine where there is a weakness in the blood supply to the cord compared with other areas (Dommisse 1975).

Clinically, apparent mechanical impairment of the sympathetic chain is often evident. Perhaps this provides an explanation for symptoms such as nausea, vague thoracic pains and headaches evoked by a SLR. Slump Tests (Ch. 7) occasionally reproduce odd symptoms such as deep abdominal pains, flushes and sweating. Upper Limb Tension Tests can cause a 'pumping feeling' in the arm and symptoms of increased sweating and colour changes in the extremity are often related to limbs with positive tension tests.

Knowledge of the anatomy and biomechanics of the sympathetic trunk opens the door to techniques of mobilising the trunk, either via the ribs, the costo-transverse joints or by combinations of nerve and joint movements. It can also help to make some sense of the kind of symptoms (sometimes rather odd) that can be reproduced by tension tests.

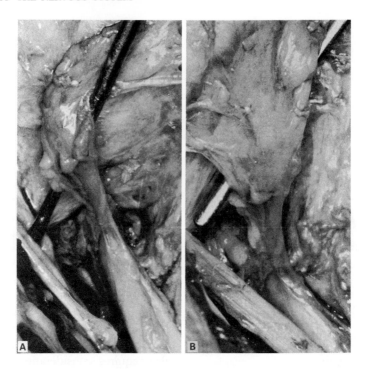

Fig. 2.15 Stretching and slackening of the lumbar sympathetic chain in the hip flexion/knee extension test. In A the ganglionic chain, together with the surrounding tissue, slackens and presents practically no resistance to displacement by a probe. In B when the hip joint is flexed and then the knee extended, the sympathetic chain is stretched. Because the chain is continuous, stretch and movement probably occurs in more rostral segments of the sympathetic nervous system. From: Breig A 1978 Adverse mechanical tension in the central nervous system. Almqvist & Wiksell, Stockholm, with permission

THE CONCEPT OF TENSION POINTS

In sections above, studies have been described, indicating that, when moving a body part or parts, the movement of the underlying nervous system is not necessarily in the same direction (Smith 1956, Reid 1960, Louis 1981). This creates points along the nervous system which apparently do not move or have minimal movement in relation to surrounding structures. Note that at these points, even though the interface may have great mobility, the nervous system 'keeps pace' with the interface. These I have termed 'tension points' and proposed that, during certain movements, they are a feature of nervous system adaptation to that movement (Butler 1989). The clinical regularity of symptoms associated with these proposed points, for example, the C6, T6 and L4 areas, and the posterior knee and anterior elbow in patients with positive tension tests, made me aware that something

special was happening at these sites. I feel these points are especially evident with tension at both ends of the nervous system (e.g., SLR with dorsiflexion, Slump Test). Repeated clinical observations have made me feel comfortable with the postulation that these points are vulnerable sites within the nervous system. Support is not only clinical but anatomical.

Clinical correlations for tension points

At the limit of the SLR test, patients (and subjects) complain of pain in varying areas. A common complaint is pain or stretch posterior to the knee or higher in the bulk of the hamstring muscles. Some complain of a 'burn' over the superior tibio-fibular joint. I believe that those who complain of this 'burn' and those who complain of pain posterior to the knee (often they can place one finger on it during the SLR) are complaining of 'tension point' pain. There are no hamstring structures at the point. At some stage in the development of an adverse tension disorder of the lower limb and spine, this sign is likely to be present.

The proposed C6, T6 and L4 tension point areas are often clinically evident. In a patient with a known lumbar disc lesion, perhaps involving irritation or tethering of the dura mater, interscapular pain and perhaps neck pain are not uncommon complaints. Clinicians with experience in treating patients with a whiplash disorder will be aware of the frequent occurrence of interscapular pain and, as a later development, lumbar pain. These spinal pains are often close to the tension point areas (Fig. 2.16) and are sometimes associated with posterior knee pain. Almost always, patients with such a presentation can be found to have a positive SLR and Slump Test (Ch. 8). In a patient with a limited SLR, palpation of the T6 vertebral level will often reveal stiffness and local pain not existing at levels above or below. In the limbs, the spread of symptoms from one area, such as the carpal tunnel to another such as the elbow, is quite common. This symptomatic dysfunction is known as the 'double crush syndrome' and is extensively discussed in the next chapter.

If the physiotherapist is applying a clinical reasoning process to his or her examination (Ch. 5), I feel a good deal of credence can be placed on reported clinical observations. After all, such a physiotherapist is continually moving, palpating and listening to patients, endeavouring to make the physical findings fit with the patients' complaints. The tension point hypothesis has come after some years of working almost entirely with patients suffering from whiplash disorders and those with repetition or overuse injuries. After a time, presentation of clear patterns of tension disorders and responses to treatment emerge.

The anatomy of tension points

The proposed tension points form one of the many mechanisms (detailed in Ch. 3) by which structural and functional inadequacies may predispose the nervous system to symptoms.

If the nervous system's adaptation to movement varies between different areas, then anatomical variations in these areas should be evident. Anatomists have not specifically looked for such variations. However, there is evidence worth extrapolating to support the concept of tension points, especially in the vascularisation and the connective tissue content.

As the nervous system is so dependant on an adequate blood supply, hypotheses as to the existence of tension points may be developed from its patterns of vascularisation. In order to adapt to different movement and tension requirements, the vascular arrangement of the nervous system differs between mobile and immobile areas. In general, extraneural vessels (feeder vessels) enter the nervous system in areas of little movement relative to the interface. These areas are often postulated tension points. In the cervical spine, the regions where most extraneural vessels enter are the C5 to C7 areas (Mannen 1966, Parke 1988). The lumbosacral plexus also has an abundant blood supply like the cervical cord (Dommisse 1986). The extraneural vessels supplying the thoracic neuraxis and meninges are less consistent, although a major artery usually enters around T9. The thoracic spine is less mobile than the lumbar and cervical spines and this probably lessens the need for feeder vessels to enter at a particular point. In the periphery, some examples are feeder vessels entering behind the hip and knee joint and flexor aspect of the elbow. In-

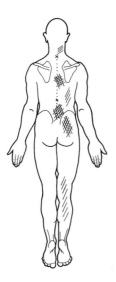

Fig. 2.16 Body chart — typical areas of pain following a lumbar disc lesion. The tension points are evident. A similar pattern may occur when the nervous system is injured in the cervical spine

traneural vessels provide nutrition for the segments of nervous system between joints. The median nerve provides a clear example. In the upper arm, feeder vessels near the elbow and shoulder supply the nerve, and in between it is almost entirely dependent on intraneural vessels. This is essentially good design because the median nerve can move up to 2 cm or more in the upper arm during movement, making it a potentially unsafe place for a feeder vessel to enter. As a generalisation, the extraneural vessels enter peripheral nerves around joints and protected areas (Sunderland 1978, Ogata & Naito 1986).

The arrangement of the connective tissue sheaths of the peripheral nervous system provides further support. The proportion of connective tissue in relation to neural tissue is different depending on the nerve and the segment of nerve examined. Where a nerve has movement as its major adaptive mechanism (such as the median nerve in the upper arm), the connective tissues occupy a smaller proportion of the cross-sectional area. Conversely, where a nerve (such as the median nerve at the wrist) is more vulnerable to compressive forces, a greater proportion of connective tissue exists. Note this relationship in Figure 2.17, where the percentages of cross sectional area of a segment of median nerve devoted to fascicles and devoted to epineurial tissue are shown. When the number of fascicles increases,

the cross sectional area devoted to them decreases. A similar relationship, although not quite as clear, exists in other nerves. Sunderland (1978) has documented the fascicular arrangement in all major nerves.

The attachments of the nervous system to surrounding structures also provides some clues. At the L4 tension point, the dura mater is firmly attached to the posterior longitudinal ligament — so firmly that it is impossible to separate the two structures (Blikna 1969, Parke & Watanabe 1990). According to Haupt & Stofft (1978), dura mater is thicker in the mid thoracic area than elsewhere in the spinal canal. However, Tencer et al (1986) differ. In their human cadaver studies they found the neural properties of elasticity were uniform throughout the length of the dura mater. The L4 and C6 regions are the approximate central levels of their respective plexuses, and the emerging spinal nerves and peripheral nerves on both sides must tether the system and limit movement up and down the spinal canal. In some areas, the peripheral nervous system is more firmly attached than elsewhere, for example, the common peroneal nerve at the head of the fibula and the radial nerve at the radio-humeral joint.

So, in summary, there is a general link between anatomy, biomechanics and blood supply (refer to Table 2.1).

Undoubtedly, the arrangement of the individual structural components and their adaptations to allow neural function during movement are complex. Table 2.1 is a broad generalisation and serves to emphasise how little we know about

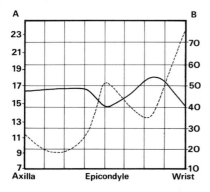

Fig. 2.17 The relationship between connective tissue and neural tissue in the median nerve. Column A is the number of fascicles (hatched line) and column B is the percentage cross sectional area of fascicles (dark line). From: Sunderland S 1978 Nerves and nerve injuries, 2nd edn. Churchill Livingstone, Edinburgh, with permission from the publishers and author

Table 2.1 The hypothesised relationship between structure and function of a particular segment of the peripheral nervous system. No. 1 is a segment where the main adaptive measure is by movement (for example, the median nerve in the mid upper arm). No. 2 is a segment where it is suggested that the main adaptive measure is by an increase in tension (for example the median nerve at the elbow).

Adaptive measure	Blood supply	Amount of connective tissue	No. of fascicles
1. Movement	Intraneural	Decreased	Decreased
2. Tension	Extraneural	Increased	Increased

neurobiomechanics. Of importance is that this pattern seems to relate to the clinical presentations of adverse tension syndromes. The nature of an injury and the location of that injury will have a bearing on the kind of altered neurobiomechanics produced. The mechanisms of these injuries are discussed in the next chapter.

FURTHER BIOMECHANICAL CONSIDERATIONS

Distribution of tension and movement

When a body is moved, the consequences for the nervous system will be spread over a greater distance than for non-neural structures. For example, dorsiflexion of the ankle will mechanically influence the nervous system in the lumbar spine and perhaps further, rostrally in the neuraxis. Muscle and joints affected by dorsiflexion will be below the knee, although fascia is probably tensed at higher levels. The spread of tension and movement in terms of distance and amplitude is not really known and will presumably be dependent on a number of factors, including the position of the rest of the body. Normative studies and pathological evidence do provide a guide as to the extent of the movement and therefore give us some basic guidelines for assessment and treatment via tension tests.

Normative studies

In Figure 2.18, the transmission of tension from the cervical cord to the lumbar cord during neck flexion is evident. Breig & Marions (1963) also provided earlier cadaveric proof that cervical flexion could influence lumbosacral nerve roots. More recent studies by Tencer et al (1986) have further supported this. In the limbs, movement of one joint will influence nerve elsewhere in the limb. Cadaver studies by Borges et al (1981) showed that plantar flexion and inversion of the foot could move and tension the sciatic nerve in the thigh. Smith (1956) and Breig & Troup (1979) demonstrated that dorsiflexion could influence the lumbosacral nerve roots, and Smith (1956) further showed that ankle dorsiflexion in

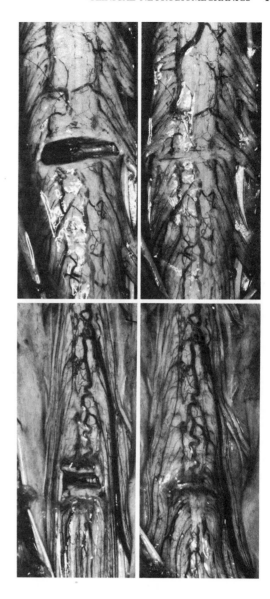

Fig. 2.18 Effects on the normal tension and relaxation of the nervous system of a transverse incision in the spinal cord at cervical (top left and right) and lumbar levels (bottom left and right). The dura has been retracted but can still transmit tension. On the left hand side, in full flexion of the cervical spine there is retraction of the wounds at the cervical and lumbar levels respectively. In the photograph on the right hand side, in the neutral position of the cervical spine moving from flexion, the wound surfaces at the cervical level come together. In the right lower picture, the wound surfaces meet when the cervical spine is fully extended. These movements of the lumbar cord have occurred with movements of the cervical spine only. From: Breig A 1978 Adverse mechanical tension in the central nervous system. Almqvist & Wiksell, Stockholm, with permission

SLR could tension the nervous system up to and including the cerebellum. In the arm, the needle studies of McLellan & Swash (1976) and cadaver studies of Shaw Wilgis & Murphy (1986) showed that wrist movement had mechanical effects on the nervous system in the upper arm. Selvaratnam (1989) studied Upper Limb Tension Test manoeuvres in cadavers and provided evidence that cervical manoeuvres, when added to elbow and wrist extension, were capable of creating strain on the nerve roots of the brachial plexus.

Some in vivo studies also provide helpful information. One of the pioneers of tension testing in the arm, Elvey (1980), claimed that movements of the contralateral arm and the Straight Leg Raise could alter symptoms provoked in an arm. In 1985, Rubenach investigated Elvey's first claim. She found that, if an ULTT (Ch. 8) was performed on one arm and the symptom response position maintained, then the addition of the same test to the other arm would result in a change of symptoms. These changes were noted in 77% of 116 young asymptomatic subjects, with the majority reporting a decrease in symptoms. Tension in the nervous system must therefore be, in part, transmitted transversely across the neuraxis. This study provides some insight into the relationship of adverse tension and bilateral carpal tunnel syndrome. Bell (1987) investigated Elvey's second claim. With the subject's ULTT maintained, it was found that, with the addition of a bilateral Straight Leg Raise, 77 out of 100 asymptomatic young volunteers experienced a change in symptoms, 67 reporting a decrease and 10 reporting an increase. These studies not only show a link between the limbs but are of interest in those disorders where the patient complains of symptoms which spread from limb to limb on the one side of the body.

Clinical correlations

Breig (1978) calls the syndrome 'sciatic brachialgia' whereby, on a SLR, the patient experiences pain in the leg and in the arm. Earlier, Torkildson (1956) observed patients who complained of sciatic pain on cervical flexion and called this 'brachialgic sciatica'. This will be a familiar finding for physiotherapists who regularly perform tension tests. Tumours around the foramen magnum are often associated with low back and sciatic pain. These symptoms may be the first sign of the tumour (Dodge et al 1956). Clinically, the level of sensitivity of the moving tissues and the mechanical compromise of the nervous system are the dominant issues. A situation could be envisaged where the dura is tethered at the T4 level. If tethered, the Passive Neck Flexion (PNF) may only tension down to the tethered level with the neuraxis structures below T4 relatively unhindered. Equally, if the neuraxis and/or its membranes are in a heightened state of irritation, PNF could easily reproduce lumbar symptoms. It is not uncommon in some severe injuries, such as the whiplash disorder, to have ankle dorsiflexion increasing neck and head symptoms and for a SLR to influence shoulder and elbow symptoms. A disease such as diabetes which raises intrafascicular pressure in all nerves may predispose to this association of apparently remote symptoms. The issue concerning the spread of symptoms is again taken up in the next chapter in the section on the double crush syndrome.

The amplitude of tension and movement distribution

The nervous system is normally under some pressure and is thus under some tension. If the nervous system is cut there will be retraction of the cut ends, resulting in some movement and tension alterations elsewhere. This has been shown experimentally in rabbit peripheral nerve (Millesi et al 1972) and is the experience of surgeons (Breig 1978, Millesi 1986, Wilgis & Murphy 1986, Lundborg 1988). Tencer et al (1985) showed that, even with the cervical spine in extension, if the dura were cut it would retract.

It appears the spread of tension and movement to other areas of the nervous system is non-uniform. That is, once a force is placed on the nervous system, this force is not equally dispersed over the whole nervous system. McLellan & Swash (1976) noted that wrist and finger extension will move the median nerve at the wrist two to four times more than at the middle upper arm. Tencer et al (1985) noted more movement occurring in cervical dura than in the lumbar dura during Passive Neck Flexion. At the site of movement, more adaptive measures will be required than elsewhere in the nervous system. So for example, in the SLR more neural responses will occur at the posterior hip and into the lumbar spine than at the calf. The greater the tension applied in one area, the greater the distance and magnitude of adaptive mechanisms elsewhere in the body. Breig (1978), however, applies St. Venant's Law to tension distribution in the neuraxis and meninges. This means that if a pulling force is placed on the rim of an elastic tube, then that force will be distributed evenly throughout the whole tube at a distance of two to three times the diameter. Clinically this does not seem correct. If it is the case, a SLR reproducing thoracic symptoms should do so equally with both left and right SLRs. This is a rare finding. I have noted in patients with cervical and head symptoms, apparently related to adverse tension, that either the left or right SLR will be more symptomatic. Apparently, the biomechanics of the various structures making up the nervous system and the complex array of attachments mean the mechanics are far more complex than that of an elastic cylinder.

Tension and compression go together in an elastic structure which interacts mechanically with a solid interface. With compression and thus an increase in local tension, any movement of the nervous system will increase that compressive force (Fig. 2.19).

Movement perpendicular to the interface

It has already been mentioned that the neuraxis and meninges do not move uniformly with the spinal canal and that all movements are not necessarily in the longitudinal axis. In spinal flexion, as well as increasing the intradural pressures, the neuraxis and meninges are pulled toward the anterior aspect of the spinal canal, i.e., the 'shortest route' (Jirout 1959, Jirout 1963, Breig 1978). However from 40 lumbar myelograms, Penning & Wilmink (1981) have shown that, during spinal flexion and extension, the lumbar dural theca moves anteriorly during extension and posteriorly during flexion (Fig. 2.20). They considered that shortening and buckling of the flaval ligaments were in part responsible.

In extension, any anterior compression is relieved although the AP diameter of the cord increases (Parke 1988). Breig (1978) has shown that, when the spinal canal is toward extension, the dural theca can lie on the side of the spinal canal in accordance with the laws of gravity. So too can the cord or cauda equina inside the dural theca. In some situations there will be antero-posterior movements, transverse movements, and combinations of these movements of the cord in relation to the theca, and the theca in relation to the spinal canal (Adams & Logue 1971, Louis 1981, Breig 1978). The Slump Test is an example. Here, although maximal tension is applied to the whole nervous system in the trunk and lower

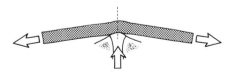

Fig. 2.19 Tension and compression go together in an elastic structure that presses on another structure. If compression increases, then tension will increase. If tension increases then compression will increase

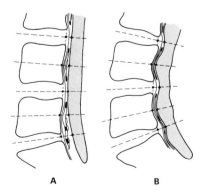

A   B

Fig. 2.20 Anteroposterior movements of the dural theca in the spinal canal during lumbar flexion (A) and extension (B). Adapted from Penning & Wilmink (1981).

limbs, the neuraxis and meninges will also move forward in the spinal canal and probably stress the dorsomedian plica.

At the elbow, the ulnar nerve slides in a dorso-medial direction from elbow extension to flexion (Apfelberg & Larsen 1973). Where a nerve is easily accessible to palpation, such as the branches of the superficial peroneal nerve in the dorsum of the foot or the median nerve in the upper arm, the nerve can be readily located and moved transversely a centimetre and more. This movement will be less when the nerve is tightened in a tension position.

Gravity and the nervous system

In the spinal canal, the weight of the neuraxis and the available spaces makes it gravity dependent to some degree. In supine, the neuraxis and meninges lie on the posterior aspect of the canal. In sidelying they lie on the down side and in prone they lie on the anterior aspect of the canal (Breig 1978). Breig (1978) clearly showed that if cervical flexion was added, the lumbar dural theca and cauda equina would rapidly return to the centre of the canal. Less movement was noted in the medullary cone as it was held more central in the theca by denticulate ligaments. The amount of laxity will depend on the limbs and head position. More laxity will be allowed in the out of tension positions such as knee flexion, hip flexion to around 30° and spinal extension.

An investigation by Miller (1987) on 100 normal young asymptomatic subjects found that a SLR performed in supine and then in side lying would produce different ranges of movement. In sidelying the lower SLR was more restricted, probably due to the lateral flexion forced upon the spine.

Due to the close proximity of the interfacing tissues, gravity is likely to have little effect on the peripheral nervous system, other than from any indirect alterations of the neuraxis and meninges.

The effect of sequence of additions and body position

If the SLR is performed by flexing the hip first and then extending the knee, the neuro-biomechanics will be different than if the knee is extended and then the hip flexed. Clinically this is quite clear. The hip flexion component takes up some of the available tension and movement first and then the knee extension is superimposed upon that. This concept may be better explained by use of the SLR and cervical flexion example. The SLR result (range of movement and pain response) will be different if the test is performed with cervical flexion or without. The cervical flexion tensions the nervous system to some degree, therefore, the tension/movement/interface relationship during the SLR will be different (Fig. 2.21). These features will be important in assessment and treatment. For example, when the SLR is performed, in order to attain an accurate reassessment, the technique should be subsequently performed with the head on the same pillow. The patient's arms should also be in the same position each time a SLR is performed. The sequence of component additions of the tension test will also influence the effectiveness of treatment via movement.

This important clinical observation was substantiated recently by Shacklock (1989). He compared the distribution of symptoms between three different methods of application of the same component movements of the SLR with plantar flexion/inversion of the foot (SLR/PFI), utilising data from studies by Mauhart (1989), Slater (1989) and Shacklock (1989). The methods were maximal SLR plus maximal PFI (Slater 1989), maximal PFI plus maximal SLR (Mauhart 1989) and minimal PFI plus maximal SLR (Shacklock 1989). The differences in the test procedures were reflected significantly in the distribution of symptoms. A higher percentage of subjects reported symptoms where the first movement was applied.

Shacklock (1989) concluded that the order and magnitude of application effected the symptom responses especially at each end of the limb. Therefore, to access the nervous system about the hip and lumbar spine best, proximal components should be taken up first (i.e., hip movements). Similarly, to test nervous system structures in the foot, the foot component should be taken up first.

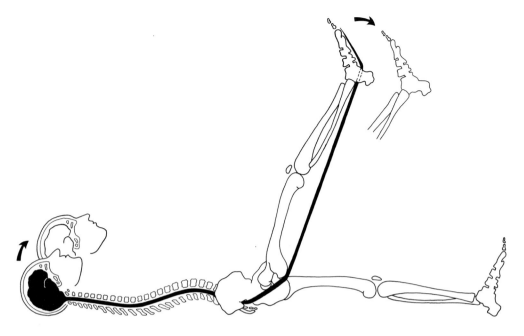

Fig. 2.21 The response to a SLR will differ depending on whether the cervical flexion is added before or after the SLR

REFERENCES

Adams C B T, Logue V 1971 Studies in cervical spondylotic myelopathy. Brain 94: 557–568

Apfelberg D B, Larsen S J 1973 Dynamic anatomy of the ulnar nerve at the elbow. Plastic and Reconstructive Surgery 51: 76–81

Babin E, Capesius P 1976 Etude radiologique des dimensions du canal rachidien cervical et de leurs variations au cours des epreuves fonctionelles. Annals of Radiology 19: 457–462

Bell A 1987 The upper limb tension test — bilateral straight leg raising — a validating manoeuvre for the upper limb tension test. In: Dalziell B A, Snowsill J C (eds) Fifth biennial conference, Manipulative Therapists Association of Australia, Melbourne

Blikna G 1969 Intradural herniated lumbar disc. Journal of Neurosurgery 31: 676–679

Bohannon R, Gajdosik R, LeVeau B F 1985 Contributions of pelvic and lower limb motion to increases in the angle of passive straight leg raising. Physical Therapy 65: 474–476

Borges L F, Hallett M, Selkoe D J, Welch K 1981 The anterior tarsal tunnel syndrome. Journal of Neurosurgery 54: 89–92

Breig A 1978 Adverse mechanical tension in the central nervous system. Almqvist & Wiksell, Stockholm

Breig A, Marions O 1963 Biomechanics of the lumbosacral nerve roots. Acta Radiologica 4: 602–604

Breig A, Troup J D C 1979 Biomechanical considerations in the straight leg raising test. Spine 4: 242–250

Butler D 1989 Adverse mechanical tension in the nervous system: a model for assessment and treatment. Australian Journal of Physiotherapy 35:–227–238

Charnley J 1951 Orthopaedic signs in the diagnosis of disc protrusion. Lancet 1: 186–192

Cyriax J 1978 Textbook of orthopaedic medicine, 7th edn. Bailliere Tindall, London, Vol 1

Dodge H W, Love J G, Gottleib C M 1956 Benign tumours at the foramen magnum: surgical considerations. Journal of Neurosurgery 13: 603–617

Dommisse G F 1975 Morphological aspects of the lumbar spine and lumbosacral region. Orthopaedic Clinics of North America: 6: 163–175

Dommisse G F 1986 The blood supply of the spinal cord. In: Grieve G P (ed) Modern manual therapy of the vertebral column. Churchill Livingstone, Edinburgh

Dyck P 1979 The stoop-test in lumbar entrapment radiculopathy. Spine 4: 89–92

Edwards B E 1987 Clinical assessment: the use of combined movements in assessment and treatment. In: Twomey L T, Taylor J R (eds) Clinics in physical therapy, Vol 13, Physical therapy of the low back. Churchill Livingstone, New York

Edwards B E 1988 Combined movement of the cervical spine in examination and treatment. In: Grant R (ed) Clinics in physical therapy, Vol 17, Physical therapy of the cervical and thoracic spine. Churchill Livingstone, New York

Elvey R L 1980 Abnormal brachial plexus tension signs. In: Proceedings, Second biennial conference, Manipulative Therapists Association of Australia, Adelaide

Fahrni W H 1966 Observations on straight leg raising with special reference to nerve root adhesions. Canadian Journal of Surgery 9: 44–48

Farfan 1975 Mechanical disorders of the low back. Lea & Febiger, Philadelphia

Goddard M D, Reid J D 1965 Movements induced by straight leg raising in the lumbosacral roots, nerves and plexuses and in the intra-pelvic section of the sciatic nerve. Journal of Neurology, Neurosurgery and Psychiatry 28: 12–18

Haupt W, Stofft E 1978 Uber die dehnbarkeit und reissfestitkeit der dura mater spinalis des menschen. Nehr Anat Ges 72: 139–142

Inman V T, Saunders J B 1942 The clinico-anatomical aspects of the lumbosacral region. Radiology 38: 669–678

Jirout J 1959 The mobility of the cervical spinal cord under normal conditions. British Journal of Radiology 32: 744–751

Jirout J 1963 Mobility of the thoracic spinal cord under normal conditions. Acta Radiologica (Diagn) 1: 729–735

Liyang D et al 1988 The effect of flexion-extension motion of the lumbar spine on the capacity of the spinal canal. Spine 14: 523–525

Louis R 1981 Vertebroradicular and vertebromedullar dynamics. Anatomica Clinica 3: 1–11

Lundborg G, Rydevik B 1973 Effects of stretching the tibial nerve of the rabbit: a preliminary study of the intraneural circulation and barrier function of the perineurium. Journal of Bone and Joint Surgery 55B: 390–401

Lundborg G 1988 Nerve injury and repair. Churchill Livingstone, Edinburgh

Macnab I 1971 The whiplash syndrome. Orthopaedic Clinics of North America 2: 389–403

Macnicol M F 1980 Mechanics of the ulnar nerve at the elbow. Journal of Bone and Joint Surgery 62B: 531–532

Maitland G D 1986 Vertebral manipulation, 5th edn. Butterworths, London

Mannen T 1966 Vascular lesions in the spinal cord of the aged. Geriatrics 21: 151–160

Mauhart D 1989 The effect of chronic inversion ankle sprains on the plantarflexion/inversion straight leg raise. Unpublished thesis, South Australian Institute of Technology, Adelaide

McKenzie R A 1981 The lumbar spine: mechanical diagnosis and therapy. Spinal Publications, Waikenae

McLellan D L, Swash M 1976 Longitudinal sliding of the median nerve during movements of the upper limb. Journal of Neurology, Neurosurgery and Psychiatry 39: 556–570

Miller A M 1987 Neuro-meningeal limitation of straight leg raising. In: Dalziel B A, Snowsill J C (eds) Manipulative Therapists Association of Australia, Fifth biennial conference, Melbourne

Millesi H 1986 The nerve gap: theory and clinical practice. Hand Clinics 2: 651–663

Millesi H, Berger C, Meissl G 1972 Experimentelle untersuchungen zur heilung durchtrennter peripherer nerven. Chirurgica Plastica 1: 174–206

Mooney V, Robertson J 1976 The facet syndrome. Clinical Orthopaedics and Related Research 115: 149–156

Nathan H 1986 Osteophytes of the spine compressing the sympathetic trunk and splanchnic nerves in the thorax. Spine 12: 527–532

Ogata K, Naito M 1986 Blood flow of peripheral nerve: effects of dissection, compression and stretching. Journal of Hand Surgery 11B: 11–14

Panjabi M M, Takata K, Goel V K 1983 Kinematics of lumbar intervertebral foramen. Spine 8: 348–357

Parke W W 1988 Correlative anatomy of cervical spondylotic neuropathy. Spine 13: 831–837

Parke W W, Watanabe R 1990 Adhesions of the ventral dura mater. Spine 15: 300–303

Pechan J, Julis F 1975 The pressure measurement in the ulnar nerve: a contribution to the pathophysiology of cubital tunnel syndrome. Journal of Biomechanics 8: 75–79

Penning L, Wilmink J T 1981 Biomechanics of the lumbosacral dural sac. Spine 6: 398–408

Reid J D 1960 Effects of flexion-extension movements of the head and spine upon the spinal cord and nerve roots. Journal of Neurology, Neurosurgery and Psychiatry 23: 214–221

Rubenach H 1987 The upper limb tension test. In: Proceedings World Congress of Physiotherapy, Sydney

Rydevik B, Lundborg G, Bagge U 1981 Effects of graded compression on intraneural blood flow, an in-vivo study on rabbit tibial nerve. Journal of Hand Surgery 6: 3–12

Schneider R C, Schemm G W 1961 Vertebral artery insufficiency in acute and chronic spinal trauma with special reference to the syndrome of acute central cervical spinal injury. Journal of Neurosurgery 18: 348–360

Selvaratnam P J, Glasgow E F, Matyas T 1989 Differential strain produced by the brachial plexus tension test on C5 to T1 nerve roots. In: Jones H M, Jones M A, Milde M R (eds) Sixth biennial conference proceedings. Manipulative Therapists Association of Australia

Shacklock M 1989 The plantarflexion/inversion straight leg raise. Unpublished thesis. South Australian Institute of Technology, Adelaide

Slater H 1989 The effect of foot and ankle position on the response to the SLR test. In: Jones H M, Jones M A, Milde M R (eds) Sixth biennial conference proceedings. Manipulative Therapists Association of Australia

Smith C G 1956 Changes in length and posture of the segments of the spinal cord with changes in posture in the monkey. Radiology 66: 259–265

Sunderland S 1978 Nerves and nerve injuries, 2nd edn. Churchill Livingstone, Edinburgh

Tencer A N, Allen B L, Ferguson R L 1985 A biomechanical study of thoraco-lumbar spine fractures with bone in the canal, Part 111, Mechanical properties of the dura and its tethering ligaments. Spine 10: 741–747

Torkildsen A 1956 Lesions of the cervical nerve roots as a possible source of pain simulating sciatica. Acta Psychiatrica Scandinavica 31: 333–344

White A A, Panjabi M M 1978 Clinical biomechanics of the spine. Lippincott, Philadelphia

Wilgis E F S & Murphy R 1986 The significance of longitudinal excursion in peripheral nerves. Hand Clinics 2: 761–766

3. Pathological processes

INJURY TO THE NERVOUS SYSTEM

The term 'trauma' evokes images of severe injury, but it comprises a wide spectrum. This chapter is about the pathological processes following injury to the nervous system. Emphasis is placed on the less severe end of the injury spectrum. Here, physiotherapy has an important role, as important as the more familiar role as part of a team, involved in rehabilitating patients suffering the consequences of severe injury to the nervous system.

In Chapter 1, the functional anatomy and some aspects of the physiology of the nervous system were discussed. This included some micro-anatomy. Together with the more obvious alterations in gross anatomy caused by trauma, alterations in the micro-environment of the nervous system also occur, and need consideration.

A definition of adverse neural tension, as this text sees it, is:

'abnormal physiological and mechanical responses produced from nervous system structures when their normal range of movement and stretch capabilities are tested'.

In the previous two chapters the considerable movement and stretch (tension) capabilities of the nervous system have been outlined. The term 'adverse neural tension' includes both movement and tension.

Sites of injury

With trauma, no part of the nervous system can be excluded from the possibility of injury. However, there are patterns to the clinical presentations of nervous system injury, even those from severe trauma. These patterns are based, in part, on vulnerable anatomic sites where an initial injury to the nervous system is most likely to occur or manifest itself after an injury elsewhere in the nervous system. These sites are:

1. Soft tissue, osseus or fibro-osseus tunnels. The median nerve in the carpal tunnel, spinal nerve in the intervertebral foramen, and the posterior interosseus nerve in the arcade of Frohse are examples of nervous system structures in tunnels where the walls are of varying structures. At a tunnel site, especially where the tunnel has unyielding walls, spatial compromise of the contained structures will be a greater possibility than elsewhere. Within a tunnel, the contained nervous system always has the potential to rub on the tunnel structures and this may create friction.

2. Where the nervous system branches. This is particularly so if the branch leaves the main trunk at an abrupt angle. To branch, a nerve sacrifices some of its gliding mechanisms and hence may become more susceptible to injury. Most branches thus occur where the nervous system has a small amount or no movement in relation to the interfacing structures. As examples of vulnerable branching, consider the union of the lateral and medial plantar nerves to form the common plantar digital nerve to the web space between the third and fourth toes. The digital nerves to the other toes can slide more freely than the common digital nerve. If traumatised, such as by enforced metatarsophalangeal extension from continued wearing of high heeled shoes, a neuroma may

result (Morton's neuroma is discussed in Chapter 12).

3. Where the system is relatively fixed. Examples of this are, the common peroneal nerve at the head of the fibula, the dura mater at the L4 vertebral segment, the attachment of the radial nerve to the head of the radius and the suprascapular nerve in the scapular notch. Neurovascular bundles such as in the popliteal fossa, may also fix the nervous system to some degree.

4. In addition to tunnel sites, the nervous system may be exposed to friction forces as it passes in close proximity to unyielding interfaces. The cords of the brachial plexus passing over the first rib, the radial nerve in the radial groove of the humerus, or where the dural sleeves run close to pedicles are examples of this situation. Fascia could be regarded as an unyielding interface, for example, where the greater occipital nerve passes through fascia at the back of the skull or the lateral femoral cutaneous nerve emerging through the fascia in the anterolateral aspect of the thigh. Any nerves in the feet passing through the plantar fascia are also vulnerable to injury.

5. Tension points. These are included in some of the above categories. However, other areas of the nervous system, such as the T6 vertebral level and the tibial nerve at the posterior aspect of the knee seem anatomically and clinically vulnerable in adverse tension disorders. There may also be various combinations of movements which create unknown tension points. Neurobiomechanics are clearly not fully understood. They are complex in the nervous system, because its various components possess differing biomechanics with attachments of various lengths and strengths to neighbouring structures.

Most of these vulnerable areas are represented in the radial nerve and its branches. See Figure 3.1. Some areas of the nervous system have many vulnerable features. For example, the tibial nerve posterior to the medial malleollus is in the posterior tarsal tunnel and branches into

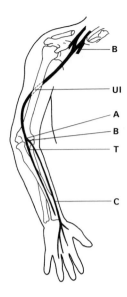

Fig. 3.1 The vulnerable anatomy of the radial nerve. A attachment, B branch, UI unyeilding interface, T tunnel, C nerve becoming cutaneous. Adapted from Lundborg (1988)

the lateral and medial plantar nerves while within the tunnel. The nervous system at the C5,6 level is in the centre of many branches and, at this level, the cervical spinal canal is at its narrowest.

Areas where the nervous system has previously been traumatised appear to be susceptible to further trauma and irritation. Even an injury that apparently did not involve the nervous system at the time would appear to predispose the nervous system to injury later. An old fracture is an example. The notion of 'subclinical entrapment', whereby an existing injury can be subclinical and then become clinical with the advent of injury elsewhere along the system, is discussed later in this chapter. Clinically, it appears that a patient can carry a subclinical injury for years. Symptoms from the old injury site may be activated by re-injury or trauma which mechanically sensitises the old injury site.

Trauma, even in a relatively non-vulnerable segment of the nervous system, will have repercussions at vulnerable sites. Ankle inversion sprains and fractures provide an example. In these injuries, the common peroneal nerve can be damaged, especially at its attachment to the fibular head (Meals 1977, Davies, 1979) or at the sciatic bifurcation in the lower part of the thigh (Nobel 1966). In these situations there has been no direct injury at the fibula head, but due to anatomical inadequacies this region is vulnerable to injury. In examination, knowledge of the vulnerable points is essential for a clear understanding, and hence treatment, of adverse tension syndromes.

Kind of injury

The most common nerve traumas encountered by physiotherapists are the mechanical and physiological consequences of friction, compression, stretch and occasionally disease. Trauma does not have to be severe — unphysiological movements, body postures and repetitive muscle contraction may be contributing factors to a nerve injury (Lundborg & Dahlin 1989). Nor is there the necessity for a direct injury to the nervous system. There could well be a secondary injury to the nervous system as a result of blood and oedema from a damaged interface or from a change in shape of the interface. Nerve anomalies, or anomalies of interfacing tissues, are likely to predispose the system to injury. These issues are expanded upon later in this chapter.

The clinical presentation of a nervous system injury will differ depending on whether the injury is acute or chronic. With the development of a chronic injury, such as an entrapment syndrome, the system has time to allow at least some adaptive measures such that conduction may only be minimally affected. However, the possibility of a more insidious effect resulting from impaired axonal transport systems should be considered. This is discussed later in this chapter.

With an acute injury, such as compression of the radial nerve in 'Saturday night palsy' or an epidural haematoma, the consequences may be more severe due to the sudden alteration in blood and axoplasm flow together with the sudden mechanical deformation of nerve fibres. The nervous system will not have had time to call upon its protective mechanisms, in particular, movement and/or reserve blood supply. There is clearly a greater urgency with treatment of the acute injury.

Another important feature for physiotherapists to recognise is that injury at one part of the nervous system is likely to have clinical repercussions elsewhere along the system. As mentioned earlier, repercussions are likely to occur at the vulnerable sites as well as at old injury sites. Examination and treatment of the local site will rarely suffice in order best to clear the signs and symptoms and prevent re-occurrences. Since the nervous system is a continuum, old and dormant injury sites are commonly exacerbated with the advent of a new injury.

Intraneural and extraneural pathology

Pathological processes that lead to adverse tension syndromes and positive tension tests can be classified as extraneural, intraneural or both. Physiotherapists are encouraged to ascertain not only the site of the disorder, but also the kind and extent of the pathological process at that site.

Intraneural pathology involves the consequences of injury involving any of the structures of the nervous system. Intraneural pathology can be considered in two ways. The first is as affecting the conducting tissues such as demyelination, neuroma formation or hypoxic nerve fibres. The other is pathology affecting the connective tissues such as scarred epineurium, arachnoiditis or irritated dura mater. Both connective tissues and neural tissues could be involved, for example, where immature regenerating axons are caught in scarred endoneurium.

Extraneural pathology involves the nerve bed or the mechanical interface. Blood in a nerve bed or epidural space, epineurium pathologically tethered to an interface, dura pathologically adhered to the posterior longitudinal ligament, and swelling of bone and muscle adjacent to a nerve trunk are examples. The narrow spinal canal is a commonly encountered extraneural situation which may lead to an adverse tension syndrome. Both extraneural and intraneural processes often occur together. However, identification of the predominant process will direct treatment. In some situations, the optimal outcome will not be reached unless both contributing kinds of pathologies are addressed.

Extraneural and intraneural pathology can be linked to the movement adaptive mechanisms of the nervous system (Ch. 2). If the location of a pathology is extraneural, it will probably affect the gross movement of the nervous system in relation to its mechanical interface. With an intraneural pathology, while the system may be free to move, the elasticity of the nervous system will be affected. A broad link can now be made between neurobiomechanics and neuropathology (Table 3.1).

As discussed, in most situations there will be a dominance of one process over the other. For example, an extraneural pathology, such as fibrosing blood in a peripheral nerve bed, could be a dominant pathology. However, there is a likelihood of some epineurial swelling and perhaps firing of the nociceptive endings of the nervi nervorum or nerve fibres located in outlying fascicles.

The clinical consequences from both extraneural and intraneural processes can be broadly considered as either pathophysiological (i.e., symptoms) or pathomechanical (i.e., loss of range of movement and elasticity). Physiotherapists can make use of the concepts of pathophysiology and pathomechanics for treatment direction (Ch. 10). In the absence of frank trauma, the initial stages of a disorder are more likely to be pathophysiological, that is, altered physiology but with none of the scarring or structural alterations that cause deformed mechanics. Pathophysiology, if not attended to, can lead to pathomechanics. There will be overlap in that it is unlikely a pathomechanical situation can exist without pathophysiology. Both situations can affect neurobiomechanics and both are treatable by appropriate movement. Thus, the term 'adverse mechanical tension in the nervous system' (Breig 1978, Butler 1989, Butler & Gifford 1989) is not entirely correct. It belittles the physiological

mechanisms occurring with nerve injury. In this text, 'adverse tension' or 'tension' could refer to either pathophysiology, pathomechanics or both.

PATHOLOGICAL PROCESSES

Two major factors in the development of nervous system pathology can be identified: vascular factors and mechanical factors. There is disagreement about which factor predominates, especially in the early stages of nerve compression. The current view is that vascular factors predominate (Sunderland 1978, Lundborg 1988, Mackinnon & Dellon 1988). In many situations both factors will co-exist. In the more minor injuries concentrated on by this text, vascular factors related to altered pressures in tissues and fluids around nerve are probably more important (Powell & Myers 1986, Lundborg 1988, Lundborg & Dahlin 1989).

Vascular factors in injury

Nerve fibres are dependent on an uninterrupted supply of blood for normal function (see Chapter 1 for a discussion of the complexity of the vascular supply including the mechanisms to allow uninterrupted supply).

Table 3.1 A postulated link between neurobiomechanics and neuropathology

Adaptive mechanisms	Location of pathology
Movement in relation to interface	Extraneural
Tension development	Intraneural

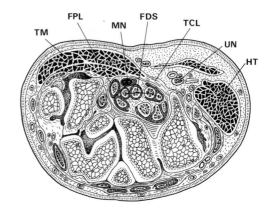

Fig. 3.2 The carpal tunnel. Note the variety of interfacing structures surrounding the median nerve. HT hypothenar muscles, FPL flexor pollicus longus, MN median nerve, TCL transverse carpal ligament, TM thenar muscles, FDS flexor digitorum superficialis tendons, UN ulnar nerve. From Lundborg G 1988 Nerve injury and repair. Churchill Livingstone, Edinburgh, with kind permission from the publishers

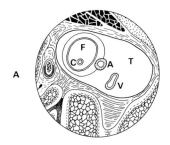

A Normal tunnel. For adequate
nerve fibre nutrition, the pressure
gradient must be:
PA>PC>PF>PV>PT

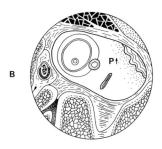

B Hypoxia. Increased tunnel
pressure→Venule collapses
Venous stasis→Hypoxic axons

Fig. 3.3 Representation of the pressure gradients in the carpal tunnel and the stages that follow alteration of the pressure gradients. For simplicity, one nerve fibre in a fascicle is represented. A arteriole, C capillary, F fascicle, P pressure, T tunnel, V venule. Adapted from the work of Sunderland (1976)

A series of pressure gradients exist in nerve and in the tissues and fluids surrounding nerve. The importance of this pressure gradient in the development of entrapment neuropathy is a well recognised medical fact (Sunderland 1976, Lundborg 1988, Lundborg & Dahlin 1989). Sunderland (1976) documented a model, based on fact and logic, that introduced alterations in pressure gradients as the basis for compression of the median nerve in the carpal tunnel. He proposed that similar events could occur in other tunnel sites. A generalisation can also be made for the neuraxis and the meninges. The nervous system is continually in a tunnel, though the structure of the walls of the tunnel repeatedly changes. Some tunnel areas are smaller and the tunnel constituents are more rigid than elsewhere. The carpal tunnel is a perfect example for the model (Fig. 3.2).

Sunderland (1976) insisted that, for adequate intrafascicular circulation and thus neural function, the pressure in structures contained within a tunnel must be greatest in the epineurial arteriole, and progressively less in the capillary, fascicles, epineurial venule and tunnel (Fig. 3.3A). Thus, the requirement for nerve nutrition is that blood must flow into the tunnel, the nerve fibre and then out of the tunnel again. A pressure gradient must therefore be maintained.

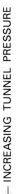

← INCREASING TUNNEL PRESSURE

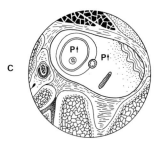

C Oedema. Venous stasis→
Deterioration of capillary
endothelium→Oedema→
↑Intrafascicular pressure

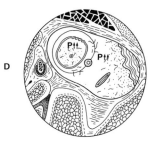

D Fibrosis. Intrafascicular
fibroblastic activity→Scar tissue→
↑Pressure, ↑Hypoxia→Segment
of nerve becomes fibrous cord→
Cycle of Irritation

If the tunnel pressure increases to greater than that in the vein, then venous drainage will be impaired or stopped (Fig. 3.3B). This situation could occur with pressures as low as 20–30 mmHg (Rydevik et al 1981, Ogata & Naito 1986). Rydevik et al (1981) used a small transparent cuff on rabbit tibial nerve to examine the response of intraneural circulation compression. A pressure of 40 mmHg altered capillary flow and, by 80 mmHg, intraneural circulation ceased. Any alteration in flow was immediately reversible, even if the compression was held for 2 hours. Some examples of situations which would increase the tunnel pressure in carpal tunnel syndrome are, flexor tendon thickening, synovial tissue hyperplasia, and oedema (Phalen 1970, Armstrong et al 1984, Faithfull et al 1985). Elsewhere in the body, impaired venous drainage may occur, for example, with blood in the epidural space of the spinal canal, and where blood and oedema surround a segment of tibial nerve after a hamstring tear. Increased compartment pressures, such as occurs with the anterior compartment syndrome in the lower leg, are possible sources of damage to nerves contained within the compartment (Mubarak et al 1989).

Sunderland (1976) details three distinct stages that may occur with persistent tunnel pressure — hypoxia, oedema and fibrosis (Fig. 3.3 B,C,D).

With venous stasis and consequent hypoxia, nerve fibre nutrition is impaired. Neuro-ischaemia is a likely source of pain and other symptoms such as paraesthesia. Large fibres suffer earlier than smaller fibres from compression and ischaemia (Gasser & Erlanger 1929, Ochoa 1980). The resultant fibre dissociation could lead to abnormal 'gating' in the cord and thus be interpreted centrally as pain.

With continuing hypoxia, damage to capillary endothelium follows and results in leakage of protein rich oedema. Mechanical pressure could also injure the capillaries (Rydevik et al 1981). The blood/nerve barriers, so effective in protecting the nerve initially, are now a disadvantage. Endoneurial fluid pressure rises, intrafascicular pressure rises, and, because the perineurium is not crossed by lymphatics, oedema cannot disperse other than longitudinally along the nerve

trunk. Further rises in intrafascicular pressure may close off the small blood vessels that pass obliquely through the perineurium (Ch. 1). The nerve can swell, usually proximal to the damaged area or where there no compressive structures such as retinacula.

From this oedematous stage, fibroblastic proliferation, enhanced by the protein rich oedema, is likely. If so, the result will be intraneural fibrosis within the nerve both in the epineurial tissues and intrafascicular. The increased volume of connective tissue again increases intraneural pressure and a self-perpetuating cycle of irritation may be established. Sunderland (1976) refers to the affected segment as becoming a 'fibrous cord', although such a sequence could occur in one fascicle and not others. This sequence is summarised in Figure 3.3. An abnormal impulse generating mechanism may be set up if components of the nerve fibre are caught in the connective tissue derangement. Clinical signs and symptoms may be more evident if immature axons or a neuroma are caught in the scar.

One possible consequence of a segment of scarred nerve is that sites of nerve friction could develop elsewhere along the tract, most likely at vulnerable tunnel sites. Sunderland (1978) considers that a 'friction fibrosis' may be more painful and damaging than the original lesion. In an area of friction fibrosis, intraneural fibrosis may be the eventual outcome of a similar sequence of events as occurred in the original lesion. This spread of symptoms is commonly encountered clinically and many of these situations could be included in the 'double crush' syndrome (Upton & McComas 1973). This syndrome is discussed in detail later in this chapter.

The vascular mechanisms, as described above, could be considered as compression from within the nerve. This situation could be maintained by extraneural damage to blood vessels. For example, an extraneural vessel could be stretched or kinked by an unphysiological movement. It could be also be caught in an extraneural scarring process. An accumulation of blood around a nerve from vessel rupture may lead to acute compression followed by an ischaemic block and consequent nerve function deficit (Sunderland 1978). Nerve traction injury (Nobel 1966, Meals 1977) can damage blood vessels associated with that nerve. A similar traumatic aneurysm can easily occur with a penetrating wound. Vasoconstriction could also be induced by irritation of the sympathetic trunk. The perineurium and epineurium are sympathetically innervated (Lundborg 1970, Selander et al 1985). Selander et al (1985) measured blood flow in rabbit sciatic nerve and found that, by stimulation of the lumbar sympathetic trunk, intraneural blood flow could be reduced to 10% of control values. An injection of noradrenaline into the aorta reduced blood flow by 40%. Lundborg (1988) suggested this mechanism may be involved in some of the chronic pain syndromes. Patients with chronic pain syndromes often adopt postures which may tense the sympathetic chain (Ch. 2) or are involved in injuries such as 'whiplash' that could injure the chain.

Another development, likely to co-exist with these vascular alterations, is extraneural scarring and tethering to interfacing structures. This could happen at the initial injury site or in the region of the friction fibrosis further along the nerve. Millesi (1986) believes that, because the nerve loses its longitudinal movement and the force distribution is only local, the tethered nerve has a greater potential for further injury and symptomatology than the intraneural process. Importantly, the kind of injury must be considered, not only for symptomatology, but also for the long term possibilities of fibre regeneration. Here, the intraneural process may lead to a worse prognosis for the patient.

Rydevik et al (1989) proposed that the tight capsule of the dorsal root ganglion (DRG) could also act to enclose and further pressurize an endoneurial oedema. They have shown in rats the ease of increasing endoneurial fluid pressure in the DRG, and have postulated that the rise in pressure decreases the blood flow to the cell bodies thus giving rise to an ischaemic situation as in a closed compartment syndrome. In a large cadaver study, Nathan (1986) has described pathological changes resulting from anterior osteophytes irritating the sympathetic ganglia and nerves. Changes such as fibrotic infiltration of the ganglia and pathological adherence to neighbouring bone were noted in 65.5% of 1000 cadavers.

Less easily understood is the relationship between vascular and mechanical factors in the neuraxis and meninges. For example, an epidural swelling or haematoma such as described by Pan et al (1988) could eventually lead to a fibrotic reaction and tethering not dissimilar to the sequelae which may follow the presence of blood around a peripheral nerve. Cord function could eventually be affected, either by the altered force distribution through the neuraxis and meninges or alterations in the ability of the CSF to percolate along the sub-arachnoid space. Uninterrupted CSF flow is a necessary condition to minimise subarachnoid scarring and spinal cord compression post injury (Oiwa 1983). In situations where the cord is tethered, it is known that altered oxidative mechanisms are responsible for the ensuing abnormalities in cord function (Pang & Wilberger 1982). Altered blood supply to the spinal cord, in association with chondro-osseus spurs and a narrow spinal canal, is considered a significant component in the development of cervical spondylitic myelopathy (Robinson et al 1977). Stretching of the cord during spinal flexion stretches the intrinsic vessels. This devascularisation will be made worse if the spinal canal is narrow and if the neuraxis is drawn up against a spur or ridge of bone (Turnbull 1971, Doppman 1975, Gooding & Hoff 1975, Breig 1978). Bohlman & Emery (1988) have reviewed the literature on the subject.

Wick catheter experiments by Szabo et al (1983) are supportive of the importance of vascular factors in nerve injury. In these experiments a wick catheter was introduced into the carpal tunnel of normal volunteers between the flexor carpi radialis tendon and the median nerve. Different levels of pressure were then effected in the carpal tunnel by a moulded template (Fig. 3.4). This allowed an accurate collaboration of subjective responses and motor and sensory latencies with varying tissue fluid pressures. Functional loss began at approximately 40 mmHg with motor and sensory responses

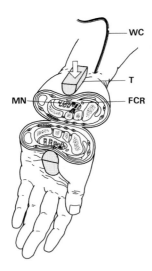

Fig. 3.4 The moulded rubber template. The template applies compression over the median nerve. The wick catheter is inserted adjacent to the flexor carpi radialis tendon. FCR flexor carpi radialis tendon, MN median nerve, T template, WC wick catheter. From Gelberman R H, Szabo R M, Hargens A R 1986 Pressure effect on human peripheral nerve. In: Hargens A R Tissue nutrition and viability. Springer Verlag, New York, with kind permission from the publishers and authors

completely blocked at 50 mmHg. Functional loss in the hypertensive group began at 60 mmHg. In normotensive and hypertensive subjects the tissue pressure threshold was consistently 30 mmHg below diastolic blood pressure. The night pain of nerve entrapments may be due to blood pressure being lower at night.

Mechanical factors in nerve injury

The nervous system can be damaged via physical force and both the connective and neural tissues are at risk. Studies by Haftek (1970) and Sunderland (1978) have found that the connective tissues of peripheral nerve require large forces before they rupture. However, such studies are of little use when considering the more minor traumas encountered clinically by physiotherapists.

The epineurium is not difficult tissue to injure, and it is a particularly reactive tissue. Slight trauma, such as mild compression or friction may result in an epineurial oedema (Triano & Luttges 1982, Rydevik et al 1984). If a nerve is rubbed slightly or warm saline applied to it, previously unnoticed blood vessels begin to function

(Lundborg 1970). Epineurial tears are common in injuries such as ankle sprains (Nitz et al 1985). Due to the perineurial diffusion barrier an epineurial injury is unlikely to affect conduction of the contained long nerve fibres unless it is severe enough to compress the fascicles and is deeply placed in the internal epineurium (Rayan et al 1988).

It would seem that symptoms are of a greater intensity and distribution from stretch of the connective tissues than compression. Stretch will involve a greater mass of tissue and more nociceptive endings of the nervi nervorum especially if these ending are caught in scarred connective tissue (Sunderland 1989). A similar rationale could be applied to stretch of the dura mater. The dura is a well innervated vascularised structure just like epineurium. Due to the arrangement of collagen fibres, the dura is far less resistant to forces transversely across the dural theca than those in the longitudinal axis.

Already in the discussion on vascular factors involved in nerve injury, the difficulty of separating the vascular and mechanical factors can be seen. The possibility of mechanical deformation of nerve fibres as a predominant factor in nerve compression pathophysiology was raised by Fowler et al (1972) and Ochoa et al (1972) following nerve compression experiments on primates. Using tourniquets, they found that most nerve fibre injury occurred at the edge of the tourniquet where the shearing forces were the greatest. On analysis, the myelin sheath was found to be stretched on one side of the node of Ranvier and invaginated on the other with the displacement towards uncompressed parts of the nerve. (Fowler & Ochoa 1975, Ochoa 1980) (Fig. 3.5). Demyelination was found to follow the displacement. Again, it is difficult to neglect vascular factors. Powell and Myers (1986) used inflatable cuffs to cause tourniquet shearing forces in rat nerve and noted Schwann cell necrosis prior to demyelination. The obvious suggestion was that local ischaemia had to be a part of the demyelination process. Rydevik et al (1987) proposed that the shear force at the edge of the cuff damaged blood vessels and the longitudinal forces distorted the myelin.

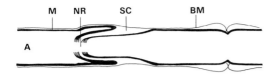

Fig. 3.5 Nodal interruption. The myelin on one side of the node becomes stretched, the myelin on the other side becomes invaginated. Displacement of the node of Ranvier is in the direction of away from the site of compression. A axon, BM basement membrane, M myelin sheath, SC Schwann cell, NR node of ranvier. Adapted from Ochoa et al 1973

All tissues of the body are under some pressure. In a structure such as the nervous system, uniform pressure is not damaging. Hence, a deep sea diver can work safely at pressures which would cause injuries, such as myelin slippage and nodal distortion if they were applied locally to a segment of nerve (Gilliat 1981).

The perineurial diffusion barrier will be affected by physical injury. Crush injury to mouse sciatic nerve can induce increased permeability through the perineurial diffusion barrier at the site of injury (Ollson & Kristensson 1973).

Mechanical stresses could also cause nerve damage by rupture of intraneural and extraneural blood vessels. Nobel (1966) reported on two cases where plantar flexion/inversion stresses at the ankle tore intraneural blood vessels in the common peroneal tract above the knee. Nobel (1966) also considered that intraneural haematomas were likely to be more common than is recognised.

With injury, both mechanical and vascular factors are likely to occur. However, it does appear that ischaemic factors are part of, or may even pre-empt, mechanical damage and in the absence of frank trauma, should be considered the ultimate neuronal pathology. What must not be forgotten, however, is the great spectrum of kinds and strengths of mechanical damage, and that vascular alterations will be inevitable with mechanical deformation.

As is usual, the peripheral nervous system is easier to study than the CNS. Also, the mechanical influences on pathology in the neuraxis are less clear. Axons in the neuraxis are probably better protected than their representatives in the peripheral nervous system. Over-

stretch of axons during movement seems likely only if there is a co-existing pathological state such as a stenotic ridge of bone in the canal or the cord is pathologically tethered. In animal studies of cervical spondylotic myelopathy, Korbrine et al (1978) felt that mechanical pressure on the cervical cord was more important in spondylotic myelopathy than vascular factors. It seems hard to differentiate the two factors. Breig (1978) has presented both mechanical and vascular mechanisms leading to adverse mechanical tension in the central nervous system. The significant effects of spinal distraction on blood flow in the spinal cord have been shown by Cusick et al (1982) in the monkey, and Dolan et al (1980) in cats.

Injury and axoplasmic flow

In Chapter 1, the basic axonal transport systems occurring within a neurone were outlined. Possible alterations in the axoplasmic transport system from nervous system injury are vital considerations for physiotherapists. The consequences of altered axoplasmic flow may be seen as trophic changes in the target tissues (such as muscle or skin), and damage to the cell body and the axon. Perhaps part of the explanation for such injuries as tennis elbow and Achilles tendon rupture lies in an understanding of axoplasmic flow.

Severe trauma will clearly effect the flow of axoplasm. In trans-section or severe injury, the axoplasm will actually 'drip' out of the cut nerve. Of more interest, however, is recent research which shows that minor injury to nerves together with changes in the micro-environment of a nerve will have consequences for the rate of axoplasmic flow and the quality of the axoplasm (Rydevik et al 1980, Dahlin et al 1984, Dahlin & McLean 1986, Dahlin et al 1986).

Like the action potential, movement of intracellular material requires an energy supply — this it gets from the blood. The flow of axoplasm will be slowed if the blood supply to the neurone is compromised. It will also slow or stop from physical constriction such as a tight band. Swelling on both sides of the constriction is evidence of the transport system running in antegrade and retrograde directions

(Mackinnon & Dellon 1988). Such constriction would also interfere with the blood supply.

Both antegrade and retrograde transports can be interrupted by mild compression of 30–50 mmHg (Rydevik et al 1980, Dahlin et al 1984, Dahlin & McLean, 1986, Dahlin et al 1986). Dahlin & McLean (1986) showed that fast axonal transport was not altered at pressures of 20 mmHg for two hours, although an accumulation occurred at the compression site after 8 hours. A pressure of 30 mmHg for a period of 2 hours led to significant slowing. These pressures are pressures similar to, or even less than, those known to cause the symptoms associated with carpal tunnel syndrome in humans (Gelberman et al 1981).

Axoplasmic flow which has stopped is reversible, at least in the experimental situation. Dahlin & McLean (1986) showed, in the experiment described above, that an axonal transport block by a pressure of 50 mmHg for 2 hours was reversible in 24 hours. Two hours of compression at 200 mmHg was reversible within 3 days and 2 hours compression at 400 mmHg was reversible within a week. The blocking is thus a graded effect and is proportional to the magnitude and duration of pressure. It is important to realise that axoplasmic transport can be altered without any structural damage to the nerve fibre.

There appears to be a relationship between slowing of the axoplasmic transport and alterations in the action potential. In an anoxic nerve, both action potentials and the axoplasmic flow will stop in approximately 15 minutes (Ochs 1975). Trophic changes in the target tissue are the result of impaired axoplasmic flow. Korr (1985) gives the example of a 'facilitated' segment of the spinal cord associated with an intervertebral joint problem. Here, high rates of afferent bombardment from the nerve endings in the facilitated segment increase the demand for energy in the affected neurones to the detriment of the axoplasmic flow. Persistent afferent bombardment may therefore lead to trophic changes in the facilitated segment.

The structural integrity of the axon will suffer if the slow transport is affected because the cytoskeletal 'maintenance' will be impaired. So too will the quality of interactions at the synapse, because transmitter materials will not arrive, or arrive in insufficient quantity, for adequate synaptic function. Lastly, and perhaps most overlooked, is that it seems the nucleus loses its information gathering mechanisms about the state of the target tissue and the neuronal environment. Hence, its ability to produce the correct neurotransmitters and cytoskeletal elements for the neurone is diminished.

FURTHER CONSEQUENCES OF NERVE INJURY

Fibrosis

Neural fibrosis is the end stage of most of the injury mechanisms. Some examples of pathological situations where neural fibrosis is involved are arachnoiditis, the development of a constant impulse generating mechanism, or a part of the obliteration of the subarachnoid space in severe spinal stenosis. Further developments are possible at the site of the original injury and also at other sites in the system. At the site of original injury, depending on the circumstances, the pathological changes may either foster additional tissue insult or be a buffer against any further injury. For example, a thickened segment of epineurium may prevent overstretch and ectopic impulse generation from some regenerating axons caught in scar. Damaged peripheral nerve in mice rapidly increases strength and stiffness and exhibits a decrease in elasticity (Beel et al 1984). A similar situation is likely in damaged human peripheral nerve according to Millesi (1986). As mentioned above, these changes in nerve may foster the development of a pathological situation where the alteration of the pressure gradients is permanent.

The development of symptoms elsewhere along the nervous system from an initial injury is likely. The basis for these symptoms can be summarised, as follows:

1. Mechanical changes in a segment of nervous system will alter tension in the whole nervous system.

2. Vascular changes will co-exist with these mechanical changes.
3. Impaired flow of axoplasm in one site will have repercussions for the whole neurone. Dahlin & McLean (1986) refer to the 'sick neurone' with repercussions for all parts of the neurone and for the target tissues.
4. A site of ectopic impulse generation may lead to altered neuronal firing elsewhere, such as in the dorsal root ganglion or in neuronal pools within the neuraxis.

Researchers who have had the opportunity to examine and reflect on the impact of altered neurobiomechanics in animals and humans have invariably emphasised that altered mechanical properties in one area of the nervous system and thus an altered relationship to the mechanical interface, could lead to further damage to the whole nerve and to the mechanical interfacing (McLellan & Swash 1976, Louis 1981, Beel et al 1984). Earlier, Lishman & Russel (1961) used a similar explanation for the regular occurrence of symptoms along nerve trunks following 'brachial neuritis' Triano & Luttges's (1982) experiments on mouse sciatic nerves suggest that intermittent mechanical agitation from longitudinal sliding of a nerve trunk across an irritant is a major factor in the production of inflammatory changes. Irritation of nerves has probably not had the scientific exposure that it seems to demand clinically. Most research has concentrated on compression, especially severe compression involving Wallerian degeneration.

Neuromatous thickening is a consequence of fibrosis and is noted in chronic nerve entrapment, usually proximal to the site of the entrapment (Gilliat & Harrison 1984). It appears that all three connective tissue constituents contribute to the thickening. Another feature is that 'Renaut bodies' (small connective tissue inclusions) are seen in increased numbers at entrapment sites (Asbury 1973, Jefferson et al 1981, Ortman et al 1983). Siqueira et al (1983) listed, as a cause of 'failed back' from disc surgery, changes in the dura mater which included fibrosis and increases in collagen content. Such changes may 'trap' the intrinsic sinuvertebral nerves causing loss of their

movement adaptive mechanisms and consequently allowing a heightened mechano-sensitivity.

Surgeons have had many opportunities to examine fibrotic reactions around nerve roots during surgery. Leyshon et al (1981) described two distinct types of involved nerve roots at surgery in 50 patients. The first was a fibrotic type where the root was 'hard, thin, white and fibrous' and the second was a 'soft pink and oedematous' root that was particularly irritable to handling. Clearly, in these two situations, the symptomatology from the first would be dominated by pathomechanics and the second by pathophysiology.

The double crush syndrome

In the vast array of literature on nerve entrapment and other forms of nerve injury, authors often express difficulty in explaining the development of symptoms elsewhere in the body or along the nervous system. In this regard, there are many references to the 'double crush' phenomenon, a concept introduced by Upton & McComas in 1973. These authors examined 115 patients with either carpal tunnel syndrome or lesions of the ulnar nerve at the elbow. They found that 81 had electrophysiological and clinical evidence of neural lesions of the neck. Upton & McComas (1973) and McComas et al (1974) proposed that minor serial impingements along a peripheral nerve could have an additive effect and cause a distal entrapment neuropathy. The basis of the distal neuropathy was considered to be altered axoplasmic flow. There is plenty of clinical support for the concept. Dyro (1983) wondered how 27% of young people (N = 50) with brachial plexus lesions could develop carpal tunnel syndrome. Electrophysiological abnormalities have been found in the ulnar nerve at the wrist in 46% (N = 63) of patients with unilateral carpal tunnel syndrome and in 88% of patients (N = 185) with bilateral carpal tunnel syndrome (Cassvan et al 1986). Similar percentages had been shown by Bendler et al (1977). In an analysis of 1000 surgical cases of carpal tunnel syndrome, 32% had bilateral CTS (Hurst et al 1985). This very large study is revealing. Patients with cervical arthritis (diagnosed by 'clinical signs and symptoms and X-rays') correlated significantly with those who had bilateral carpal tunnel syndrome. Diabetics form 1.7% of the population, yet in the study by Hurst et al, 7% of the unilateral carpal tunnel syndrome patients had diabetes and 34% of the bilateral carpal tunnel group had diabetes. The most commonly studied double crush syndrome is the carpal tunnel syndrome-cervical spine injury. Combinations of these two disorders are often seen together (Guyon & Honet 1977, Massey et al 1981, Pfeffer & Osterman 1986). I have noticed that the occurrence of unexplained hand and finger symptoms for example, pain in the trapezio/first metacarpal joint, with cervical spine symptoms, is more common than a clearly defined carpal tunnel syndrome/cervical spine association.

The double crush syndrome presents useful clinical support for the hypotheses suggested in Chapter 2. It also links in with the notion of vulnerable areas of the nervous system discussed earlier in this chapter. As well as double crush, a 'reversed crush' is noted by Lundborg (1988) and is clinically very evident. Here, the initial injury is distal, such as a carpal tunnel syndrome and then the next 'crush' is proximal, such as an entrapment of the median nerve at the elbow. Cherington (1974) presented 72 patients (90 limbs) with carpal tunnel syndrome who had symptoms proximal to the wrist. Of the 49 patients who had surgical decompression of the carpal tunnel, 46 experienced disappearance of the proximal symptoms. Lundborg (1988) proposes that the retrograde axoplasmic flow is altered and therefore does not deliver material synthesised by the target tissues. There are reports of 'triple crush' and 'multiple crush' syndromes (Mackinnon & Dellon 1988). These 'crush' disorders, or certainly disorders with a similar advent of symptomatology, can be commonly seen in physiotherapy practice; more so if the patient population involves the treatment of chronic disorders. Often these symptoms, presumably neurogenic in origin, can be reproduced by the tension tests outlined later in this text. Further clinical support for the relationship of such symptoms is evident from surgery. Double crush provides a basis for the surgical observations that some patients with carpal tunnel

syndrome may require a proximal decompression as well as a distal decompression (Mackinnon & Dellon 1988). The term 'crush' to describe the symptoms could be improved. The symptomatic dysfunction that we are discussing may not be a crush but an irritative injury. The term 'crush' evokes thoughts of compression.

'Underlying subclinical neuropathy' is often blamed for the double crush syndrome (Sedal et al 1973, Neary et al 1975, Silver et al 1985). Upton & McComas (1973) proposed that the underlying mechanisms were based upon altered axoplasmic flow at one site making the rest of the axon susceptible to entrapment. This idea of the 'sick neurone' predisposing other areas of the nervous system to injury is consistently reported in the literature. There is some experimental support using banded rat sciatic nerves (Seiler et al 1983). These authors showed that, if a proximal part of the nerve was banded at a compressive level insufficient to alter electrical activity, it made the nerve more susceptible to distal compression. A similar experiment (Mackinnon & Dellon 1988) showed that distal compressive banding made proximal segments of the nerve more susceptible to entrapment. Altered axoplasmic flow mechanisms in the double crush syndrome are summarised in Figure 3.6.

Aligned with the proposals of altered axoplasmic transport, the possibility of loss of normal mechanics of the nervous system resulting in unusual or incongruent nerve interfacing relationships elsewhere along the nervous system, also needs heeding. In Figure 3.7, I have made an attempt to illustrate a possible mechanical mechanism for the double crush syndrome. Impaired axoplasmic flow could be a consequence of the mechanical deformation or may predispose areas to deformation. This concept fits neatly with the vascular based scenario mentioned earlier (Sunderland 1976) whereby an initial entrapment at one site has the potential to cause a 'friction fibrosis' elsewhere along the track. Lundborg (1988) also raises the possibility that an isolated nerve entrapment could lead to decreased use of the extremity, thus contributing to an oedematous limb that predisposes nerves to entrapment. There is still the possibility of the existence of a generalised, perhaps subclinical neuropathy, such

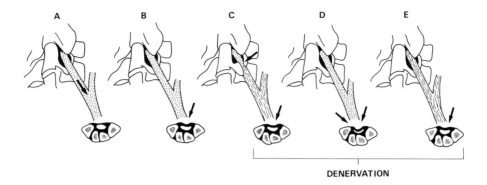

Fig. 3.6 The 'double crush syndrome' based on alteration of the axonal transport systems. A Normal cervical spine, median nerve and carpal tunnel, large arrow represents antegrade axoplasmic flow. B Symptomatic threshold not reached despite a mild compression at the carpal tunnel. C Impingement of cervical root plus the carpal tunnel compression; the serial compression results in symptomatology and denervation because the symptomatic threshold has been surpassed. D Normal cervical spine but severe carpal tunnel compression results in symptomatic carpal tunnel. E Mild carpal tunnel compression plus diabetes results in symptomatology. From: Hurst L C, Weissberg D, Carroll, R E 1985 The relationship of double crush to carpal tunnel syndrome: an analysis of 1,000 cases of carpal tunnel syndrome. Journal of Hand Surgery 10B: 202–204 with kind permission of the publishers and authors.

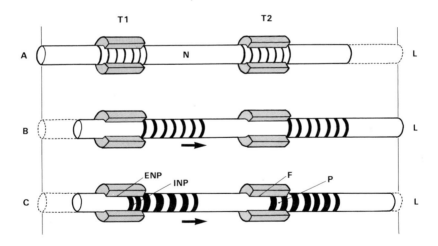

Fig. 3.7 The 'double crush syndrome' Postulated mechanical contribution to the development of symptoms elsewhere along nerve tracts following an initial injury. ENP extraneural pathology, INP intraneural pathology, N nerve, T1 tunnel one, T2 tunnel two, L limit of movement of nerve possible, P pressure, F friction. Striped area represents the surface of the nerve that remains in contact with T during movement, i.e, it has a relationship with the interface.
A. Neutral
B. N has ben pulled to the right. The striped area moves in relation to the interface and tension is generated in the nerve
C. With pathology at T1 (intraneural or extraneural), for the nerve to adapt to the same movement as in B, at T2, more pressure (P) will develop and a segment of N will not leave T2, therefore creating an area of increased friction (F)

as diabetes. Such a disease raises the intra-fascicular pressure throughout the body (Myers & Powell 1981) and could consequently predispose the entire nervous system to entrapment.

Most nerve entrapment studies rely on electrodiagnosis to show some form of neuropathy. I would suggest that, if there is evidence of altered conduction, then pathological alterations in the connective tissues are likely. Perhaps this may precede the neurophysiological changes. Recent experiments on mice are revealing. With a unilateral nerve entrapment, changes in structural proteins in the contralateral nerve have been found (Luttges et al 1976). The contralateral nerve will also have altered biomechanics (Beel et al 1984). No such alterations in biomechanics or structure have been shown in the intervening nerve roots (Beel et al 1986, Stodieck & Luttges 1986) and spinal cord (Sodieck & Luttges 1983). There is also the possibility, especially with the more trivial injury, that minor changes to nerve fibres will not register as abnormal with electrodiagnostic testing. A neuropathy could reside in one fascicle only and electrodiagnosis cannot be fascicle specific (Mackinnon & Dellon 1988). Hurst el at (1985) showed that, while the asymptomatic wrist in human carpal tunnel syndrome may have normal electromyographic scores, they are in the upper limits of normality.

Double crush is now well documented in the peripheral nervous system but what of the neuraxis where there appears to be a form of double crush as well? A common pattern of disorder presentation is where a patient complains of lumbar symptoms from an injury with likely spinal canal trespass, such as a discogenic trauma. Then, over time, they complain of T6 area symptoms and perhaps even cervical symptoms. With a whiplash injury, patients often complain of thoracic and even lumbar symptoms, most often around the tension point areas. These areas also seem vulnerable to symptomatology following injury to the peripheral nervous system.

Abnormal impulse generating mechanisms

In addition to sites along the nervous system rendered vulnerable by the nature of the surrounding anatomy, there are also sites within the nervous system where symptoms are more likely to originate. These are the impulse generating sites such as the dorsal root ganglia, sympathetic ganglia, neuronal pools in the spinal cord, brain and neuromuscular junctions. Most of the nervous system is designed for impulse transmission, not generation. For a segment of the nervous system, such as mid peripheral nerve trunk or mid tract in the cord, to become an impulse generator, there must be some pathoanatomical changes in the nerve fibres and in the endoneurial or the perineurial connective tissues. The exact pathological bases to such a development are unknown, but must involve a combination of some of the mechanical and vascular mechanisms mentioned earlier in this chapter. Note that the nervi nervorum could be caught in epineurial scar or the sinuvertebral nerves caught in dural scar, and as well that the primary nerve fibres contained in the nervous system could be caught up in abnormal surrounding connective tissue. There are symptom possibilities from minor demyelination (Calvin et al 1982), sensitive immature axons and neuromas (Wall & Gutnik 1974) and hypoxic nerve fibres (Howe et al 1976,77). The primary stimulus to ectopic impulse generation would be mechanical, although there could be spontaneous generation. There may be an abnormal chemosensitivity to sympathetic efferent discharge and to other released chemicals in the area. Such activity will increase the mechano-sensitivity of the abnormal impulse generator (Devor 1983).

An insight into the equivalent abnormal impulse generating mechanisms in the neuraxis can be gained from the effects of multiple sclerosis, where sensory disturbances often occur in response to movement. Smith & McDonald (1980) produced a demyelinating lesion in the dorsal columns of 9 cats and found that small deformations of less than 1 mm increased the firing rate of normally spontaneously active units together with recruiting previously silent units. They also considered that such a lesion could be a cause of transient paraplegia on neck flexion.

Contracture of the nervous system

As a further consequence of neural fibrosis and resultant disuse, there is the possibility of contractures developing in both the connective and neural tissue components of the nervous system. The idea is hardly addressed in the literature, although Seddon (1975) was in no doubt of this possibility, either from severe trauma or failed surgery.

Contracture of the structures in the spinal canal is possible after severe injury and, in some cases, after spinal surgery. The 'rats tail' formation seen in myelograms of severely stenotic and scarred spinal canals could be placed under the category of contracture. Spasticity and frozen shoulder could also lead to nerve contractures. In these disorders, the amount of reversibility of signs and symptoms, that manual therapy can achieve is clearly limited.

MINOR NERVE INJURY

Subclinical entrapment

Nervous system contracture and fibrosis are at the severe end of the injury spectrum. At the other end are the subclinical entrapments. Pathological changes in the nervous system are likely to be evident before the patient complains of symptoms, although substantial proof of this assertion is lacking. Neary et al 1975 studied twelve postmortem specimens of median and ulnar nerves, unaffected by any known medical or neurological process that may effect the peripheral nervous system. Alterations in the normal anatomy such as a pathological distortion of the connective tissue elements, myelin slippage, demyelination, and an increase in the number of Renaut bodies were evident. Similar changes to that found in Neary's study have been reported by Chang et al (1963) in the ulnar nerve at the elbow, Nathan (1960) in the lateral femoral cutaneous nerve at the thigh, and Castelli et al (1980) in the median nerve in the carpal tunnel. There is no evidence to suggest that similar processes do not occur in the neuraxis and the meninges. The possibility that some of these changes are a part of the normal ageing process should also be entertained.

With testing the nervous system via movement, it seems likely that a pathological process in either connective or neural tissues will have occurred before tension testing registers as positive. A skill in handling and interpretation is therefore necessary and encouraged (Part II).

I believe that skilled tension testing will reveal altered nervous system mechanics and related neuropathies earlier than any other form of testing. So often clinically, the idea of subclinical entrapment appears when patients complain of old symptoms 'reactivated' by a new injury.

The notion of potential entrapment is worthy of consideration. Certain situations, such as increased compartment pressure, oedema around a nerve and plaster of Paris casts are examples of potential nervous system injury situations. This issue is discussed further in Chapter 9.

Denervation supersensitivity

Gunn (1980) raises and gives some support to the interesting issue of 'prespondylosis'. This term is used to describe the early and insidious effects of spondylitic attrition of peripheral nerves. This condition is usually painless, although there may be early and subtle changes in a significant number of young people. A further development is denervation supersensitivity of receptor organs and also hyperreactive internuncial neuronal pools, one of the main avenues of effect being through altered axoplasmic flow. Gunn's partly supported hypothesis has been further supported by the recent studies discussed above showing that axoplasmic flow can be altered by very minimal distortion of a peripheral nerve. As well as trophic changes in the target tissues, increased sensitivity in autonomic pathways can increase blood vessel tone and deprive structures of blood, potentially weakening them. I believe that skilled tension testing will reveal many of these 'prespondylitic' conditions.

OTHER FACTORS IN ADVERSE TENSION PROCESSES

Anomalies and adverse tension

Like other structures, nervous system anatomy is rarely exactly as the textbooks would have it. As well as anomalous neural anatomy, anomalies in innervation fields, blood supply and in mechanical interfaces are important considerations. There is some evidence and it is a logical assumption, that an anomaly in the nervous system and/or its interfacing structures could predispose to an adverse tension syndrome such as a nerve entrapment or irritation. Injury to an area with so called normal anatomy may not be as clinically significant as if the same area had an anomaly.

Anomalous anatomy means a greater likelihood of bizarre symptomatology and consequently more difficulty in interpretation. It can also be presumed that the prognosis may not be as good for the patient who has a neuropathic disorder that involves the anomalous area. Without electrodiagnosis it is difficult to be aware of the presence of any anomalies and the physiotherapist, in most instances, can only guess. Palpation techniques (Ch. 9) can be of some help. Treatment techniques may not be as effective, especially if treatment is directed solely at anatomy and biomechanics rather than signs and symptoms.

Nervous system anomalies are quite common and estimates of their incidence vary. From many studies it appears that at least 10% of the population will have a common form of anomaly. It would be interesting to know if this group has a disproportionate representation in those who attend for treatment. However one such anomaly is the Martin-Gruber anastamosis, whereby motor and sensory links between the ulnar and the median nerves in the forearm have been reported. This occurs in up to 25% of the population (Piersol 1907, Guttman 1977) (Fig. 3.8).

Around 15% of the population have anomalous lumbosacral nerve roots (Kadish & Simmons 1984) (Fig. 3.9). The most frequent lumbar nerve root anomalies reported in this study were common dural sleeves of two roots and two roots exiting via one foramen. Marzo et al (1987) found intradural connections between adjacent cervical nerve roots to be so common that they regarded them as normal variations rather than anomalies. The furcal nerve, a nerve arising from the L4 and L5 roots, has attracted little attention, yet by contributing to the femoral and obturator nerves and the lumbosacral trunk, it may be instrumental in some of the atypical sensory deficits and symptom areas seen (Kikuchi et al 1984).

Two examples of mechanical interface anom-

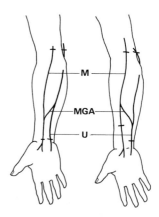

Fig. 3.8 The Martin Gruber anastamosis. M median nerve, U ulnar nerve, MGA Martin Gruber anastamosis. From: Sunderland S 1978 Nerves and nerve injuries, 2nd edn. Churchill Livingstone, Edinburgh, with kind permission of the publishers and author

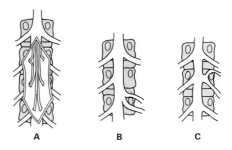

Fig. 3.9 .Examples of lumbosacral nerve root anomalies. A. intradural connections, B. closely adjacent nerve roots, C. extradural division. From: Kadish L J, Simmons E H 1984 Anomalies of the lumbosacral nerve roots. Journal of Bone and Joint Surgery 66B: 411–416, with kind permission from the publishers and authors

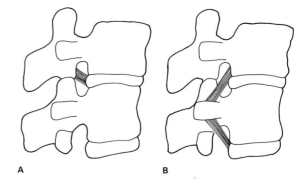

Fig. 3.10 Examples of transforaminal ligaments. From: Bogduk N, Twomey L T 1987 Clinical biomechanics of the lumbar spine, with kind permission of the publisher and authors

alies are, transforaminal ligaments (Golub & Silverman, 1969) (Fig. 3.10 A,B) and variations in the size and strength of the lumbosacral ligaments. (Nathan et al 1982).

There is some support for the notion that an anomalous nervous system predisposes an individual to injury. Werner et al (1985) demonstrated, in 9 patients, that pronator syndrome (high median nerve compression) was far more common when the median nerve pierced the humeral head of the pronator teres muscle rather than its usual passage between the humeral and ulnar heads of the muscle.

Temporal factors in nerve injury

The time elapsed following a nervous system injury is crucial to both the pathological processes and the clinical manifestations.

On one end of the scale, the nervous system adapts very well to long term sustained tension or pressure without loss, or only minimal loss of function. It appears that the system, especially the peripheral nervous system has considerable plasticity and hence the ability to adapt over a period of time. Nerve roots can be flattened to ribbons in stenotic foramina and still conduct. In spinal stenosis and stenotic root canals it has been noted that apparent severe root damage (constriction to 25% of the usual diameter) may only cause a slight neural deficit (Watanabe & Park 1986). At the other end of the scale, if an

injury is sudden, it is more likely there will be more severe damage to the system. Shear stresses from rapid nerve deformation will be less with a slower (say 20 secs) advent of pressure (Olmarker et al 1989). Simply, there is no time to call upon all the tension deployment mechanisms and spare vascular channels. An extreme example is that of a bullet injury. If a bullet passes through a limb yet misses a nerve, the forces and pressure waves that the bullet causes in surrounding tissues may result in severe damage to that nerve (Seddon 1975, Sunderland 1978). Of course, there is likely to be indirect damage from the injury to the other structures around the nerve. In this regard, a whiplash injury is an injury involving rapid velocity changes. The clinical consequences from such an injury are often severe.

With the slower process, the connective tissues of the nervous system allow some protection for the contained nerve fibres. It takes time for the perineurium to be breached and for a reaction to become intrafascicular. It also raises the prospect of irreversibility of the disorder. Once an intraneural fibrosis is established, there may be an irreversible component to the disorder and treatment may be more difficult. This potential irreversibility exists in nerve roots (Murphy 1977) and nerve trunks (Ford & Ali 1985). Fernandez & Pallini (1986) demonstrated the proliferation of intradural connective tissue of mice once an inflammatory process gained access to the dura mater.

REFERENCES

Armstrong T J, Castelli W A, Evans F G et al 1984 Some histological changes in carpal tunnel contents and their biomechanical implications. Journal of Occupational Medicine 26: 197–200

Asbury A K 1973 Renaut bodies: a forgotten endoneurial structure. Journal of Neuropathology and Experimental Neurology 32: 334–343

Beel J A, Groswald D E, Luttges M W 1984 Alterations in the mechanical properties of peripheral nerve following crush injury. Journal of Biomechanics 17: 185–193

Beel J A, Stodieck L S, Luttges M W 1986 Structural properties of spinal nerve roots: biomechanics. Experimental Neurology 91: 30–40

Bendler E M, Greenspun D O, Yu J et al 1977 The bilaterality of carpal tunnel syndrome. Archives of Physical Medicine and Rehabilitation 58: 362–368

Bogduk N, Twomey L T 1987 Clinical anatomy of the lumbar spine. Churchill Livingstone, Melbourne

Bohlman H H, Emery S E 1988 The pathophysiology of cervical spondylosis and myelopathy. Spine 13: 843–846

Breig A 1978 Adverse mechanical tension in the central nervous system. Almqvist & Wiksell, Stockholm

Butler D S 1989 Adverse mechanical tension in the nervous system: a model for assessment and treatment. Australian Journal of Physiotherapy 35: 227–238

Butler D S, Gifford L S 1989 The concept of adverse mechanical tension in the nervous system, Part 1, Testing for 'dural tension'. Physiotherapy 75: 622–629

Calvin W H, Devor M, Howe J F 1982 Can neuralgias arise from minor demyelination? Spontaneous firing, mechanosensitivity and afterdischarge from conducting axons. Experimental Neurology 75: 755–763

Castelli W A, Evans F G, Diaz-Perez R et al 1980 Intraneural connective tissue proliferation of the median nerve in the carpal tunnel. Archives of Physical Medicine and Rehabilitation 60: 418–422

Cassvan A, Rosenberg A, Rivers L F 1986 Ulnar nerve

involvement in carpal tunnel syndrome. Archives of Physical Medicine and Rehabilitation 67: 290–292

Chang K S F, Low W D, Chan S T et al 1963 Enlargement of the ulnar nerve behind the medial epicondyle. Anatomical Record 145: 149–153

Cherington M 1974 Proximal pain in carpal tunnel syndrome. Archives of Surgery 108: 69

Cusick J F, Mycklebust J, Zyvoloski M et al 1982 Effects of vertebral column distraction in the monkey. Journal of Neurosurgery 57: 185–659

Dahlin L B, Rydevik B, McLean W G et al 1984 Changes in fast axonal transport during experimental nerve compression at low pressures. Experimental Neurology 84: 29–36

Dahlin L B, McLean W G 1986 Effects of graded experimental compression on slow and fast axonal transport in rabbit vagus nerve. Journal of the Neurological Sciences. 72: 19–30

Dahlin L B, Sjostrand J, McLean W G 1986 Graded inhibition of retrograde axonal transport by compression of rabbit vagus nerve. Journal of the Neurological Sciences 76: 221–230

Davies J A 1979 Peroneal compartment syndrome secondary to rupture of the peroneus longus. Journal of Bone and Joint Surgery 61A: 783–784

Devor M 1983 Nerve pathophysiology and mechanisms of pain in causalgia. Journal of the Autonomic Nervous System 7: 371–384

Dolan E J, Transfeldt E E, Tator C H et al 1980 The effect of spinal distraction on regional spinal cord blood flow in cats. Journal of Neurosurgery 53; 756–764

Doppman J L 1975 The mechanism of ischemia in anteroposterior compression of the spinal cord. Investigative Radiology 10: 543–551

Dyro F M 1983 Peripheral entrapments following brachial plexus lesions. Electromyography and Clinical Neurophysiology 23: 251–256

Faithfull D K, Moir D H, Ireland J 1985 The micropathology of the typical carpal tunnel syndrome. Journal of Hand Surgery 11B: 131–132

Fernandez E, Pallini R 1986 Connective tissue scarring in experimental spinal cord lesions: significance of dural continuity and the role of epidural tissues. Acta Neurochirurgica 76: 145–148

Ford D J, Ali M S 1985 Acute carpal tunnel syndrome. The Journal of Bone and Joint Surgery 65B: 758–759

Fowler T J, Danta G, Gilliat R W 1972 Recovery of nerve conduction after a pneumatic tourniquet: observations on the hind limb of the baboon. Journal of Neurology, Neurosurgery and Psychiatry 35: 638–647

Fowler T J, Ochoa J 1975 Unmyelinated fibres in normal and compressed peripheral nerves of the baboon: a quantitative electron microscopic study. Neuropathology and Applied Neurobiology 1: 247–265

Gasser H S, Erlanger J 1929 The role of fibre size in the establishment of a nerve block by pressure or cocaine. American Journal of Physiology 88: 581–591

Gelberman R H, Hergenroeder P T, Hargens A R et al 1981 The carpal tunnel syndrome: a study of carpal canal pressures. The Journal of Bone and Joint Surgery 63A: 380–383

Gilliatt R W 1981 Physical injury to peripheral nerves: physiologic and electrodiagnostic aspects. Mayo Clinic Proceedings 56: 361–370

Golub B S, Silverman B 1969 Transforaminal ligaments of the lumbar spine. Journal of Bone and Joint Surgery 51A: 947–956

Gooding M R, Wilson C B, Hoff J T 1975 Experimental cervical myelopathy: effects of ischaemia and compression of the canine cervical spinal cord. Journal of Neurosurgery 43: 9–17

Gunn C C 1980 Prespondylosis and some pain syndromes following denervation supersensitivity. Spine 5: 185–192

Guttman L 1977 Median-ulnar nerve communications and carpal tunnel syndrome. Journal of Neurology Neurosurgery and Psychiatry 40: 982–986

Guyon M A, Honet J C 1977 CTS or trigger finger associated with neck injury in automobile accidents. Archives of Physical Medicine and Rehabilitation 58: 325–327

Haftek J 1970 Stretch injury of peripheral nerve: acute effects of stretching on rabbit nerve. Journal of Bone and Joint Surgery 52B: 354–365

Howe J F, Calvin W H, Loeser J D 1976 Impulses reflected from dorsal root ganglia and from focal nerve injuries. Brain Research. 116: 139–144

Howe J F, Loeser J D, Calvin W H 1977 Mechanosensitivity of dorsal root ganglia and chronically injured axons: a physiological basis for the radicular pain of nerve root compression. Pain 3: 25–41

Hurst L C, Weissberg D, Carroll R E 1985 The relationship of double crush to carpal tunnel syndrome (an analysis of 1,000 cases of carpal tunnel syndrome). Journal of Hand Surgery 10B: 202–204

Jefferson D, Neary D, Eames R A 1981 Renaut body distribution at sites of human peripheral nerve entrapment. Journal of the Neurological Sciences 49: 19–29

Kadish L J, Simmons E H 1984 Anomalies of the lumbosacral nerve roots. Journal of Bone and Joint Surgery 66B: 411–416

Kikuchi S, Hasue M, Nishiyama K, Tsukasa I 1984 Anatomic and clinical studies of radicular symptoms. Spine 9: 23–30

Kobrine A I, Evans D E, Rizzoli H 1978 Correlation of spinal cord blood flow and function in experimental compression. Surgical Neurology 10: 54–59

Korr I M 1985 Neurochemical and neurotrophic consequences of nerve deformation. In: Glasgow E F et al (eds) Aspects of manipulative therapy, 2nd edn. Churchill Livingstone, Melbourne

Leyshon A, Kirwan, E O G, Wynn Parry C B 1981 Electrical studies in the diagnosis of compression of the lumbar root. Journal of Bone and Joint Surgery 63B: 71–75

Lishman W A, Russel W K 1961 The brachial neuropathies. Lancet 2: 941–947

Louis R 1981 Vertebroradicular and vertebromedullar dynamics. Anatomica Clinica 3: 1–11

Lundborg G 1970 Ischemic nerve injury: experimental studies on intraneural microvascular pathophysiology and nerve function in a limb, subjected to temporary circulatory arrest. Scandinavian Journal of Plastic and Reconstructive Surgery (Suppl) 6: 1–113

Lundborg G 1988 Nerve injury and repair. Churchill Livingstone, Edinburgh

Lundborg G, Dahlin L B 1989 Pathophysiology of nerve

compression. In: Szabo R M (ed) Nerve compression syndromes. Slack, Thorofare

Luttges M W, Kelly P T, Gerren R A 1976 Degenerative changes in mouse sciatic nerve: electrophoretic and electrophysiological characterisations. Experimental Neurology 50: 706–33

Mackinnon S E, Dellon A L 1988 Surgery of the peripheral nerve. Thieme, New York

Marzo J M, Simmons E H, Kallen F 1987 Intradural connections between adjacent cervical nerve roots. Spine 12: 964–968

Massey E W, Riley T L, Pleet A B 1981 Coexistant carpal tunnel syndrome and cervical radiculopathy (double crush syndrome). Southern Medical Journal 74: 957–959

McComas A J, Jorgensen P B, Upton A R M 1974 The neuropraxic lesion: a clinical contribution to the study of trophic mechanisms. The Canadian Journal of Neurological Sciences 1: 170–179

McLellan D C, Swash M 1976 Longitudinal sliding of the median nerve during movements of the upper limb. Journal of Neurology, Neurosurgery and Psychiatry 39: 556–570

Meals R A 1977 Peroneal nerve palsy complicating ankle sprain. Journal of Bone and Joint Surgery 59A: 966–968

Millesi H 1986 The nerve gap. Hand Clinics 2: 651–663

Mubarak S J, Pedowitz R A, Hargens A R 1989 Compartment syndromes. Current Orthopaedics 3: 36–40

Murphy R W 1977 Nerve roots and spinal nerves in degenerative disc disease. Clinical Orthopaedics and Related Research 129: 46–60

Myers R, Powell H 1981 Endoneurial fluid pressure in peripheral neuropathies. In: Hargens A (ed) Tissue fluid pressure and composition. Williams & Wilkins, Baltimore

Nathan H 1960 Gangliform enlargement on the lateral cutaneous nerve of the thigh. Journal of Neurosurgery 17: 843–849

Nathan H 1986 Osteophytes of the spine compressing the sympathetic trunk and splanchnic nerves in the thorax. Spine 12: 527–532

Neary D, Ochoa J, Gilliat R W 1975 Sub-clinical entrapment neuropathy in man. Journal of the Neurological Sciences 24: 283–298

Nitz A J, Dobner J J, Kersey D 1985 Nerve injury and grade II and III ankle sprains. The American Journal of Sports Medicine 13: 177–182

Nobel W 1966 Peroneal palsy due to haematoma in the common peroneal nerve sheath after distal torsional fractures and inversion ankle sprains. Journal of Bone and Joint Surgery 48A: 1484–1495

Ochoa J, Fowler T J, Gilliat R W 1972 Anatomical changes in peripheral nerves compressed by a pneumatic tourniquet. Journal of Anatomy. 113: 433–455

Ochoa J 1980 Nerve fibre pathology in acute and chronic compression. In: Omer G E, Spinner M (eds) Management of peripheral nerve problems. Saunders, Philadephia

Ochs S 1975 Axoplasmic transport. In: Tower D (ed) The nervous system. Raven Press, New York, vol 1

Ogata K, Naito M 1986 Blood flow of peripheral nerve: effects of dissection, stretching and compression. Journal of Hand Surgery 11B: 10–14

Oiwa T 1983 Experimental study on post laminectomy deterioration in cervical spondylotic myelopathy-influences of the meningeal treatment of persistent

spinal cord block. Nippon Seikeigeka Gakkai Zashi 57: 577–592

Olsson Y, Kristensson K 1973 The perineurium as a diffusion barrier to protein tracers follwing trauma to nerves. Acta Neuropathologica 23: 105–111

Olmarker K, Rydevik B, Holm S 1989 Edema formed in spinal nerve roots induced by experimental graded compression. Spine 14: 569–573

Ortman J A, Zarife S, Mendell J R 1983 The experimental production of renaut bodies in response to mechanical stress. Journal of the Neurological Sciences. 62: 233–241

Pan G, Kulkarni M, MacDougall D J, Miner M E 1988 Traumatic epidural haematoma of the cervical spine: diagnosis with magnetic resonsnce imaging. Journal of Neurosurgery 68: 798–801

Pang D, Wilberger J E 1982 Tethered cord syndrome in adults. Journal of Neurosurgery 57: 32–47

Pfeffer G, Osterman A L 1986 Double crush syndrome: cervical radiculopathy and carpal tunnel syndrome (abstract). Journal of Hand Surgery 11A: 766

Phalen G S 1970 Reflections on 21 years experience with the carpal tunnel syndrome. Journal of the American Medical Association 212: 8: 1365–1367

Piersol G A 1907 Human anatomy, 3rd edn. Lippincott, Philadelphia

Powell H C, Myers R R 1986 Pathology of experimental nerve compression. Laboratory Investigations 55: 91–100

Rayan G M, Pitha J V, Wisdom P et al 1988 Histologic and electrophysiologic changes following subepineurial haematoma induction in rat sciatic nerve. Clinical Orthopaedics and Related Research 229: 257–264

Robinson R A et al 1977 Cervical spondylotic myelopathy: etiology and treatment concepts. Spine 2: 89–99

Rydevik B et al 1980 Blockage of axonal transport induced by acute graded compression of the rabbit vagus nerve. Journal of Neurology, Neurosurgery and Psychiatry 43: 690–698

Rydevik B, Lundborg G, Bagge U 1981 Effects of graded compression on intraneural blood flow. Journal of Hand Surgery 6: 3–12

Rydevik B, Brown M D, Lundborg G 1984 Pathoanatomy and pathophysiology of nerve root compression. Spine 9: 7–15

Rydevik B L, Myers R R, Powell H C 1989 Pressure increase in the dorsal root ganglion following mechanical compression. Spine 14: 574–576

Seddon H 1975 Surgical disorders of the peripheral nerves, 2nd edn. Churchill Livingstone, Edinburgh

Selander D, Mansson L G, Karlsson L et al 1985 Adrenergetic vasoconstriction in peripheral nerves in the rabbit. Anesthesiology 62: 6–10

Sedal L, McLeod J G, Walsh J C 1973 Ulnar nerve lesions associated with the carpal tunnel syndrome. Journal of Neurology, Neurosurgery and Psychiatry 36: 118–123

Selier W A et al 1983 The double crush syndrome: experimental model in the rat. Surgical Forum 34: 596–598

Silver M A, Gelberman R H, Gellman H et al 1985 Carpal tunnel syndrome: associated abnormalities in ulnar nerve function and the effect of carpal tunnel release on these abnormalities. Journal of Hand Surgery 10A: 710–713

Siqueira E B, Kranzler L I, Dhakar D P 1983 Fibrosis of

the dura mater: a cause of failed back syndrome. Surgical Neurology 19: 168–70

Smith K J, McDonald W I 1980 Spontaneous and mechanically evoked activity due to central demyelinating lesion. Nature 286: 154–155

Stodieck L S, Luttges M W 1983 Protein composition and synthesis in the adult mouse spinal cord. Neurochemical Research 8: 599–619

Stodieck L S, Luttges M W 1986 Structural properties of spinal nerve roots: protein composition. Experimental Neurology 19: 41–51

Sunderland S 1976 The nerve lesion in carpal tunnel syndrome. Journal of Neurology Neurosurgery and Psychiatry 39: 615–626

Sunderland S 1978 Nerves and nerve injuries, 2nd edn. Churchill Livingstone, Edinburgh

Sunderland S 1989 The mischievous fibroblast: friction trauma, fibrosis and adhesions. In: Jones H M, Jones M A, Milde M R (eds) Sixth biennial conference proceedings, Manipulative Therapists Association of Australia, Adelaide

Szabo R M, Gelberman R H, Williamson R V et al 1983 Effects of systemic blood pressure on the tissue fluid threshold of peripheral nerve. Journal of Orthopaedic Research. 1: 172–178

Triano J J, Luttges M W 1982 Nerve irritation: a possible model of sciatic neuritis. Spine 7: 129–136

Turnbull I M 1971 Micro vasculature of the human spinal cord. Journal of Neurosurgery 35: 141–147

Upton A R M, McComas A J 1973 The double crush in nerve entrapment syndromes. Lancet 2: 359–362

Wall P D, Gutnik M 1974 Properties of afferent nerve impulses originating from a neuroma. Nature 248: 740–743

Werner C O, Rosen I, Thorngren K G 1985 Clinical and neurophysiological characteristics of the pronator syndrome. Clinical Orthopaedics and Related Research 197: 231–236

Watanabe R, Parke W W 1986 Vascular and neural pathology of lumbosacral spinal stenosis. Journal of Neurosurgery 64: 64–70

4. The clinical consequences of injury to the nervous system

WHERE CAN THE PAIN COME FROM?

Prior to a discussion of the possible array of signs and symptoms which may emerge when the nervous system is involved in an adverse tension syndrome, it is worth attempting to answer the question, 'if the nervous system is injured, where can the pain come from'? The answer is difficult for a number of reasons:

1. Compared to the normal nervous system, the injured nervous system is hardly studied.

2. Most studies are on animals.

3. Most studies are on compression of the nervous system, few are on stretch or irritation of the nervous system.

4. Inevitably, an injury to the nervous system will necessitate injury to a surrounding structure. For example the pain pattern that might be originating from an injured nerve root may also have contributions from an injured zygapophyseal joint. Ultimately, an injury to the nervous system will cause denervation in the non-neural tissues innervated by the damaged segment.

5. An injury to the nervous system will rarely be limited to one segment or structure of the nervous system. The connective tissues and the conducting tissues are intimately related. Therefore, expressions of the injury elsewhere along the nervous system are possible physiologically and, ultimately, mechanically.

6. Perhaps the bottom line is that some nerve injuries hurt and some do not; the reasons for this are not known.

Pain associated with the nervous system can be categorised in terms of physiological mechanisms into central, neurogenic and nociceptive. Central pain is generated in the second order neurones in the central nervous system, neurogenic pain is caused by a process that affects and triggers peripheral axons. Nociceptive pain arises from stimulation of peripheral nociceptors (Bogduk 1989).

The question of the origin of pain from the nervous system can be best answered by considering the connective tissue elements of the nervous system and the transmitting elements.

The connective tissues of the nervous system

In Chapter 1, the innervation of the connective tissues was outlined. The kind of symptoms resulting from this innervation can only be inferred from clinical observations and a few rare studies. The most common symptom is pain. Note that this pain could be considered a nociceptive pain, that is, there is no injury to the conducting elements of the nervous system.

Dural pain

The concept of dural pain was introduced by Cyriax (1942) and further expanded upon in his many editioned 'Textbook of Orthopaedic Medicine' (1982). His thoughts are based on extrapolation of literature and his many years of clinical experience. On the basis of its innervation by the sinuvertebral nerve, dura mater as a source of primary pain has also been suggested by Edgar & Nundy (1966), Murphy (1977), Bogduk (1983) and Cuatico et al (1988). There is some experimental support for the concept. Smyth & Wright (1958) attached sutures to the dural sleeves of lumbar nerve roots of humans during laminectomy procedures. By pulling on them, back and thigh pain could be produced. As well as demonstrating mechanosensitivity, the dura is also chemosensitive. If the dura is bathed in hypertonic saline, back pain can be evoked (El Mahdi et al 1981). This pain can be abolished by applying xylocaine to the dura.

Cyriax proposed a body chart (Fig. 4.1) showing 'the limits of dural reference'. Whilst this is the only attempt in the literature to define some of the features of dural pain, some elements of this concept may be usefully criticised.

1. The name 'dural pain' is unfortunate. It is in common usage amongst physiotherapists and there is some danger of the dogma

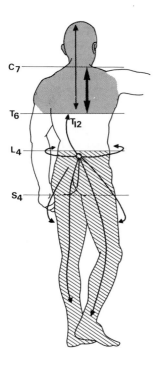

Fig. 4.1 Extrasegmental referral of pain from the dura mater according to Cyriax (1982). Cyriax considered that low lumbar dural pain could spread to the legs, the abdomen and to the mid-thoracic spine. The cervical dura mater could refer pain to the head and to the mid thoracic spine. Adapted from Cyriax (1982)

persisting that tension tests are solely tests of dura mechanics. It implies that symptoms arising from structures within the spinal canal are due to the dura mater exclusively. Symptoms may well emanate from dural attachments or other structures within the canal, such as blood vessels, pia mater, denticulate ligaments or the spinal cord.

2. Some confusion is possible because tests, such as the Straight Leg Raise and Passive Neck Flexion used by Cyriax, have the potential to provoke symptoms from other attached structures. A test such as Passive Neck Flexion could be, via normal meninges, placing tension and movement on an irritated segment of posterior longitudinal ligament or posterior annulus fibrosis. There is too much uncertainty about the nature of evoked symptoms from different structures to conclusively make one structure culpable.

3. 'Dural pain' is also misleading as it implies that pain is the only symptom coming from the neuraxis and its membranes. In a clinical study, muscle stiffness, paraesthesia and feelings of warmth and cold were symptoms which could be altered (usually eased) by a paravertebral block at the third lumbar ganglion of the sympathetic chain (El Mahdi et al 1981). Further, sinuvertebral nerves have a sympathetic component and thus it is quite possible that an irritated or depressed sympathetic nervous system is responsible for aspects of some syndromes. El Mahdi et al (1981) take up this issue, noting that the back pain caused by a SLR is dull, vague and difficult to localise. They also note that the surgical correlation of the level of a disc protrusion with dermatomal pain distribution is under 50% (Lansche & Ford 1960, Edgar & Park 1974). This they use as evidence for an autonomic pain component. Some support comes from Meglio et al (1981) who have shown that electrical epidural stimulation has a beneficial effect on vascular insufficiencies. From clinical observations, I feel that complaints of stiffness may relate to the dura mater.

Cyriax's diagram includes the feet but does not include the arms and hands. There is no neurological basis for one extremity to be involved and not the other and it is also difficult to accept clinically.

Nevertheless, there are many aspects of Cyriax's interpretation of dural pain that are very relevant and useful in assessment and treatment. Cyriax (1982) observed that the dura mater does 'not obey the rules of segmental reference'. That is, it does not follow the familiar dermatomal or myotomal reference. Cyriax expands this statement by saying 'false localising symptoms are commonplace' and makes the suggestion that attention should be focussed on the dura mater when the patient's description of pain is theoretically impossible. This is excellent advice. Perhaps it could be taken further to suggest that the nervous system, rather than just the dura mater, should be suspected as a possible source of symptoms when there is no localising value to the patients symptoms. Cyriax (1982) also made the observation that the pain was usually in the posterior trunk and could be central or either side.

In these matters, an open mind must be kept when considering those structures not innervated, or where an innervation has not yet been discovered. The glia, pia mater, denticulate ligaments, dural ligaments and subarachnoid trabeculae are examples. Even if a structure is devoid of nerve endings it can still be instrumental in symptom production. For example, scarred posterior dura mater will affect the biomechanics of the more richly innervated anterior dura, or axons in the cord may be trapped in scarred glia.

Surely part of the explanation for the characteristics of dural pain lies in the innervation characteristics of the sinuvertebral nerve; especially the wide distribution and overlap of individual nerves and its somatic and autonomic components (Ch. 1).

Peripheral nerve trunk pain

Due to the nervi nervorum, it can be inferred that injury or irritation to the sheaths and capsules of the peripheral nervous system may cause symptoms. The possibilities of this have been noted by authorities such as Sunderland (1978), Thomas (1982) and Pratt (1986).

An interesting hypothesis was presented by Asbury & Fields (1984). These neurologists distinguished two types of pain in peripheral nerve disorders — dysesthetic pain from the nerve fibres and nerve trunk pain. They postulated that nerve trunk pain was due to the innervated connective tissues. Table 4.1 summarises their clinical impressions. This table is a rarity in the literature in that it attempts to link symptoms with pathoanatomy. Although this hypothesis needs proof, for physiotherapists using tension tests and attempting interpretations of symptoms, it is helpful and fits with what is found clinically. Perhaps a useful way of thinking would be to consider symptoms from the connective tissues to be the same as symptoms from innervated connective tissues anywhere in the body. On the other hand, if the primary neurones were involved, the patient would complain of different symptoms, unfamiliar and perhaps bizarre, such as 'burning' or 'crawling'. Classifying the symptoms is difficult. Nerve trunk pain could be considered nociceptive and the symptoms from

Table 4.1 Characteristics of two major forms of neurogenic pain (modified from Asbury & Fields 1984)

	Dysesthetic pain	Nerve trunk pain
Description	Burning, tingling, raw, searing, crawling, drawing, electric	Aching, knifelike, tender
Recognition	Unfamiliar, never experienced before	Familiar, like a 'toothache'
Distribution	Cutaneous or subcutaneous, in the area innervated by the nerve	Deep, along the nerve trunk
Constancy	Variable, jabbing, intermittent, lancinating, shooting	Usually continuous, waxes and wanes
Aggravate/ Ease	Activity worsens hard to ease	Worse with movement, stretch, palpation, ease with rest or positioning
Examples	Causalgia, small fibre neuropathy (e.g., diabetes), post herpetic neuralgia	Spinal root compression brachial neuritis, leprosy neuritis

the nerve fibres as neurogenic, although I have used the term neurogenic in this book to include both.

The possibility of referral from peripheral nerve connective tissues should be entertained. There are similarities between the innervation of the connective tissues of the peripheral nerve and the dura mater, in that, they both have sympathetic and somatic innervation. Referred pain from the dura is accepted. There is no reason why the connective tissue sheaths cannot refer symptoms, from either irritation of nervi nervorum or mechanical distortion of nervi nervorum caught in scar. Given the extra-segmental referral from dura mater, it seems reasonable enough that such referred symptoms may also be extrasegmental, and thus not in any familiar pattern such as a dermatome. The connective tissue capsules of the autonomic trunks and ganglia must also be considered as symptom sources. The nature of these possible symptoms is unknown. However, there is no shortage of unexplained pains in symptomatology. Some patients with adverse tension disorders complain of 'lines of pain', sometimes along a nerve such as in the inner arm, or at other times more parallel to the nerve trunk. Common examples are lines of pain over the deltoid muscle, in the buttock from a focus of pain in the lumbar spine, superior to the wrist, and along the trapezius muscle. Having noted that these symptoms are often associated with positive tension tests, I feel they may be an example of referred pain from peripheral nerve connective tissues.

The neural tissues

The pain mechanisms related to the impulse conducting tissues of the nervous system are more complex. Readers are directed to the many relevant chapters in Wall & Melzack's 'Textbook of Pain' (1985), also review articles by Sweet (1987) and Wolff (1987).

In peripheral nerve there are a number of hypotheses suggesting nerve fibre as a source of pain when the injury is 'in continuity'; that

is, the nerve has not been separated. These mechanisms are listed below:

1. 'Ectopic impulses from compression, stretch or vascular insult' (Howe et al, 1976,1977). This may be from localised sites, or the whole nerve may become an ectopic generator (Ochoa and Torebjork, 1981). Symptoms will depend on the type (sensory, motor or autonomic) and size of nerve fibre affected. To be a consistent site of ectopic impulse generation, there would need to be an injury of some kind.

2. 'Spontaneous discharge from neuroma formation' (Wall & Gutnik 1974). Neuromas are mechanosensitive and chemosensitive. Large segments of a nerve could be involved in a neuroma. Devor (1985) suggested that individual axons may form 'microneuromas' scattered throughout the trunk. Within the neuroma, immature axon sprouts have been identified as the source of the discharge (Wall & Gutnik 1974) although minor demyelination is another possibility (Calvin et al 1982).

3. Where there is damage affecting the large fibres, excess C fibre activity or an excess of C fibres may lead to 'fibre dissociation'. This is part of the now partly disproven gate control theory (Noordenbos 1959, Melzack & Wall 1965).

4. If the endoneurial tubes and the Schwann-myelin complex of neighbouring axons are disrupted, the formation of abnormal or ephaptic synapses can ensue (Granit & Skoglund (1945). With these false synapses, for example if a sensory fibre synapsed on an autonomic fibre, there would be potential for bizarre symptomatology. This process is known colloquially as 'crosstalk'.

Combinations of these suggested mechanisms probably occur and, in combination with scarred connective tissue sheaths, may lead to the development of an abnormal impulse generating site at an injury site (discussed in the previous chapter). For example, immature axon sprouts may be caught in endoneurial scar. These sites could occur anywhere in the nervous system including the central nervous system. Smith & McDonald (1980) produced a demyelinating lesion in the dorsal column of cats. From this they could demonstrate that small deformations of the injured site increased the firing rate of normally spontaneously active units together with the recruitment of previously silent units. There is also clinical evidence of the mechanosensitivity of the nervous system in demyelinating disorders such as multiple sclerosis.

Abnormal impulse generating mechanisms could occur anywhere in the nervous system, not just in major nerve trunks, nerve roots or the neuraxis. For example, injury could occur in a sinuvertebral nerve, in the end branch of a cutaneous nerve just before a receptor organ, in a sympathetic ganglia, or in a cranial nerve. Clearly, a mechanically compromised segment of nervous system will have co-existing vascular compromise, and part of the symptomatology could be due to metabolic insufficiency.

Other clinical consequences of neural injury

The major concern of this text is injury to the nervous system itself, but clinically there must be other concerns. If there is an injury to the transmitting tissues of the nervous system then information to and from the non-neural structures will be affected. In the symptom dominant approach used by physiotherapists, this is an important consideration . For example, if a patient's injured foot is passively mobilised and the physiotherapist is basing treatment on the patient's descriptions of symptoms, that description may not be accurate if there is some injury along the nervous system distorting information. The treatment's effectiveness may be adversely affected.

The other important consequence is that trophic changes in the target tissues of the damaged nerve may lead to signs and symptoms from that tissue. This has been discussed in Chapter 3 and emphasis has been placed on the fact that only minimal injury to the nervous system is required

to make an alteration in the axonal transport systems.

SIGNS AND SYMPTOMS FOLLOWING NEURAL INJURY

If the nervous system has been badly damaged, such as by severe crush or transection, a neuropathic basis for pain is quite obvious and easily proven, although the exact mechanisms of pain may not be known. In contrast, the symptomatology from the more minor injuries to which this text is directed is less clear, less reported and consequently open to argument. It is not any easy thing to state that symptoms are neurogenic in origin.

This chapter is a combination of reports in the literature and the clinical observations by myself and others of patients presenting with physical signs of altered nervous system mechanics, i.e., positive tension tests (Ch. 7 & Ch. 8).

I believe that physiotherapists who are skilled in questioning patients, possess good handling skills, and can relate physical findings to subjective findings have much to contribute in this area. In this regard, the clinical reasoning processes inherent in the Maitland approach (Maitland 1986, Grant et al 1988, refer to next chapter) have allowed subjective information to be linked with purported pathoanatomy. It has also allowed confident reporting on previously unreported implied neuropathic symptoms. However, with any new information or different logic, these assertions should be immediately challenged.

General

Patients will always have a ready array of subjective and physical clues that, on analysis, can tell the examiner if the nervous system is mechanically or physiologically involved. Further, these clues can be interpreted to supply the physiotherapist with such information as:

1. Level of involvement (e.g., upper motor neurone, lower motor neurone, segmental level)

2. Severity of involvement
3. The tissue components involved (neural tissue or connective tissues of the nervous system)
4. If from local sources or from remote sources
5. Whether an intraneural or extraneural process is evident
6. The stage of the disorder (acute/chronic)
7. The progression of the disorder.

The clinical spectrum

In recent years it has become apparent that adverse neural tension is a component of most disorders encountered by physiotherapists. How much of a component and the clinical importance of the component is not yet really known. The initial anecdotal and unreported findings by those practitioners seeking better results for their patients have slowly been followed by clinical studies. There have been normative studies of tension tests (discussed in Ch. 7 & Ch. 8) and recently clinical studies and case studies linking positive tension tests and various disorders such as hamstring tears (Kornberg & Lew 1989), repetition strain injury (Elvey et al 1986), whiplash (Quintner 1989) and hand hypersensitivity following surgery or trauma (Sweeney & Harms 1990).

The advent of tension testing has made many physiotherapists question the structural basis of a number of disorders presented to them for treatment. Examples of such disorders are tennis elbow, de Quervain's tenosynovitis or the symptoms related to disc degeneration. Any disorders with the name 'syndrome' tacked on the end, such as thoracic outlet syndrome, is immediately up for question. Not only physiotherapists are questioning but so too are some neurosurgeons. De Quervain's tenosynovitis is a good example. Saplys et al (1987) treated 71 patients for radial sensory nerve entrapment and 82 patients for neuromas of the lateral antebrachial and radial sensory nerves. In the first group, 17 had been diagnosed as de Quervain's disease as had 24 in the second group. Release of the first extensor compartment had not helped the condition or they developed neuromas of

one of the dorso-radial sensory nerves. These authors, including Mackinnon & Dellon (1988), Kopell & Thompson (1963), Sunderland (1978) and Loeser (1985) all present strong arguments to the effect that injury to the peripheral nervous system is underestimated. The spectrum must spread to the neuraxis as well. Here, minor injury is hardly considered compared with the peripheral nervous system. The idea of a neuropraxic cord lesion has only been recently raised (Torg et al 1986). Although the cord is very well protected, there is the likelihood of minor injuries being treated by movement by doctors and physiotherapists unaware of the injury. As in the peripheral nervous system, I feel the consequences of altered tension in the central nervous system are understated. It is worth quoting Breig (1978):

I have found that many neurological disorders in which no mechanical component has ever been suspected do in fact have their origin in tension in the nervous tissue; we are at present only just beginning to recognize the histological and neurophysiological sequelae of this tension.'

As well as being a familiar and significant component of such well known syndromes as the acute and chronic nerve root syndromes or the nerve entrapment syndromes, many bizarre, unexplained and even spot pains can be inferred by physical examination, with support from treatment responses, to have their origin in altered nervous system physiology and/or mechanics. Many of these disorders are discussed in Part IV.

I believe it is useful to think in terms of patterns of symptom presentation. Once the physiotherapist can pick up a certain pattern of symptoms, the clinical reasoning process (Ch. 5), which should be inherent in the examination, is made easier. Hypotheses can be proven or disproven.

AREA OF SYMPTOMS

Due to the multilayered mesh of nervous system in the body and the referral potential of the system, no area of the body will be exempt from symptoms arising from injury to the nervous system.

There are, however, patterns of symptom area distribution which give valuable clues to the nature of the injury. Some can be linked up with the pathological processes such as the 'double crush', outlined in the previous chapter. It should go without saying that, for an examiner to make use of symptomatology, he/she must be prepared to firstly believe the patient and secondly to ask about symptoms away from the patient's main complaint, and about symptoms further away than the known referral sites.

1. Such symptoms include those over vulnerable nervous system areas such as the carpal tunnel, the head of the fibula, the intervertebral foramina, the T6 area. Areas of the body where the nervous system is vulnerable are outlined in Chapter 3.

2. Symptoms that do not fit familiar patterns such as a dermatomal or myotomal distribution are also relevant. Most physiotherapists are familiar with patterns of symptom presentation from joints or muscles. The idea of symptom presentation from the nervous system is rather new and hence unfamiliar. It is again worth remembering Cyriax's statement (1982), based on his clinical experience: 'suspect the dura mater when the symptoms have no localising value'. Cyriax was referring to the extrasegmental pain referral patterns from the dura. This can be taken further to suspicion of the entire nervous system when the symptoms have no localising value. The clinical features of neurogenic pain are not clear and the suggestion to think of the nervous system when symptoms are a bit obscure is good advice. When symptoms do not fit familiar patterns, some clinicians lose interest in the patient and, sadly, begin to suspect the validity of the complaints.

3. Symptoms that fit with nerve anatomy are significant. This includes symptoms in an area of the cutaneous distribution of a nerve, in a dermatome or along a nerve trunk. Where symptoms are in a field of innervation it is a logical inference that the conducting tissues are injured or abnormal in some way.

4. Symptoms may link up. For example,

'double crush' type symptoms such as coexistent tennis elbow and carpal tunnel syndrome, bilateral symptoms such as bilateral carpal tunnel syndrome or bilateral 'shin splints' must immediately raise the suspicion of altered nervous system mechanics. A high index of suspicion must be given to co-existing presentations of low cervical symptoms and mid thoracic symptoms, for wrist pain that has spread to the shoulder, or shoulder pain that has spread to the wrist. Once the idea of the double crush becomes understood, it is obvious in many of the patients who present to physiotherapists. Even the 'multiple crush' kind of patient should now be entitled to more of a clinical hearing than they may be accustomed to.

Symptom 'link up' can be of two kinds. Firstly in a behavioral sense when the symptoms may come on together with certain activities or where the patient may complain of one symptom only when the other is absent. Secondly, a link between a number of symptoms can be made historically. Here, the patient notices that the second symptom did in fact start at about the same time as the first symptom, or perhaps after a re-injury of the initial problem. There is also a pattern where symptoms 'jump' from area to area. For example, one day the symptom might be in the lumbar spine and the next it could be in the knee. Often these patients invite disbelief in the existence of an organic basis for their symptoms. With persistent questioning, perhaps over a number of treatment sessions, a pattern of symptom presentation, though complex, invariably emerges.

It is hoped, however, that once the practitioner gets a feel for adverse tension syndromes, then familiar patterns will emerge; just as there are accepted patterns for joint injury (Cyriax 1982, Maitland 1986) and for muscle injury (Janda 1978, 1986). Some of these patterns have become accepted dogma. Patterns from the nervous system may lead to a challenge of some of this dogma.

5. 'Lines' and 'clumps' of pain or symptoms may occur. These features are regularly seen in patients and should raise the

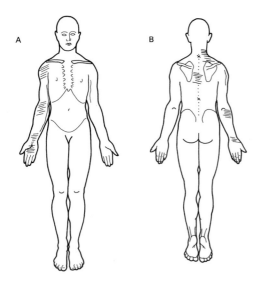

Fig. 4.2. An example from case notes illustrating 'lines and clumps' of pain. This patient suffered from an overuse syndrome of 6 months duration. The areas of symptoms were limited to the right arm and the spine, although on the initial assessment this patient complained of some 'twinges' in the opposite arm

index of suspicion regarding the possibility of their relationship to some form of neuropathy. Clinically, this can be a useful way to make some of the more bizarre symptoms make sense. If patients complain of lines of pain, they are often along peripheral nerves. Common clinical examples are lines of pain in the forearm in carpal tunnel syndrome or lines of pain in the hamstrings in sciatica. Lines often go with a description of 'strings pulling' and, if the patient is questioned, these lines are sometimes only a centimetre or two wide. Clumps of pain appear more around joints or tension points. The area is often vague and the patient will place their whole hand over the area or refer to it as a focus of symptoms. In some situations, both clumps and lines co-exist. Figure 4.2 A,B is an example taken from my case-notes of a patient suffering from an upper limb overuse disorder and exhibiting lines and clumps of pain.

KINDS OF SYMPTOM

There are certain patterns of behaviour and also certain kinds of symptom which implicate the nervous system.

Remember that pain and undesirable sensations are not easy to describe and the descriptions that emerge from patients are influenced by many factors other than the actual injury. Pain is not a necessary symptom. While a pain-only situation could be envisaged from the dura or the epineurium, there are no mechanisms whereby only nociceptive axons can be irritated or compressed without affecting fibres that convey other sensations. Although pain is usually the dominant symptom, there are others such as weakness, paralysis, paraesthesia and anaesthesia. A complaint of pain may need clarifying. Pain to the patient could mean 'ache', 'tiredness', 'dragging' etc. The major presenting symptom could be an alteration in normal movement, for example, an inability to pinch correctly, perhaps indicating a paralysis of the anterior interosseus nerve in the forearm.

1. Presumed neuropathic pain elicits a wide vocabulary from patients. The pain may be described as 'vague', 'deep', 'burning', 'heaviness', 'aching', 'searing' and many other terms. It can be in an entire limb or there may be catches or painful arcs during movement. Burning is a common complaint associated with nervous system involvement. There may be more bizarre complaints such as 'strings pulling', 'strangling', 'wooden' or 'dead'. I recall a patient with an upper limb overuse syndrome telling me that her arm felt 'pickled'. The patient's description of symptoms is useful for treatment — it is an indication of how far their discomfort needs changing and this could be part of the measure of treatment success. The kind of symptoms described may help to locate the site of the nervous system injury. Some of these are have been described in Table 4.1. A discussion of further analysis in terms of extraneural and intraneural pathologies may be found in Chapter 9.

An important distinction to be made is whether the symptoms are constant or intermittent. Constant symptoms may indicate an inflammatory involvement or a process that has gained access deep into the nerve associated with, or contributing to, maintained increased intrafascicular pressure.

2. Sensations of swelling, especially in extremity regions such as the feet, the metacarpophalangeal row and the web space, are not uncommon. On examination, it often appears that there is not enough swelling to warrant such a complaint. While there can actually be swelling, in the minor injuries it is more often a complaint of swelling. Perhaps this a clue to an autonomic nervous system component in the disorder. This may be due to irritation or loss of the normal movement of the sympathetic trunks and ganglia. As well as a clue to the presence of an adverse tension syndrome, it should also direct the physiotherapist to examine the spine.

3. Paraesthesia and anaesthesia are two symptoms allowing instant recognition of involvement of the nervous system. These symptoms may exist with or without pain. Macnab (1972) has reported that experimental compression of normal lumbar nerve roots using a catheter inserted into the intervertebral foramen did not cause pain but elicited paraesthesia and numbness.

The distribution of these sensations can be of some help in locating the source. Figures of dermatomes and cutaneous fields of innervation are shown in Chapter 6. However, with anomalies and the inclusion of pathology, the neat anatomical innervation fields illustrated by textbooks are not often seen. The clarity of the field of sensation loss could be impaired if the area is affected by pain from another site.

4. Weakness as a complaint does arise and it can do so for a number of reasons. There could be paralysis of movement when efferent impulses are impaired. There could also be a pain-inhibited weakness. In this, muscle disuse may occur, or at a cortical level the patient refuses to allow a desired movement because of the knowledge that the movement will hurt.

5. Symptoms may be worse at night. This is a well known symptom of peripheral entrapment syndromes (Dawson et al 1983) and could be related to the lower blood pressure experienced at night, perhaps in combination with certain postures. For example, sleeping on a protracted shoulder girdle could tension the suprascapular nerve,

or the wrist flexion postures adopted by some people during sleep could worsen carpal tunnel syndrome symptoms by increasing the pressure inside the carpal tunnel. Patients who are tucked tightly into bed with sheets holding their feet in plantar flexion and inversion could be risking injury to the peroneal nerves. Another consideration is that the neuraxis and meninges lie on the downside of the spinal canal during sidelying. In some situations, the movement might be symptomatic — perhaps irritated dura lying on an osteophyte, for example.

6. Symptoms may be worse at the end of the day. This is a common feature of chronic nerve root irritation. It may be related to muscle weakness, sustained posture throughout the day or simply overuse.

Thomas (1982) has provided a summary of symptomatology expected and noticed in various neuropathies involving disease processes.

HISTORY

The history of the mechanisms of injury, previous injuries, previous treatment, other contributing factors and the state of the disorder since the original injury provides useful information. Sometimes it may direct the examiner to the likelihood of a nervous system source of symptoms.

Previous history and predisposing factors

I feel that the nervous system never 'forgets' an injury. Many patients seen with adverse tension syndromes give a history which involves a known nervous system injuring situation. This may be many years before. Commonly, a car accident or velocity accident (such as a fall from a horse or out of a tree) is reported. It is proposed that this may lead to increased tension in the nervous system and thus allow the development of symptoms earlier than in a less tensioned individual. Some patients are engaged in occupations such as keyboard operation or playing a musical instrument such as a violin which involve some repetitious movements while other body parts are held static. Once the nervous system tension is increased in one area, there is potential for injury elsewhere along the system. This issue has been discussed in Chapter 3.

Chronicity of symptoms

It seems a feature of adverse tension syndromes is the chronicity of the disorders. There are a number of reasons for this. Firstly, if the nervous system is injured, especially if injury reactions have penetrated deep within the nerve or is inside the dural theca, there is potential for irreversibility. Secondly, I feel that altered nerve mechanics and physiology are not picked up early enough to address them adequately. In many cases, by the time the patient presents to a physiotherapist, a significant component of this disorder could be irreversible and surgery the only option. Carpal tunnel syndrome is an outstanding example here. Thirdly, most practitioners approach a neuro-orthopaedic problem via one structure (usually the joint tissue). Such an approach may not be getting at all the structures involved. Often patients will give a history of many kinds of treatment such as electrotherapy, chiropractic, and joint mobilisation, with partial or no relief. Simply, in many of these cases the nervous system has not been adequately addressed.

POSTURAL AND MOVEMENT PATTERNS

Patterns of movement and associated symptom reproduction from tension testing are described in Chapters 7 and 8.

Postural patterns

When a person loses the normal mechanics of the nervous system, certain dynamic and static postural patterns emerge to allow that patient to best cope with the neural movement loss.

An antalgic nervous system posture is evident. An extreme example can be seen such as in Figure 4.3. Here, all possible movements are combined to get pressure off the nervous system. This patient's history is from my case notes. Briefly, she fell backwards, with her lumbar

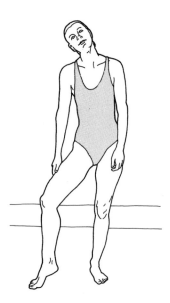

Fig. 4.3 An antalgic tension posture. Note the foot in neutral and towards plantar flexion, knee flexion, hip flexion, abduction and lateral rotation and the cervical spine laterally flexed towards the side of pain

spine over a 6 inch pipe. At the time she was holding a 15 kg weight in her arms. On examination, there were no neurological signs of altered conduction. In her most painfree position, as seen in the figure, her foot was in neutral towards plantar flexion, her knee was flexed, her hip was abducted and laterally rotated, and her spine, including the cervical spine, was laterally flexed towards the painful side. If I dorsiflexed her foot a little, she immediately laterally flexed her neck further. All positions are anti-tension. This is an extreme example. Another example of an antalgic nervous system posture is the patient who holds his/her arm above his/her head to avoid tension on the middle cervical nerve roots.

The subtle postural variations are more common. This may be a raised shoulder girdle, or a hip held in some lateral rotation. Lower limb postures can be nicely checked as the patient walks. The 'poked chin' posture could be in part antalgic to the nervous system, since in this position, the upper cervical spine is extended thus taking tension away and perhaps allowing some relief of symptoms (Fig. 4.4). I have also encountered a posture where, in

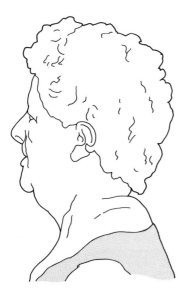

Fig. 4.4 The fixed forward head posture

Movement patterns

1. Symptoms are usually worse with known tension increasing manoeuvres, e.g., reading long sitting in bed (Straight Leg Raise position), getting into a car (Slump and Straight Leg Raise position), reaching up to a clothes-line (shoulder abduction and elbow extension), shoulder girdle depression. Nordin et al (1984) reported paraesthesias worsening on movement in five patients. This increase was associated with abnormal ectopic impulses measured by microelectrodes in skin nerve fascicles. The five cases were:

- When Tinel's sign was elicited in a patient with entrapment of the ulnar nerve at the elbow.
- When paraesthesia was provoked by elevation of the arm in a patient with symptoms consistent with a thoracic outlet syndrome.
- Passive Neck Flexion manoeuvres in a patient with an S1 syndrome due to a herniated lumbar disc.
- During a Straight Leg Raise in a patient with an S1 syndrome due to root fibrosis.
- When Lhermitte's sign (Ch. 5) was elicited in a patient with multiple sclerosis.

All five examples are involved with tension increasing manoeuvres.

2. Symptoms can usually be eased by 'out of tension positions'. Just as certain combinations of movement place tension on the nervous system, so too combinations of movement exist, such as those discussed in the section on posture, that are antalgic. There are some exceptions however. Some forms of chronic nervous system pain with spontaneous impulse generation may not ease. There is also a group of patients who get pain on easing of a tension manoeuvre, for example, on release of a Straight Leg Raise. It is my interpretation that this pain is caused by an abnormality in the normal nerve/interface relationship, but only manifests when the movement is one way (Fig. 4.5). In this situation the structure around the nervous system will probably need treating.

sitting, the patient leans back with elbow straight and wrist flexed, shoulder externally rotated with the weight of the body forcing some elevation of the shoulder girdle. The common physical sign in these patients is an abnormal neural tension in the thoracic region with apparent sympathetic epiphenomena. Scoliosis could also be an antalgic nervous system posture (Boyling 1988). In patients with thoracic adverse tension involvement, a flat, even lordotic, thoracic spine can be evident.

Another postural consideration is the effect of certain forced postures on the nervous system, where some gross deformation of the interfacing structures inevitably has an effect on the nervous system. For example, Breig (1978) outlined the mechanisms where stretch and anterior displacement of the neuraxis and meninges from a thoracic kyphosis can cause adverse tension. According to Breig (1978) scoliosis alone rarely generates neurological manifestations.

Early morning stiffness seems to be an associated symptom with altered nervous system mechanics. There are some patients who, on waking in the morning and taking their first few steps, require some time before they can get their heel to the floor. Tension tests that include the foot, are often positive in this kind of patient.

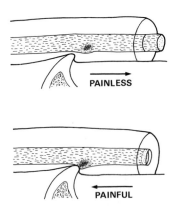

Fig. 4.5 A hypothetical situation where a segment of scarred epineurium will only be symptomatic when the nerve moves in one direction against a pathological interface

3. A common movement pattern associated with symptoms is that of small repetitive movements, or what I feel is an overuse of a small part of the nervous system's range of movement. Some examples related to occupation are the use of a keyboard, playing a musical instrument or a particular repetitive action used in sport. In these situations there seems to be a particular nerve/interface relationship that may be symptom provocative. It is common for these patients to report that perhaps half an hour on a keyboard or playing an instrument is enough to reproduce symptoms. Yet, they can accomplish movements where the nervous system is taken through a greater range and variety of movement such as a different sport or even an apparently vigorous activity. I refer to this situation as 'activity specific mechanosensitivity'.

4. The movement patterns could be dominated by the pathology at the mechanical interface. A bulging disc, for example, could further narrow the spinal canal during spinal flexion. A cervical zygapophyseal joint could close down on rotation or lateral flexion to the same side, or the cubital tunnel cross-sectional area may become smaller on flexion of the elbow.

In these matters the role of a static resisted contraction is raised. A muscle contraction could squeeze an irritated nerve and produce symptoms from that nerve. This mechanism may inhibit an effective contraction of the muscle.

Some areas of the body have a more important relationship with the nervous system than elsewhere, for example, the superior tibio-fibula joint, the L4, T6 and C6 areas, the first rib, the radiohumeral joint, the transverse carpal ligament, the scalenes and the supinator muscle. These are all vulnerable areas for the nervous system.

5. If a combined movements model is followed, such as that described by Edwards (1987, 1988), irregular patterns of movements provoking symptoms may indicate involvement of structures other than the joint. The movements may be 'out of pattern' for a coupled movement. For example, if cervical rotation produced cervical pain, it would be expected that lateral flexion to the same side would give a similar response. If not, there may be other structures involved. Muscles and nerves come immediately to mind.

6. Maitland (1986) places great store on the examination of spinal intervertebral movements by passive accessory intervertebral movement (PAIVM). These allow an interpretation of resistance through range and its association with symptoms. I also place great importance on this part of examination. However, I feel that the tissue resistance encountered during these examination techniques can give some indication of the structures involved. A joint feel has resistance usually associated with symptoms and this can change as it is mobilised. When other structures are involved in the disorder and have effect on the joint movement, the palpation feel is 'rubbery', there is a through range stiffness and it will not change with mobilisation. Readers may need some appreciation of the palpation skills required by the Maitland concept to make greater use of these ideas.

7. Palpation. When the nervous system is injured or sensitised, it may be abnormally responsive to palpation. This is an important skill. Uses and analysis of the findings from nervous system palpation are discussed in Chapter 9.

REFERENCES

Asbury A K, Fields H L 1984 Pain due to peripheral nerve damage: an hypothesis. Neurology (Cleveland) 34: 1587–1590

Bogduk N 1983 The innervation of the lumbar spine. Spine 8: 286–293

Bogduk N 1989 The anatomy of headache. In: Dalton M (ed) Proceedings of headache and face pain symposium, Manipulative Physiotherapists Association of Australia, Brisbane

Boyling J 1988 Idiopathic scoliosis: a study of mobility, muscle length and neural tissue tension. In: Proceedings, International Federation of Orthopaedic Manipulative Therapists Congress, Cambridge

Breig A 1978 Adverse mechanical tension in the central nervous system. Almqvist & Wiksell, Stockholm

Calvin W H, Devor M, Howe J F 1982 Can neuralgias arise from minor demyelination? Spontaneous firing, mechanosensitivity and afterdischarge from conducting axons. Experimental Neurology 75: 755–763

Dawson D M, Hallett M, Millender L H 1983 Entrapment neuropathies. Little, Brown, Boston

Cuatico W, Parker J C, Pappert E et al 1988 An anatomical and clinical investigation of spinal meningeal nerves. Acta Neurochirurgica 90: 139–143

Cyriax J 1942 Perineuritis. British Medical Journal 570–580

Cyriax J 1982 Textbook of Orthopaedic Medicine, 8th edn. Baillierre Tindall, London, vol 1

Devor M 1985 The pathophysiology and anatomy of damaged nerve. In: Wall P D, Melzack R (eds) Textbook of pain. Churchill Livingstone, Edinburgh

Edgar M A, Nundy S 1966 Innervation of the spinal dura mater. Journal of Neurology, Neurosurgery and Psychiatry 29: 530–534

Edgar M A, Park W M 1974 Induced pain patterns on passive straight leg raising in lower lumbar disc protrusion. Journal of Bone and Joint Surgery 56B: 658–667

Edwards B E 1987 Clinical assessment: the use of combined movements in assessment and treatment. In: Twomey L T & Taylor J R (eds) Clinics in physical therapy, Vol 13, Physical therapy of the low back. Churchill Livingstone, New York

Edwards B E 1988 Combined movement of the cervical spine in examination and treatment. In: Grant R (ed) Clinics in physical therapy, Vol 17, Physical therapy of the cervical and thoracic spine. Churchill Livingstone, New York

El Mahdi M A, Latif F Y A, Janko M 1981 The spinal nerve root innervation, and a new concept of the clinicopathological interrelations in back pain and sciatica. Neurochirurgia 24: 137–141

Elvey R L, Quintner J L, Thomas A N 1986 A clinical study of RSI. Australian Family Physician 15: 1314–1319

Granit R, Skoglund C R 1945 Facilitation, inhibition and depression at the artificial synapse formed by the cut end of a mammalian nerve. Journal of Physiology 103: 435–448

Howe J F, Calvin W H, Loeser J D 1976 Impulses reflected from dorsal root ganglia and from focal nerve injuries. Brain Research 116: 139–144

Howe J F, Loeser J D, Calvin W H 1977 Mechanosensitivity of dorsal root ganglia and chronically

injured axons: a physiological basis for the radicular pain of nerve root compression. Pain 3: 25–41

Janda V 1978 Muscles, central nervous regulation and back problems. In: Korr I M (ed) Neurobiologic mechanisms in manipulative therapy. Plenum, New York.

Janda V 1986 Muscle weakness and inhibition (pseudoparesis) in low back pain syndromes. In: Grieve G P (ed) Modern manual therapy of the vertebral column. Churchill Livingstone, Edinburgh

Kopell H P, Thompson W A L 1963 Peripheral entrapment neuropathies. Williams & Wilkins, Baltimore

Kornberg C, Lew P 1989 The effect of stretching neural structures on grade I hamstring injuries. The Journal of Orthopaedic and Sports Physical Therapy. June: 481–487

Lansche W E, Ford L T 1960 Correlation of the myelogram with the clinical and operative findings in lumbar disc lesions. Journal of Bone and Joint Surgery 42A: 193–206

Loeser J D 1985 Pain due to nerve injury. Spine 10: 232–235

Mackinnon S E, Dellon A L 1988 Surgery of the peripheral nerve. Thieme, New York

Macnab I 1972 The mechanism of spondylogenic pain. In: Hirsch C, Zotterman Y (eds) Cervical pain. Pergamon, Oxford

Maitland G D 1986 Vertebral Manipulation, 5th edn. Butterworths, London

Maitland G D 1990 Peripheral manipulation, 3rd edn. Butterworths, London (in press)

Meglio C, Cioni B, Del Lago A et al 1981 Pain control and improvement of peripheral blood flow following spinal cord stimulation. Journal of Neurosurgery 54: 821–823

Melzack R, Wall P D 1965 Pain mechanisms: a new theory. Science 150: 971–978

Murphy R W 1977 Nerve roots and spinal nerves in degenerative disc disease. Clinical Orthopaedics and Related Research 129: 46–60

Noordenbos W 1959 Pain. Elsevier, Amsterdam

Nordin M, Nystrom B, Wallin U et al K 1984 Ectopic sensory discharges and paresthesiae in patients with disorders of peripheral nerves, dorsal roots and dorsal columns. Pain 20: 231–245

Ochoa J, Torebjork H W 1981 Paraesthesiae from ectopic impulse generation in human sensory nerves. Brain 103: 835–853

Pratt N E 1986 Neurovascular entrapments in the regions of the shoulder and posterior triangle of the neck. Physical Therapy 66: 1894–1900

Quintner J L 1989 A study of upper limb pain and paraesthesiae following neck injury in motor vehicle accidents: assessment of the brachial plexus tension test of Elvey. British Journal of Rheumatology 28: 528–533

Saplys R, Mackinnon S E, Dellon A L 1987 The relationship between nerve entrapment versus neuroma complications and the misdiagnosis of de Quervain's disease. Contemporary Orthopaedics 15: 51–57

Smith K J, McDonald 1980 Spontaneous and mechanically evoked activity due to central demyelinating lesion. Nature 286: 154–155

Smyth M J, Wright V 1958 Sciatica and the intervertebral disc: an experimental study. The Journal of Bone and Joint Surgery 40A: 1401–1418

Sunderland S 1978 Nerves and nerve injuries. Churchill Livingstone, Edinburgh

Sweeney J E, Harms A D 1990 Hand hypersensitivity and the upper limb tension test: another angle. Pain (Suppl) 5, S466

Sweet W H 1988 Deafferentation pain in man. Applied Neurophysiology 51: 117–127

Thomas P K 1982 Pain in peripheral neuropathy : clinical and morphological aspects. In: Culp W J, Ochoa J (eds) Abnormal nerves and muscles as impulse generators. Oxford University Press

Torg J S, Pavlov H, Genuario S E et al 1986 Neuropraxia of the cervical spinal cord with transient quadriplegia. The Journal of Bone and Joint Surgery 68A: 1354–1370

Wall P D., Gutnik M 1974 Properties of afferent nerve impulses originating from a neuroma. Nature 248: 740–743

Wall P D, Melzack R 1985 Textbook of pain. Churchill Livingstone, Edinburgh

Wolff C J 1987 Physiological, inflammatory and neuropathic pain. Advances in Technical Standards in Neurosurgery 15: 39–62

PART II

Examination

5. Clinical reasoning

Mark Jones and David Butler

INTRODUCTION

Too often attention is given only to examination and treatment techniques without the reasoning behind them. Exactly where techniques fit in, when to vary the routine and how to use the information gained are frequently neglected. Physiotherapists are taught a routine examination as students, and experience and further training should develop this further. A routine examination collecting information without 'reasoning' is inadequate. While it may suffice to solve a simple patient problem, it will be ineffective when the physiotherapist is confronted with a complex one.

The various approaches to patient examination and treatment taught around the world appear to be seeking different information from patients. Yet they all reach a decision on what and how to treat. How should that decision be reached? Are the approaches really that different?

What should guide a physiotherapist's questions? Are there standard questions asked of all patients, or should questions vary depending on the individual patient's history and presentation? How far should a line of questioning be pursued? Should standard techniques be used to examine every shoulder or low back, for example? How many examination techniques should be used? What should be done with all the information obtained, and what if it does not make sense?

The thinking process or clinical reasoning behind patient examination and management is the key combined with a knowledge of clinical patterns. Understanding clinical reasoning will improve one's own thinking through patients' problems and broaden the repertoire of clinical patterns one recognises.

All clinicians approach their patients with the same aim: to solve the patient's problem whether it be pain, stiffness, weakness, etc. or some functional complaint with combinations of all these things. We, as physiotherapists, have at our disposal, a multitude of treatment options including advice, passive and active movement, exercise, supports, therapeutic modalities and referral to other disciplines for medical, surgical or psychological consultation. To achieve the aim of solving the patient's problem efficiently and safely, physiotherapists must acquire information regarding the following basic issues:

- What is the source of the symptoms and/or dysfunction?
- Are there contributing factors?
- What are the precautions and contraindications to physical examination and treatment?
- What is the prognosis?
- What treatment should be selected and what progression is likely?

Information regarding these basic issues should be sought with all patients regardless of their presenting complaint. Most questions and examination techniques of the various manual therapy approaches around the world can be linked to one or more of these issues. The information enabling appropriate hypotheses to be made about these basic issues is obtained and tested during the subjective and physical examination as well as the ongoing treatment. It is gained from scanning different aspects of the patient's presentation. Examples include site and behaviour of symptoms, general health, investigations, medications, history, posture, behaviour of symptoms and quality of movement during active and passive physiological, and passive accessory, movements, and muscle integrity including quality of contraction, length, strength, and endurance.

Obtaining information on these aspects of the patient's presentation above may be considered 'routine'. However, the depth and detail of examination should be tailored to each individual patient.

This chapter does not attempt to cover all the questions or physical tests that could or should be considered when examining a patient. Rather, it emphasises the importance of clinical reasoning throughout examination and ongoing treatment. A discussion follows of various inquiry and advanced examination strategies which assist in understanding a patient's problem and enable one to arrive at the most effective treatment. Lastly, precautions and contraindications to examination and treatment of the nervous system are presented.

THE CLINICAL REASONING PROCESS

Clinical reasoning can be defined as the application of relevant knowledge (facts, procedures, concepts and principles) and clinical skills to the evaluation, diagnosis and management of a patient problem. The clinical reasoning process describes the steps taken by a clinician to reach a diagnostic and management decision.

Extensive research has been carried out in medicine and other fields to describe the clinical reasoning process of experts and novices (Chi et al 1981, Chi et al 1988, Muzzin et al 1983, Feltovich et al 1984, Patel et al 1986, Barrows & Feltovich 1987). One line of research, where clinicians' thoughts (e.g., perceptions, interpretations, plans) were analysed retrospectively as they thought aloud, through a video or audio playback of a patient examination just completed, or concurrently as they read a patient's unfolding clinical history, has lead to a better understanding of our clinical reasoning process and what differentiates levels of expertise. This process is illustrated in Figure 5.1 adapted from Barrows & Tamblyn (1980).

The process begins with the physiotherapist's perception and interpretation of initial cues from the patient. Even in the opening moments of greeting a patient, the physiotherapist perceives specific cues, such as a movement pattern, facial expression or resting posture, which are recognised and interpreted. For example, a patient complaining of 'shoulder pain' with guarded upper limb movement and a grimace, while removing his jacket in such a way so as to take the uninvolved arm out first, and then the involved arm, to avoid any shoulder elevation or elbow extension, should elicit a number of different hypotheses. In this example there will be hypotheses regarding potential sources of the pain and guarded movement, its severity, the degree of limitation in movement, and even an initial clue as to prognosis. Does the guarded movement fit a low cervical nerve root lesion which is made less painful by that position, or is the patient avoiding shoulder elevation and perhaps rotation to protect a local shoulder structure? Perhaps the elbow is held flexed as it too is involved, or maybe it is as a means of decreasing stress on either the two joint muscles of the upper limb, or on neural and surrounding tissues. These conjectures represent only a sample of the possibilities here.

Hypotheses regarding sources must be kept very broad at this early stage. In this example, they would include any structure(s) within the upper quadrant capable of producing such symptoms and signs. The indication that the symptoms are severe (at least with regards to that movement) represents one important factor affecting the physiotherapist's hypothesis of precautions to physical examination and treatment. This, as with all initial clues, will need to be tested and pursued with other important factors in the subjective examination before the hypothesis is acted on. Both the apparent severity and degree of limitation also represent potential negative indicators of prognosis. To state the prognosis for resolving a patient's problem as 'good' or 'bad' is too simplified. While one

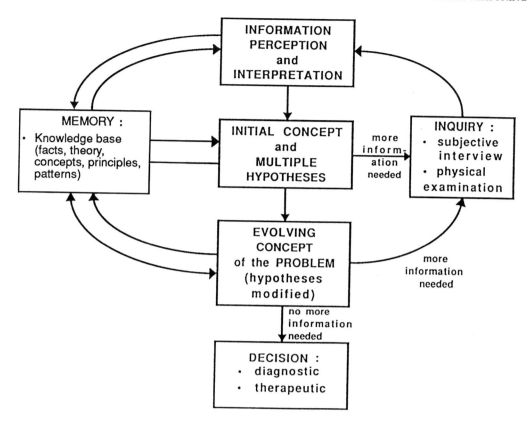

Fig. 5.1 The clinical reasoning process in physiotherapy (adapted from Barrows & Tamblyn 1980)

may come to that decision, it is only after consideration of both positive and negative factors, which will often be weighted sufficiently one way or the other to make a firm decision that the problem will or will not be helped by your treatment, and give some indication of the length of treatment required. Clinical reasoning in formulating a prognosis is discussed in Chapter 10.

When 'shoulder pain' in the example is clarified and localised to a line of pain extending from just below the anterior acromion to approximately mid biceps, and, importantly, other areas carefully cleared as having no symptoms, the initial hypotheses as to potential sources of the symptoms can be made more specific (e.g., long head of biceps, subacromial structures, glenohumeral periarticular structures, C5/6 somatic referred, neural and surrounding tissues). Obviously, the physiotherapist has insufficient information at this stage to reach a diagnostic

or management decision. Thus further information is sought through ongoing inquiry (both subjective and physical examination).

The important point is that the inquiry is not simply a routine set of questions and physical tests. Certain aspects of the patient's presentation may be scanned with all patients as suggested earlier (e.g., site, behaviour and history of symptoms, active, passive and resistive tests, etc.). However, the search for details at any time should be related to the issues listed above.

Hypotheses are formed even within the opening moments of a patient examination as seen in the above example. As the examination continues, hypotheses are refined, reranked, ruled out and new ones added. Thus, the physiotherapist should have an evolving understanding of the patient's problem. A good test of whether one is actively reasoning through an examination, or simply collecting information is to stop at any point and summarise one's impression thus far. The student who is concentrating on not omitting any parts of a newly learned examination technique will tend to recite specific details as expressed by the patient. In contrast, the experienced physiotherapist will be able to interpret information while it is being obtained and organise this information into the different appropriate hypotheses. In the above example, after learning that the patient's 'shoulder pain' is constant and that, if not careful with even the single activity of taking his jacket off, it can be made much worse, taking ¾ hour to settle, a summary of the experienced physiotherapist's thinking may simply be:

This disorder is definitely severe and irritable with a likely inflammatory presentation, I'll need to be very careful in my handling and probably limit my physical examination. Cervical, local shoulder and neural tissues are all implicated by that area and movement but he doesn't have any subjective indications of nerve root involvement. I should get a better idea of the source of symptoms with further questioning of what aggravates and eases his pain.

Further questioning would seek out, in part, which movements and/or positions specifically aggravated and eased the shoulder pain. Were these movements spinal, shoulder, elbow or even wrist, or combinations of any? Which directions were most troublesome? This information should be interpreted with regard to the ongoing hypothesis development. For example, if this patient, when asked whether there was anything he could do to ease the symptoms, said that the only way he could get relief was to put his arm up behind his head, it would lend support to neural involvement and weaken the hypothesis of local upper limb joints as the principal source. The key words here are 'support' and 'weaken'. Subjective information such as this provides valuable clues, however the clues must add up, and this information must fit with other clues obtained through the subjective examination.

The process of inquiry continues with new information constantly being interpreted for its correlation with information previously obtained and with hypotheses under consideration. When information does not fit, clarification is required and the line of questioning should be pursued further. The subjective examination stops when the clinician has gained sufficient information to determine what structures require physical examination and how far this examination can be taken to obtain the most useful information while ensuring the disorder is not worsened. The hypotheses are then subjected to specific testing through the physical examination, culminating in a decision on diagnosis and treatment. The effect of the treatment itself then provides additional confirmation. An effective treatment in itself does not ensure effective clinical reasoning, but effective clinical reasoning will ensure the most effective treatment is identified. In this way, potential sources have been logically and systematically eliminated or incriminated and treatment options explored.

Why is such attention to clinical reasoning so important? You may be thinking that you have never thought in this way, or stopped to consider how you actually do think through a patient's problem. Your own routine may have served you well so far. However, following a routine examination and fixed treatment prescriptions will never allow the recognition of new patterns. On the other hand, reasoning through a patient's problem, as described here, allows the physiotherapist to be constantly testing patterns previously learned and in turn to recognise the existence of other patterns. This requires attention, not only to those features that fit a previously recognised pattern, but also to those that are absent. For example, some clinicians are quick to label a disorder as discogenic if the patient complains of central low back pain and difficulty sitting. But variations of that pattern are common, and these two features may be present in other non-discogenic disorders. Medical research into errors of reasoning has shown that failure to attend to features which are missing and overemphasis on features which support the clinician's 'favorite hypothesis' are the most common errors made (Elstein et al 1978, Barrows & Tamblyn 1980). This probably occurs similarly with physiotherapists, where clinicians lock into a diagnosis based on a few recognised features too early, taking little notice of features missing from the pattern, or of features that are present but do not fit. In the above example central low back pain which is immediately made worse with sitting, it would not fit the hypothesis of disc involvement alone if, on examination of lumbar flexion, the patient had full pain free movement. A rigid thinking style will limit one's effectiveness with the more complex patient presentations and hinder the opportunity to broaden one's repertoire of clinical patterns recognised.

The clinical patterns of interest include those associated with various syndromes or particular structures (eg., impingement or intraneural tension respectively). Other sorts of patterns also exist and should be understood. These include inflammatory, mechanical, irritability, stability, postural, and biomechanical patterns.

CHARACTERISTICS OF EXPERTISE

There has been considerable research conducted in medicine and other fields investigating differences between experts and novices. Early expert/novice studies were conducted in chess comparing the thought processes and representation of knowledge of chess masters to that of novices (DeGroot 1965, Chase & Simon 1973). Short term memory experiments revealed that experts have a remarkable ability to reconstruct a chess position almost perfectly after viewing it for only seconds. In contrast, there was a dramatic drop off of this ability below the master level. No differences were found between the expert and novice with the same experiment using randomly placed chess pieces, precluding the results being attributed to superior memory. With experts and novices constrained by the same short term memory, the authors concluded that experts have a superior ability to perceive patterns in chess positions and encode these as chunks in their memory.

The DeGroot (1965) and Chase & Simon (1973) studies have since been replicated in medicine with similar findings as to experts' and novices' representation of knowledge (Muzzin et al 1983, Patel & Frederiksen 1984, Patel et al 1986). Patel et al (1986) showed that expert clinicians recalled more information in patterns and made significantly more inferences about the clinically relevant information, while novices made more verbatim recall of the surface features and remembered more details that were irrelevant. These authors proposed that expert clinicians have a more highly developed knowledge base that includes a store of patterns that can be recognised. Thus, patient cues are interpreted and collated through an inductive process until a pattern is recognised. This pattern is then tested through a deductive process and the original hypotheses are modified accordingly.

The effectiveness of physiotherapists' clinical reasoning is, in part, dependent on the organisation of their knowledge base. Less experienced physiotherapists would have less developed and fewer variations of patterns stored in their memory causing them difficulty in selecting relevant and discarding irrelevant information. The inexperience of the novice leaves him/her with only those patterns which have been learned through texts. Thus, the patterns recognised by the novice are excessively rigid and the inability to recognise relevant information causes them to either close a line of questioning too soon or indiscriminately act on every detail. Hypotheses are accepted prematurely and the opportunity for learning is hindered. With a less developed knowledge base, the novice's clinical reasoning is more demanding cognitively and inefficient.

The organisation of knowledge relevant to physiotherapy includes the facts (e.g., anatomy, pathology, etc.), procedures (eg., examination and treatment techniques), concepts (e.g., irritability, adverse neural tension) and patterns of presentation. It is utilised with the assistance of rules or principles (e.g., selection of grade of passive movement technique) to acquire, interpret, infer, and collate information. This is likely to allow the expert physiotherapist to solve a typical problem almost automatically through recognition of clinical patterns. However, when faced with an atypical problem, the expert, like the novice, must rely more on the hypothetico-deductive method of reasoning (i.e., hypotheses testing) to solve it.

It should be apparent that solution of a patient's problem is not derived from simple application of a clinical reasoning process, nor a vast knowledge of facts. Rather, it is dependent on the physiotherapist's organisation of knowledge as it relates to that problem. This includes the facts, procedures, concepts, patterns of presentation, and principles or rules. Therefore, we as physiotherapists, in order to improve our clinical reasoning, should attempt to improve our organisation of knowledge. As was depicted in the clinical reasoning process diagram (Fig. 5.1), this organisation of knowledge contained in our memory will influence all aspects of our reasoning from our initial perceptions to our diagnostic and treatment decisions. The double arrows highlight a crucial feature in this relationship between knowledge and the process. That is, experience in years alone will not ensure one's organisation of knowledge will grow. It requires experience using a clinical reasoning process that is founded in the logic of hypothesis testing while encouraging open-mindedness and lateral thinking. Our challenge should be to identify the patterns we recognise and continually test these patterns to substantiate their existence. When clinical incongruities occur, further inquiry is indicated to understand better any discrepancies that may exist. In this way we can continually test our present understanding of different patterns and acquire new ones. Expertise in physiotherapy comes, not only from years of experience or superior handling skills, but from highly developed knowledge bases acquired through advanced clinical reasoning where critical thinking, as advocated here, has allowed the acquisition of a more comprehensive repertoire of clinical patterns.

This book is an attempt to broaden your recognition of clinical patterns. It should challenge some of your previously recognised patterns and encourage the discovery of new ones. The information put forward in this book will be most useful if used with a clinical reasoning process that is both logical and open-minded.

ANALYSING STRUCTURES AND CONTRIBUTING FACTORS

Adopting a hypothesis testing approach to your clinical reasoning will enhance your ability to solve the patient's problem and expand your own clinical knowledge. While it is suggested that this clinical reasoning approach should be used by all manual therapists regardless of their different training around the world, differences will exist with regards to the hypotheses physiotherapists are prepared to consider. If we consider the 'source of the symptoms', the potential sources should include any structure under the area of symptoms and any structure capable of referring to that area of symptoms. Thus, a patient's complaint of lateral elbow pain could be emanating from local structures under the area of pain such as the radiohumeral joint or from remote structures capable of referring to the lateral aspect of the elbow such as the C5/6 zygapophyseal joint. With 'contributing factors', one would have to consider any structural, biomechanical, environmental or behavioural predisposing factors. The following discussion will focus on the structures which the physiotherapist must consider and be prepared to examine. In the example of lateral elbow pain, remote structures such as the scalenei muscles become relevant when one considers their relationship to the lower trunks of the brachial plexus. Entrapment or irritation, particularly of the middle and lower nerve trunks as they travel through the scaleni, could be a contributing factor to lateral elbow pain. This might occur through the development of local common extensor muscle facilitation, the direct referral of neurogenic pain or through a process such as the 'double crush' (Ch. 3). With this in mind, it is easy to appreciate how alteration of any structure sufficient to alter the stresses and demands placed on local elbow structures (e.g., stiff wrist creating excessive extensor muscle activity), or capable of affecting neural and surrounding tissues (e.g., tight pectoralis minor or carpal tunnel syndrome affecting nerve mechanics) can contribute, if not directly cause a separate area of symptoms as in this case of lateral elbow pain.

The potential complexity of structure involvement is evident when one considers the close proximity of multiple structures about the lateral elbow. The radial nerve lies anterior, often attached to the radiohumeral joint and inferior and medial to the common extensor muscles.

Thus injury to any of these structures can result in inflammatory changes sufficient to involve neighbouring structures including the radial nerve. Concurrent involvement could also exist with the C5/6 zygapophyseal joint referring pain to the lateral elbow. Additionally, if by being pathologically adhered to an emerging spinal nerve, this too can contribute to altered neural tension at the elbow. See Table 5.1 for an example of the sources of symptoms and contributing factors to lateral elbow pain. Sources are differentiated into local and remote.

The pathological and biomechanical mechanisms involved in nervous system injury are presented in Chapters 2 and 3. This provides an additional basis on which the patient's subjective and physical presentation can be considered and hypotheses formulated. The patient with widespread areas of symptoms associated with lateral elbow pain, for example, cervical and thoracic pain and perhaps lateral elbow pain in the other arm, will have a far longer list of possible sources and contributing factors to be considered. It will take the physiotherapist longer to examine (both subjectively and through physical testing) all possible structures/components and determine their involvement. Remember, from Chapter 3, injury at a local site has the potential to set up secondary injury sites, be they at a vulnerable point or possibly at the site of an old injury. How far to examine can be a dilemma. How often do lumbar laminectomy patients present with tennis elbows?

If there are symptoms elsewhere, anywhere in the body including the legs, then they require examination and perhaps treatment to test their potential contribution. Some neurosurgeons operating on nerve entrapments emphasise that, if there is a dual lesion ('double crush') present, then treatment will need to be directed at both sites (Massey et al 1981, Mackinnon & Dellon 1988). The initial statement in this text that the nervous system is continuous mechanically, electrically and chemically throughout the body cannot be forgotten. Consideration of all potential sources (both local and remote) and contributing factors will assist one's reasoning, especially in those more complex patient presentations with widespread areas of symptoms as can occur in a whiplash syndrome. The idea of remote and local structures linked in part by the nervous system and including contributing factors, provides a logical and testable mechanism to what was, perhaps, previously considered an illogical presentation of symptoms.

As stated previously, clues to potential sources and contributing factors will emerge through the subjective examination and these hypotheses are then tested in the physical examination. In considering potential intra- and extra-neural structures, it is useful to 'think along the trunks and tracts' of the nervous system. This is not only to seek familiar referral sites but also those sites that can mechanically compromise the nervous system, such as the previous example of the scalenei. The clinician will require skills

Table 5.1 Possible neuro-orthopaedic sources and contributing factors relating to lateral elbow pain

	Local	Remote	Contributing Factors
Muscle	Common extensor origin, tendons		e.g., scalenei, pectorals wrist flexors
Joint	Radio-humeral Superior radio-ulnar Annular ligament	Cervical disc Zygapophyseal joint (especially 5, 6)	Wrist joint Shoulder girdle joints
Nerve	Radial nerve and branches Musculocutaneous nerve	Nerve root Dura mater Dural sleeves Neuraxis Brain	Entrapment elsewhere (double crush) Sympathetic epiphenomena Cortical interpretations
Other	Fascia Blood vessels Bone (periosteum, radial head)		

to analyse whether the potential sources and contributing factors are relevant. There must be clear physical signs that can be retested after a treatment. A potential source is supported only when specific testing reveals abnormalities such as soft tissue changes and/or positive joint, muscle or neural tests locally at the site of symptoms or at a remote structure capable of referring such symptoms. Similarly, a potential contributing factor must reveal some abnormality such as muscle dysfunction (e.g., tightness or imbalance) or joint stiffness. The hypothesis for a structure's involvement is supported when physical examination reveals a relevant abnormality. The hypothesis is only truly accepted, however, once treatment has altered the structure in question and the patient's signs and symptoms have improved. Thus, if specific scalenei stretches result in improved lateral elbow signs and symptoms, then the hypothesis of scalenei as a contributing factor is accepted. It is essential at this point of one's reasoning not to interpret improvement as absolute confirmation of the hypothesis. To do this would be to inhibit further development of one's repertoire of clinical patterns. It may be that the scalenei were, in fact, not the contributing factor and concurrently our scalenei stretches mobilised a previously undetected stiff C5/6 zygapophyseal joint. We need to remain open-minded and critical with continual hypothesis testing to ensure the expansion and refinement of clinical patterns we recognise.

INQUIRY STRATEGIES

While use of an hypothesis-testing clinical reasoning process encourages critical and open-minded thinking, the quality/usefulness of the information we obtain from our patients is largely a function of our ability to extract that information — our 'inquiry strategies'. The term 'maximising principles' has been coined in the medical education literature to describe the inquiry strategies used by expert clinicians to elicit the most useful information in the most efficient way in order to narrow down the possibilities that must be considered (Kleinmuntz 1968, Barrows & Tamblyn 1980). Inquiry strategies that maximise the quality of information obtained are similarly available to physiotherapists (Maitland 1986, Grant et al 1988). Maitland has contributed enormously to the development and refinement of these inquiry strategies, and their use will provide the optimal information to which the clinical reasoning process can be applied.

Communication

The patient is the most valuable source of information and our ability to extract that information will determine our depth of understanding and, subsequently, our ability to manage the patient's problem. However, the patient will not know what is, and is not, important and cannot be expected to know what we do, and do not, need to know. This is important as we need to be skilled in helping patients through the accounts of their problems and virtually teach patients how to listen to their own bodies and inform us of the relevant information. We can achieve this through a combination of open and directed questions, active listening and selective encouragement as to what information is most useful to us. Establishing rapport with the patient is essential to obtaining this information, and will be built on a developing patient-therapist relationship of interest and belief. That is, we need to communicate to patients our interest and belief in what they tell us. Often a patient's account of his/her problem that seems implausible is more a reflection of our own limited knowledge and repertoire of clinical patterns recognised. Sunderland (1978) puts it succinctly when he says 'the patient will always have one witness and the clinician has none.' Opportunities for detection of unreliable information are available and will become clearer throughout this text. Maitland (1986) provides a thorough discussion of the value of communication and describes the inquiry strategies he utilises to obtain the most useful information in the most efficient manner; examples of these strategies are outlined below.

Frame of reference

Both the patient and the physiotherapist have their own unique backgrounds with individual experiences that have conditioned how they perceive, interpret, and respond to both their own sensations (e.g., pain), and the appearance and behaviour of others. Attention to the natural human bias will assist the physiotherapist in avoiding misinterpretations of information.

Non-verbal communication

The reflexive character of non-verbal signals makes them less easily controlled than words and therefore, frequently more informative. The physiotherapist must be aware when nuances of behaviour shown by the patient do, and do not, match the verbal message.

Spontaneous information

Questions should be asked in such a way as to provide opportunities for spontaneous comments from the patient. This provides insight into how the patient views the symptoms, and what the patient feels is important.

Use of the patient's own words

Sensitivity to the patient's frame of reference, in this case adopting the words chosen by the patient to describe a symptom, will enhance therapist-patient rapport and thereby the quality of information forthcoming.

Avoiding assumptions

The variations of presentations possible in a given disorder do not allow the presence or absence of any particular feature to be assumed. Further, language differences necessitate that interpretation of patient response be clarified. For example, the patient's description of pain as constant may mean it is present throughout the day and night, or instead that the pain is constant when it is present, but it is not present all day.

The body's capacity to inform

The patient's body can tell the patient things related to the disorder which will frequently provide valuable clues as to the choice of treatment. It can be useful to ask a patient 'What does it feel like in there?', or 'What do you feel it needs to get it better?'. Many patients are surprised by such a question, but with a little prompting they can often give an answer, although the answer may not come until the second or third treatment. It is likely that no-one has given them such responsibility for their problem. Some will say it is just swollen, for example, and others will give extremely helpful answers such as 'It needs a stretch in this direction'. This information needs to be weighed up along with other features of the disorder presentation, but should be taken seriously as it often surprisingly accurate.

'Make the features fit' (Maitland 1986)

This is an inquiry strategy that is fundamental to an hypothesis testing approach. Hypotheses formulated throughout the examination and treatment are either supported or not depending on their 'fit' with the unfolding patient story and physical presentation. It is when features do not fit that clarification and further inquiry/examination are indicated. Thus after a subjective examination, the physiotherapist should have a good idea about what to expect on the physical examination. The quality and amount of movement exhibited by various structures during the physical examination should fit with the physiotherapist's hypotheses from the subjective examination. If features do not fit, the physiotherapist should have a heightened index of suspicion for something missed. This is ultimately the method of inquiry which leads to the discovery of new clinical patterns. Below is an example of how this strategy led to Maitland's development of the Slump Test.

The dialogue with the patient would have been long forgotten and has not been recorded, but it may have gone something like this:

Maitland: When do you get your low back pain?

Patient: I get it when I bend over
Maitland: Is there a particular way you bend that is worse than others?
Patient: No, not really, I just go to get into the car and it really hurts my back.
Maitland: I see — what is it about getting into the car that hurts so much?
Patient: It's a bit odd, but I can get my leg into the car with just a little bit of back pain, but it's when I go to put my head down to get right into the car, that my back really hurts.
Maitland: Thank you, that's helpful information. Tell me, is it when you get into the driver's side or the passenger side that you have the most problems?
Patient: Only the driver's side.
Maitland: Could you show me how you do it? Pretend this chair is the driver's seat . . .

This conversation would have gone on as there is still much valuable information to be gained. But the crucial thought is that this does not quite fit — it's the neck movement that makes the back worse, thus there must be something more than just the lumbar spine implicated in this disorder. Hence, from this patient and undoubtedly from many others, the Slump Test was born (Maitland 1978). Such reasoning is now obvious to many physiotherapists, but 10 years ago it was not. There may have even been some disbelief in the existence of organic pathology in such a patient.

Two clinical situations that further exemplify the need for the inquiry strategy 'make the features fit' are given below.

• During a subjective examination, all information may be pointing to the shoulder joint as a source of symptoms — pain deep in the shoulder, difficulties reaching and using the shoulder, even radiographic changes in the shoulder joint — when the patient volunteers the information that the tip of his index finger and thumb have recently gone numb. This information should immediately register with the physiotherapist that there may be more than shoulder structures involved in this disorder. The anaesthesia in the thumb does not fit a shoulder joint disorder and thus, by necessity, the examination needs to be taken further.

• A patient returns after a treatment, and declares that he/she is '80% improved'. However an examination of the relevant signs (e.g., stiff intervertebral movement) reveals that they are only minimally changed since last treatment. The physiotherapist must think 'the features do not fit' and then attempt to work out why the patient is subjectively better and whether the significance of other signs (e.g., neural or muscle) have been underestimated and possibly altered by the intervertebral joint treatment.

This inquiry strategy combined with the knowledge that mobile structures other than joints are also innervated, for example, muscles, fascia and the nervous system itself has prompted a closer look at nervous system mechanics. The thought process involved in making features fit needs to include knowledge of pathoanatomy, pathophysiology and biomechanics. It is this background knowledge and the continual attempt to make features fit which is largely responsible for the evolving ideas regarding the nervous system put forward in this text.

'A technique is the brainchild of ingenuity' (Maitland 1986)

Techniques (examination and treatment) can be made up or borrowed from any source be they chiropractic, osteopathic, Kaltenborn, Cyriax or any other system of manual, or other form of physical, therapy. There are no set techniques for a particular disorder and the physiotherapist must always be flexible enough to vary techniques depending on physical attributes of both the physiotherapist and patient, severity, irritability, stability of the disorder and knowledge of the patient's pathology. Techniques listed in this book are techniques that have been found useful. Handling skills will develop after mastery of a number of techniques as described in texts and only then can the physiotherapist pursue different and perhaps better combinations. Any manual therapy technique applied to a particular patient will never be repeated in another with exactly the same force, direction, duration, and with the same communication. Hence there should be no 'recipes', 'treatment packages', or insistence on dogma that, in the long run, can only limit the physiotherapist's treatment options.

'A technique is the brainchild of ingenuity' is an important strategy for the ongoing development of nervous system examination and treatment techniques. At this stage, the best handling combinations and skills are still being developed. Once physiotherapists become adept at the base tests, they must explore. It would be a most unusual patient if a simple base test (say SLR) was the best test for reproducing symptoms. More likely there will need to be a combination of tests such as SLR/hip adduction/ankle plantarflexion/spinal lateral flexion. Some of the techniques in this text came from the principal author's students and course participants fiddling and experimenting with combinations of movements and handling. It is early days yet for mobilisation of the nervous system and one should feel that, in perhaps every situation, there is a better way of getting at the problem.

Reassessment

Reassessment is crucial to the testing of examination hypotheses, the progression of ongoing management, the confirmation of existing clinical patterns recognised and the acquisition of new ones. It is of little use merely applying a treatment without seeing if it works there and then. A physiotherapist's examination skills should be such that the most minute alterations in range and quality of movement can be detected if needed. This validation of treatment by reassessment should continually question and reaffirm the hypotheses already formulated. Both subjective and physical reassessments are required. Patients should be asked how they feel as well as being physically re-examined. Both responses should fit. For example, if a patient has had a cervical manipulation and said 'that feels better, my headache is lifting', it would fit that the physical signs of joint restriction were also better. Improvement produced must also be repeatable as often any intervention will produce an initial favorable change, but only the correct treatment will lead to continued improvement. Evaluating the degree of change then enables the physiotherapist to progress the treatment accordingly. Therefore, it is reassessment that determines when a change in technique, or management in general, is necessary and as such provides an impetus for technique modification and development. This requires disciplined reassessment of the most significant physical sign associated with each potential component. For example, following mobilisation of the nervous system using components of the Upper Limb Tension Test, reassessment may include cervical physiological lateral flexion, passive accessory movement tests at the appropriate levels, active shoulder flexion, resisted shoulder abduction, passive shoulder quadrant and the relevant upper limb tension test. Constant monitoring of signs associated with potential components in this way allows the physiotherapist to systematically compare the effect of treating different potential components and using different treatment techniques.

Many physiotherapists armed with a battery of techniques that have been proven successful in the past will stop at that. There is no guarantee that, just because a treatment helped last time, it will be the treatment of choice for the same patient having an apparent recurrence of the same problem, or for another patient with an apparently similar problem. It is impossible to say whether the treatment you delivered is the optimum treatment. Whilst it may be a tried and accepted technique, there are others which may also work, perhaps better, and these will not be learned unless they are tried and the patient reassessed. If they fail, the original technique can always be used. Further discussion of the range of variables that can be altered once reassessment has confirmed the need for a change in treatment will be presented along with examples of different techniques in later chapters. Additional details on reassessment, such as assessment during a technique and retrospective assessment, can be found in the Maitland references given above.

STRUCTURAL DIFFERENTIATION

While there may appear to be routine physical examination tests performed on each part of the body, these should be performed to test hypotheses formed through the subjective examination, and varied as indicated by clues unique to the patient's presentation. For example, a patient may describe a functional activity or specific position which reproduces his or her symptoms. While not considered part of your routine examination, this activity or position should be observed and carefully examined to differentiate physically what component of the activity/position is responsible for the symptoms and, where possible, what structure is most implicated. For example, if the disorder were not irritable, our earlier patient with anterior shoulder pain could be asked to assume the position in removing his jacket where the pain was first felt to increase. With careful handling, his neck position could be altered, ensuring no movement of his shoulder and vice versa. This would give further support to the broad hypotheses of either cervical or local shoulder involvement. However as both movements can alter neural tension, further differentiation in this position would still be necessary. Returning to the same starting position, at the first increase in pain, and ensuring there had been no build up of discomfort from the two previous movements, the patient's wrist could then be extended. An increase in shoulder pain with this isolated movement would clearly implicate neural tension involvement. Differentiation such as this, using the patient's functional aggravating activity or position, provides a quick and informative indication of potential components involved. These findings are then matched against those of the subjective and routine physical examination to further refine the hypotheses considered.

Routine physical tests can be difficult to interpret as, quite commonly, more than one structure will be moved or stressed in the test movement. The ability to decide on the primary tissue at fault is a valuable skill. Structural differentiation is an advanced examination strategy which assists to further refine one's hypotheses. It involves altering the pain provoking position or movement in such a way that one structure is incriminated as a source while another is eliminated from contention (Trott 1985). This is analogous to the reasoning behind the simple differentiation tests commonly used to assess muscle versus joint involvement when finger flexion is limited. There are two aspects to structural differentiation. Firstly, between structures i.e., joint/muscle/nerve other and then differentiation further within a structure. For example, within the shoulder joint, differentiation between the glenohumeral and the acromiohumeral joint (Trott 1985) or within nerve between extraneural and intraneural sources (Chs 3 and 9). Because the nervous system is a continuum, it provides excellent opportunities to differentiate nervous system 'injury' in the presenting disorder. For example, when we go to examine our patient discussed earlier who is cradling his right arm and find that passive shoulder abduction reproduces his shoulder pain, we know this could well be coming from a number of sources, local peripheral nerve structures being just one of them. If the shoulder position is held stable and then the elbow extended, resulting in a worsening of the shoulder pain, the position is a little clearer. The faulty structure could still be nerve as it is tightened further with elbow extension. However it could be related to the biceps muscle as well which has also been stretched due to attachments to both shoulder and elbow. A much clearer situation exists if the shoulder and elbow positions are maintained, and then wrist extension added to see if this alters the symptoms. If, in this position, wrist movement alters the shoulder pain, then one can clinically infer that the shoulder pain is at least partially neurogenic in origin. In this situation, the only structure being directly altered at the shoulder is the nervous system. In many of the disorders where the use of tension tests reproduces patients' symptoms, a neurogenic source of symptoms can often be incriminated via differentiation. Differentiation is a powerful tool. For many disorders, there may only be minor injury to the nervous system and for minor injuries neuropathological evidence is extremely difficult to get. At this stage, structural differentiation is the major tool we have. While validation is needed for the concept of structural differentiation, once this is achieved, the process of scientific validation of tension testing will be easier.

Usually when tension testing, it is possible to further clarify the source of symptoms by testing other limbs. Perhaps an Upper Limb Tension Test (ULTT) performed on the contra-lateral arm will change the shoulder pain, or even a SLR might change the shoulder pain. Often there are many directions to take the limb. It does not have to be a tension increasing manoeuvre; clarification could come by relieving tension. For example, if in an Upper Limb Tension Test position (Ch. 8) reproducing wrist pain, the addition of cervical lateral flexion towards the test side (Fig. 5.2) decreases the wrist symptoms, again there are clear indications that the pain is neurogenic.

There are many examples of neural differen-tiation. If a Straight Leg Raise were to provoke buttock pain, it does not exclusively implicate the nervous system. The pain sensitive source could be hip joint, ischial bursa or lumbar spinal joints, for example. But if the pain pro-voked could be made worse by dorsiflexion or plantarflexion of the ankle or by flexion of the cervical spine, then abnormal mechanics in the nervous system are likely.

With regards to structural differentiation and the nervous system, the following points need considering:

• Symptoms do not have to worsen when differentiating. A decrease or change in symptoms can still implicate the nervous system.

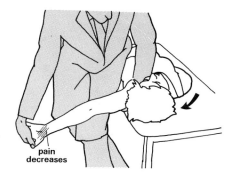

Fig. 5.2 In the ULTT position, if cervical lateral flexion towards the test side decreases wrist symptoms, the inference is that the wrist symptoms are neurogenic

pain decreases

• It is possible to alter tension of a healthy, normal nervous system and get a change in symptoms because of the nervous system's attachment to a sensitive or pathological structure.

• There are continuous fascial planes and blood vessels, both of which are innervated. Information gleaned from differentiation cannot be used alone, without details gathered during the subjective and physical examination. It is useful to consider during tests 'Is it fitting that this pain comes from the nervous system'.

• Depending on the stage of the disorder, findings will differ. For example, if a patient's range of shoulder abduction is limited by a stiff joint capsule at half normal range, the stiff joint component could be 'protecting' the nerve component from being adequately examined. If the shoulder range of movement were to improve, the nervous system would become more available for examination.

• For the clearest indictment of nervous system involvement, symptoms should be altered by movement of a remote part unlikely to alter the local tissues physically at the site of symptoms (e.g., moving cervical spine for wrist pain or wrist movements for shoulder pain).

• Careful and meticulous handling is essential to valid and reliable differentiation.

Structural differentiation as discussed thus far has referred to physical differentiation manoeuvres which can be used to incriminate a component or source of symptoms when more than one structure is involved in the test movement. By the end of the physical examination the physiotherapist is typically still left with several potential sources and contributing factors which can only be retrospectively differentiated following reassessment after treatment. Consider the ex-ample of a neck disorder with physical signs including tight left upper trapezius and levator scapulae plus zygapophyseal joint stiffness of 'opening' on the left. The muscle could be treated, the effect on muscle length, physio-logical movements and accessory joint signs reassessed and then compared to the effect of treating the joint directly. The primary structure at fault will eventually be recognised.

PRECAUTIONS AND CONTRAINDICATIONS

If physiotherapists are conscious of the incompleteness of scientific understanding in this area, they will always be suspicious of the possible pathological processes involved in the patients presenting for treatment.

As in physical therapy of any structure, there are inherent dangers in mobilising the nervous system. There will always be some aspect of the unknown, be it unknown pathology or the variable responses particular to the human psyche. This is precisely why 'precautions and contraindications to physical examination and treatment' is a basic issue which should be investigated and understood prior to initiating the physical examination or treatment.

Physiotherapists should be well acquainted with lists of precautions and contraindications as found in Grieve (1981) (1988), Corrigan and Maitland (1983) and Maitland (1986). Known precautions and contraindications are part of the clinical reasoning process guiding the extent and force of examination and treatment which can be conducted safely so as to minimise the risk of exacerbating the patient's symptoms or worsening the disorder. Those listed below are particularly relevant to the nervous system. The greatest precaution, however, is that the physiotherapist is adequately trained.

Precautions

1. Other structures involved in testing.
For example, injured lumbar discs are at risk during the flexion component of the Slump Test, as are injured zygapophyseal joints of the cervical spine during neck movements in the Upper Limb Tension Tests (ULTT). The tension tests are complex and involve many components that are often spread all over the body. The Slump Test and the ULTTs are particularly complex tests. It is sometimes easy to forget the other structures that tension testing traverses and that these structures could be injured or aggravated by the testing itself. Care is required with known spinal stenosis and or spondylosis, as a neural response is more likely to occur earlier during testing.

2. Irritability related to the nervous system.
Irritability is based on three variables:

(a) How much activity the patient can perform before being stopped by symptoms
(b) The severity (intensity and physical restriction) and distribution of symptoms
(c) How long it takes for the symptoms to subside to its original level.

An irritated segment of nervous system can be particularly reactive, possessing an inherent mechano- and chemo-sensitivity different to other structures. This is probably due not only to the conduction properties of nerve, but also to the complexity and number of structures involved. Often there will be more than one site of irritation or injury. Clinically, it seems easier to aggravate arm symptoms than leg. This may be related to the greater complexity of nerve anatomy in the arm, the proximity of upper limb peripheral nerves to the exterior compared with the leg, or to the greater mobility of upper limb interfacing structures and associated inter structure friction. Friction can be a symptom provoker and is a common part of the repetitious activities that many modern occupations demand.

3. Worsening disorder. Of interest is whether the disorder is worsening and, if so, what is its rate of deterioration. A patient's complaint of low back pain spreading posteriorly down the thigh and calf which has only gradually developed over the last nine months will require less precaution in one's physical handling than would a disorder with the same site of pain which had developed in the last 24 hours.

4. The presence of neurological signs.
The presence of neurological signs should not preclude examination or treatment by passive movement (but see contraindications list). As long as the disorder is chronic and the neurological changes are stable, and not indicative of any active disease process, then with constant reassessment, the nervous system can be mobilised.

5. General health problems. Great respect should be given to pathologies that affect the nervous system, although manual treatment may be appropriate for some of the symptoms evoked. Diabetes, leprosy, AIDS, and multiple sclerosis are some examples of disease process that weaken the nervous system. The presence of neoplastic disease of the nervous system causing positive tension signs is always a possibility. Elvey (1986) warns that the ULTT could also be positive due to a Pancoast's tumour. Patients with intermedullary tumours may present with scolioses and minimal neurological signs (Citron et al 1984). The questioning involved in the subjective examination should be sensitive to the presence of disease processes and if 'features are made to fit' then the physiotherapist may identify those very occasional patients that slip through the medical net.

6. Dizziness. Hopefully, all physiotherapists are aware that dizziness related to vertebrobasilar insufficiency is a contraindication to cervical manipulation and, in some cases, mobilisation (Grant 1988). Dizziness should also be a precaution when mobilising the nervous system. The Slump Test, Passive Neck Flexion and the depression components of the ULTTs are manoeuvres that must tense the blood vessels in the neck. Dizziness itself is a symptom that can be analysed just like pain and paraesthesia. Nervous system mobilisation may well be a low risk method of mobilising the cervical spine with minimal interference to joints and vertebral arteries.

7. Circulatory disturbances. In many regions of the body, the circulatory system is closely connected to the nervous system, forming a neurovascular bundle. Like the nervous system, the circulatory system is a continuous structure throughout the body and must move and elongate during body movements. However, compared to nerve, the circulatory system runs a more tortuous course, is quite elastic and with blood as the only content, is far more compressible than the more solid nervous system. The normative responses noted from tension testing are more related to nerve than circulation. Nevertheless, an awareness of the fact that the circulatory system is being mobilised as well should place limitations in the presence of any symptoms or signs of circulatory disturbance.

8. Frank cord injury. While frank cord injury is a contraindication to mobilisation in most situations, it seems likely that patients could present with minor cord injuries that go undetected and probably benefit from mobilisation. If minor cord injury is suspected, a good rationale would be to do less than the patient would be doing in normal daily activities. Torg et al (1986) defined the syndrome of cord neuropraxia with transient quadriplegia. Thirty-two male athletes were presented. Physiotherapists examining and treating the nervous system, particularly via the Slump manoeuvre, should be aware of it. The sensory changes involved in the clinical entity were burning pain, numbness, tingling and loss of sensation. The motor changes ranged from weakness to complete paralysis. These were transient episodes with recovery in 10–15 minutes though gradual resolution could be over 48 hours. A significant percentage of this group were found to have cervical instability, stenosis, disc protrusion or a decrease in the anteroposterior dimensions of the spinal canal. While there was no evidence that such an injury predisposes an individual to further neurological injury, great care should be taken with Slump Tests, or the technique should not be performed at all. It seem likely that minor cord injury is probably more common than is diagnosed (Hopkins & Rudge 1973).

Contraindications

These contraindications listed are specific to the nervous system. Malignancy involving the nervous system, the vertebral column or any acute inflammatory infection are definite contraindications. Where other structures are used to test the mechanics of the nervous system (e.g., flexion of the vertebral column in the Slump Test, there may be contraindications (e.g., instability) to testing these structures.

1. Recent onset of, or worsening, neurological signs. Disorders which are acute, or have neurological signs that are unstable enough to require a daily neurological examination are contraindications to mobilisation of the nervous system.

2. Cauda equina lesions. Alterations in bladder and bowel function plus alterations in perineal sensation related to the spine can be surgical emergencies.

3. Injury to the spinal cord. There is a syndrome known as tethered cord syndrome, where the cord is tethered to the dura mater which may in turn be tethered to the spinal canal. This is usually congenital and is associated with some form of spinal dysraphism. There is also increasing evidence that an adult version of tethered cord syndrome is not as infrequent as was once thought (Pang & Wilberger 1982). If the cord is tethered, then forces from spinal movements that would usually be transmitted away from the cord via the denticulate ligaments, meninges and nerve roots are transmitted directly to the cord. The result could be a segment of anoxic cord. There is no benefit to be gained by mobilising the nervous system in these patients and they require a surgical option. Clues as to a possible tethered cord may come from hair tufts, dermal sinuses in the lumbar spine, and a myelogram or magnetic resonance imaging. Physiotherapists should always be wary of the young patient with tight calves and hamstrings. These patients usually have tight muscles but the possibility of cord injury also exists. With a history of enuresis and any cord symptoms (Ch. 6) such a patient should be investigated further.

REFERENCES

Barrows H S, Feltovich P J 1987 The clinical reasoning process. Medical Education 21: 86–91

Barrows H S and Tamblyn R M 1980 Problem-based learning: an approach to medical education. Springer, New York

Chase W G and Simon H A 1973 Perception in chess. Cognitive Psychology 4: 55–81

Chi M T, Feltovich P J, Glaser R 1981 Categorization and representation of physics problems by experts and novices. Cognitive Psychology 5: 121–152

Chi M T, Glaser R, Farr M J 1988 The nature of expertise. Lawrence Erlbaum Associates, Hillsdale

Citron N, Edgar M A, Sheehy J, et al 1984 Intramedullary spinal cord tumours presenting as scoliosis. Journal of Bone and Joint Surgery 66B: 513–517

Corrigan R, Maitland G D 1983 Practical orthopaedic medicine. Butterworths, London

DeGroot A D 1965 Thought and choice in chess. Basic Books, New York

Elstein A S, Shulman L S, Sprafka S S 1978 An analysis of clinical reasoning. Harvard, Cambridge

Elvey R L 1986 Treatment of arm pain associated with abnormal brachial plexus tension. Australian Journal of Physiotherapy 32: 225–230

Feltovich P J, Johnson P E, Moller J H, Swanson D B 1984 LCS: The role and development of medical knowledge in diagnostic expertise. In: Clancey W J, Shortliffe E H (eds) Readings in medical artificial intelligence: the first decade. Addison-Wesley, Reading

Grant R 1988 Dizziness testing and manipulation of the cervical spine. In: Grant R (ed) Physical therapy of the cervical and thoracic spine: Clinics in physical therapy 17. Churchill Livingstone, New York

Grant R, Jones M, Maitland G D 1988 Clinical decision making in upper quadrant dysfunction. In: Grant R (ed) Physical therapy of the cervical and thoracic spine: Clinics in physical therapy 17. Churchill Livingstone, New York

Grieve G P 1981 Common vertebral joint problems. Churchill Livingstone, Edinburgh.

Hopkins A, Rudge P 1973 Hyperpathia in the central cervical cord syndrome. Journal of Neurology, Neurosurgery and Psychiatry 36: 637–642

Kleinmuntz B 1968 The processing of clinical information by man and machine. In: Kleinmuntz B (ed) The formal representation of human judgement. John Wiley, New York

Mackinnon S E, Dellon A L 1988 Surgery of the peripheral nerve. Thieme, New York

Maitland G D 1978 Movement of pain sensitive structures in the vertebral canal in a group of physiotherapy students. In: Proceedings, Inaugural congress of the Manipulative Therapists Association of Australia, Sydney

Maitland G D 1986 Vertebral manipulation, 5th edn. Butterworths, London

Massey E W, Riley T L, Pleet A B 1981 Co-existent carpal tunnel syndrome and cervical radiculopathy (double crush syndrome). Southern Medical Journal 74: 957–959

Muzzin L J, Norman G R Feightner J W, Tugwell P, Guyatt G 1983 Expertise in recall of clinical protocols in two specialty areas. Proceedings 22nd Conference on Research in Medical Education, Washington, 122–127

Pang D, Wilberger J E 1982 Tethered cord syndrome in adults. Journal of Neurosurgery 57: 32–47.

Patel V L, Frederiksen C H 1984 Cognitive processes in comprehension and knowledge acquisition by medical students and physicians. In: Schmidt J G and DeVolder M L (eds) Tutorials in problem-based learning. Van Borcum, Assen/Maastricht

Patel V L, Groen G J, Frederiksen C H 1986 Differences between medical students and doctors in memory for clinical cases. Medical Education 20: 3–9

Sunderland S 1978 Nerves and nerve injuries. Churchill Livingstone, Edinburgh

Torg J S, Pavlov H, Genuario S E et al 1986 Neuropraxia of the cervical spinal cord with transient quadriplegia. The Journal of Bone and Joint Surgery 68A: 1354–1370

Trott P 1985 Differential mechanical diagnosis of shoulder pain. In: Proceedings Manipulative Therapists Association of Australia, 4th biennial conference, Brisbane

6. Examination of nerve conduction

Physiotherapists can examine the nervous system in a number of ways:

• Conduction can be examined. This is achieved by a subjective examination, physical tests and observation of structures served by the innervation. Few patients will require or have access to electrodiagnostic tests.
• The movement and elasticity of the nervous system can be examined. This utilises the tension tests described in the next two chapters.
• The nervous system can be palpated. In many areas of the body, especially in the extremities, the nervous system is accessible to palpation (Ch. 9).

This chapter concentrates on the manual examination of nerve conduction. Greater scope, and in some areas, different material on the examination of conduction, can be found in texts by the Mayo Clinic (1981), Bickerstaff & Spillane (1989) and McLeod & Lance (1989) among others.

GENERAL POINTS

1. The connective and neural tissue constituents of the nervous system are intimately related. Examination of one will require examination of the other. Any relationship between altered nervous system mechanics, i.e., positive tension tests and impaired conduction, must ascertained.

2. The manual tests for conduction are rather simple. While an inadequate means for research into sensory and motor mechanisms, they are adequate for detecting and evaluating conduction changes, localising the site of the injury, and monitoring recovery (Seddon 1972, Sunderland 1978). They are also easily repeatable tests and thus useful for monitoring the progress of a disorder.

3. The status of conduction must be known and recorded before and after treatment. It will determine the choice of treatment technique, the vigour of the technique and, in some situations, contraindicate treatment. The orthopaedic schools of manual therapy have always stressed the importance of the neurological examination. Clearly it is even more applicable with the selective nervous system mobilisation encouraged by this text.

4. There is an art to a good neurological examination. It requires a combination of adept handling and patient communication skills, together with an underlying basic knowledge of neuroanatomy. Physiotherapists should be well placed in all these areas. Those with experience assessing and treating neurological disease and injury will be even better placed. In some patients, the examination of conduction can be difficult due to communication difficulties or the complexity of the innervation changes.

5. The majority of patients seen by physiotherapists will not have undergone any electrodiagnostic testing such as nerve conduction tests or electromyography, nor will they require testing. Manual examination is usually the only available method of testing neurological status. Consequently it is clinically more relevant for the type of patient that most physiotherapists are likely to see. As injuries are usually not severe in such cases,

expertise in handling and interpretation is vital. Injuries may only lead to minor changes in nerve conduction which may be undetectable.

6. One key to effective testing is to bear in mind the contributions of non-neural structures to the examination findings. Possible complicating features such as muscle weakness from muscle injury, joint stiffness, pain from non-neural structures, patient apprehension, attention and state of memory patterns need interpretation. For example, the neurological examination of a patient who has just come out of a plaster of Paris cast would be have to be interpreted in the light of muscle weakness from disuse, pain, skin changes and altered movement memory patterns. Be well aware that the influences of the central nervous system cannot be measured, only guessed at.

7. A neurological examination should be performed before any treatment via mobilising the nervous system. There are also certain pathologies where a neurological examination is necessary because the nervous system could be ultimately involved. Examples of this situation are an acute disc lesion that could crowd the spinal canal, and compartment syndromes.

Physiotherapists should do a neurological examination when warranted for a number of reasons:

(a) The safety factor. Worsening neurological signs or neurological symptoms and signs that do not fit the overall clinical picture should be a precaution and perhaps a contraindication for assessment and treatment. Any alterations in central nervous system conduction should be initially taken as a contraindication to manual therapy (though see Ch. 13). It is desirable that all patients with a degree of nerve injury, regardless of how minor, have been examined by an understanding medical practitioner.

(b) Neurological examinations aid in the treatment and prognostic decision. An accurate neurological examination can provide information about the site, nature, stage and prognosis of the disorder. For example, a loss of sensation in a dermatomal distribution implies some sort of conduction alteration at spinal nerve or nerve root level; a delineated loss of sensation in a cutaneous nerve distribution implies that loss of conduction may be in the nerve trunk. Levels of entrapment can be gauged by selective muscle loss. A poorer prognosis could be indicated with marked changes in conduction.

(c) Objective neurological changes are an excellent reassessment after treatment. They can be reassessed after one treatment and then also assessed retrospectively, say after 2 weeks or more of treatment.

SUBJECTIVE NEUROLOGICAL EXAMINATION

All symptoms, including pain, may be thought of as neurological symptoms. Even if they originate from non-neural tissue, the nervous system has a large part in conveying, interpreting and expressing the impulses related to that symptom. A neurological examination should not be seen as merely a series of physical tests to be performed.

The Maitland approach to examination that this text follows requires knowledge of the area, behaviour, nature and history of all relevant presenting symptoms. Information is also gleaned regarding the relationship between presenting symptoms. In this regard, not only is information about pain necessary, but also such symptoms as paraesthesia, heaviness, feelings of swelling, coldness and any others. Area of neurological symptoms such as pain, paraesthesia, anaesthesia, sensory changes, feeling of weakness etc. should be clearly defined and marked onto a body chart such as that in Chapters 4 or 13. With a clear understanding of the area of symptoms and the relationship between the symptoms, an analysis of the behaviour and history can follow (Maitland 1986).

Patients may need help with the subjective neurological examination. What they mean by 'numbness' or 'heavy leg' may not be how the physiotherapist interprets it. Clarification is often needed. The previous chapter discusses aspects of communication.

Further subjective neurological information may be gained by asking a series of mandatory questions. Maitland (1986) refers to a section of questioning as special questions, better thought of as precautionary questions. This involves questions about possible vertebral artery insufficiency, general health questions, medication including use of steroids and anticoagulants, involvement of the spinal cord and the cauda equina, and other tests such as X-rays or myelograms.

To allow for the safest and most effective selective nervous system treatment, further precautionary questions are suggested, and some of the original precautionary questions become more relevant. Note however that these are not necessarily contraindications.

1. Dizziness. Dizziness is usually associated with vertebro-basilar insufficiency, the middle ear or the upper cervical spine. It is possible that dizziness may be associated with tension testing or may come on in a position of tension. If a SLR causes dizziness it may well be the effect of a dural attachment pulling on sensitised zygapophysial joints in the upper cervical spine. Depression of the shoulder may cause tension on the subclavian and the vertebral artery and perhaps be related to a symptom of dizziness.

2. Involvement of the cauda equina. It is routine in all spinal patients to ask about the function of the bladder, bowels, perianal and genital sensation. If there is any disturbance then this should be related to any spinal disturbance; e.g., 'Do you notice that your bladder problem is worse when your back pain is worse?' Many physiotherapists are not accustomed to urogenital questioning, nor are patients. It should be encouraged unless it greatly interferes with patient communication. A medical opinion and perhaps treatment is necessary if the cauda equina is involved. Disturbances in sexual function are often associated with cauda equina lesions. It is often difficult to discuss with patients and it is a rare patient that offers impotence as a symptom. Physiotherapists are encouraged to seek out all the signs and symptoms of any disorder they treat.

3. Cord symptoms. These are discussed later in this chapter. However the tethered cord

syndrome is of particular relevance (see Ch. 5). If the spinal cord is tethered to the dura mater and then perhaps the dura to the spinal canal, any forces placed along the neuraxis will not be dispersed the usual way via the denticulate ligaments and nerve roots. Consequently there is the possibility of further cord damage. Great care should be taken with those who have sustained a previous transient cord neuropraxia following forced spinal flexion as described by Torg et al (1986). A question like "Have there been any occasions when your limbs have gone completely numb?" is suggested.

4. General health. There are some pathologies which effect the nervous system; either weakening the connective tissues, damaging the impulse transmission mechanisms or altering the axonal transport mechanisms. Diabetes is probably the most commonly encountered disease, but AIDS, multiple sclerosis and the various inflammatory polyneuropathies are examples of others. While mobilisation may offer a method of treating the symptoms and minimising any post inflammatory scarring, much greater care will be required. The underlying pathology cannot be changed.

5. Other tests. Any available tests of the nervous system, such as thermography, computerised tomography, magnetic resonance imaging and electrodiagnostic tests should be utilised if available. In these days of complex and varied diagnostic tests, patients can often be confused about what tests have been performed and some time may be required to get the desired information.

PHYSICAL EXAMINATION OF SENSATION

A few simple pieces of equipment are required. It is essential to have a percussion hammer, a flagged pin and some cotton wool or a tissue. Also useful are a two point discriminator, and a vibration fork (256 cycles per second). If available, an objective measure of muscle power such as a dynamometer can be utilised. I also think that a readily available anatomy textbook is valuable. Joint domination of manipulative therapy may have diminished the importance of the nervous system and such aspects as dermatomes, cutaneous fields of innervation and location of nerves may need review.

Light touch

The sensation of light touch is examined to assess involvement of the nervous system together with the level of involvement. Repeated examination will assist in determining whether a disorder is worsening or improving.

The fascicles of each ventral ramus, on entering a plexus, split and contribute to any number of emerging peripheral nerve branches. Each peripheral nerve thus contains nerve fibres originating from a number of ventral rami. This allows each spinal nerve to contribute to a skin segment of the body, referred to as a 'dermatome'. Figure 6.1 is an example of the fascicular splitting that occurs in the brachial plexus and is worth consideration before too much emphasis is placed on dermatomes. However, reasonably consistent patterns emerge, despite all the possible variations (Figs 6.2 A,B).

The cutaneous innervation fields are different from the dermatomes except in the trunk, where the lack of plexus formations means that the spinal nerve continues as the peripheral nerve. There is overlap with the cutaneous nerve supply — this is obvious because loss of conduction in a peripheral nerve will cause greater numbness in the centre of the innervation field than in the periphery. These central zones may also be regarded as autonomous zones for peripheral nerves. Anomalies in neuroanatomy are very common and may lead to odd results from a neurological examination. Some of these anomalies are discussed in Chapter 3. Areas of

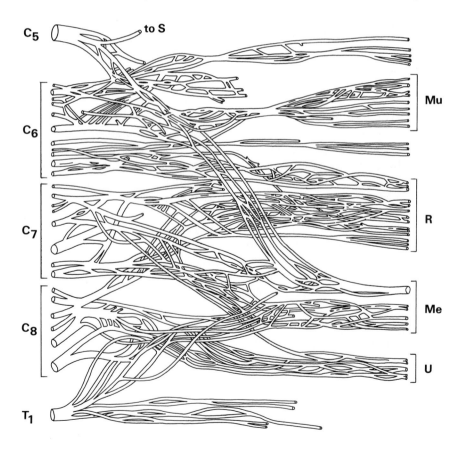

Fig. 6.1 Internal and external plexus formations in the brachial plexus. Adapted from Kerr (1918). Me median, Mu musculocutaneous, R radial, S suprascapular, U ulnar

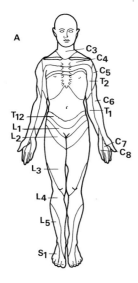

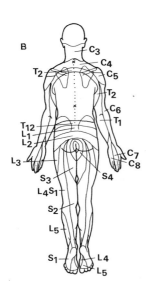

Fig. 6.2 The dermatomes A anterior view, B posterior view

it is deficient. The patient should also be told that minimal changes could be of interest to you; however, this may vary depending on the complexity of the neurological changes.

2. The patient's eyes must be closed throughout the test.

3. A base sensation response is needed so responses can be compared. This may be the opposite limb or even the abdomen. Where possible, when seeking a comparison, the tested parts should be matched to similarly sensitive areas. For example, the ventral aspect of the forearm is much more sensitive than the dorsal aspect therefore a comparison is difficult.

4. Commence distally on the limb, comparing the sensation in the digits to each other and to the digits on the other limb. Also test along the digits (Fig. 6.4) and mark the site of any sensory changes. Pay great attention to areas of sensory change complained of in the subjective examination.

5. For the rest of the limb, test for light touch by going around the limb to traverse as many dermatomes and cutaneous innervation fields as possible (Fig. 6.5).

The impulses conveying sensations of light touch travel in large myelinated fibres in peripheral nerves with cell bodies in the dorsal root ganglia. In the cord, they ascend mainly in the dorsal columns.

Pinprick

Pinprick tests the sensation of superficial pain. A flagged pin is suggested. Some institutions may prefer disposable pins. A flagged pin can easily be constructed by placing a piece of sticking plaster around the end of a large pin. The examiner uses the pin by holding the flag. This prevents anything more than just a light tapping of the skin (Fig. 6.6) A similar method to light touch is employed, whereby a pinprick in one limb is compared to one in the other limb and then changes within the limb are assessed. More emphasis is likely to be placed on the extremities and it is a good idea to mark areas of altered sensation

cutaneous nerve supply are shown in Figures 6.3 A, B, C, D and E.

To test sensation, the patient must wear the most minimal clothing that age, sex and culture dictate. Socks and stockings in particular need to be removed. For testing light touch, a tissue or a piece of cotton wool should be used. The technique suggested is as follows:

1. Describe the test to the patient and establish a clear means of communication such as 'yes' when sensation is normal or 'no' when

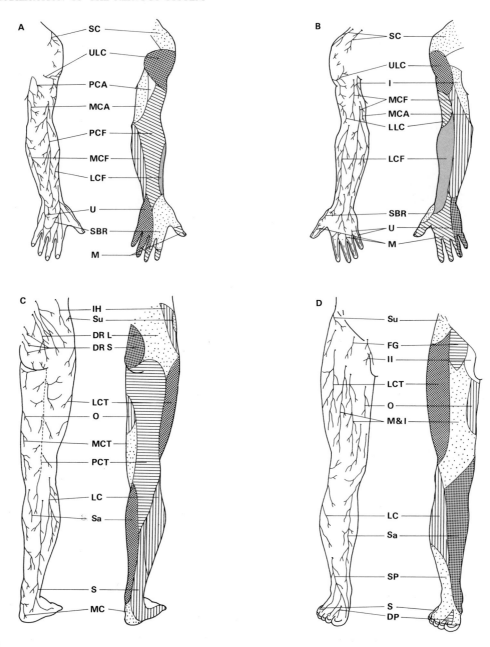

Fig. 6.3

with a pen. The bases of the nails are the most sensitive part of the fingers to test.

With tests of sensation it is useful to try and 'make features fit'. For example, with an apparent C6 nerve root or spinal nerve irritation/compression and symptoms in the C6 dermatome, I would expect that the tip of the thumb would be deprived of some sensation.

Testing can thus be biased towards the expected findings. In the examination of motor function in the example given, it would fit the pattern if the biceps jerk rather than the triceps jerk was altered.

Be aware too that trophic changes in skin may contribute to altered sensation. These changes may arise from the same injury, although

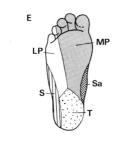

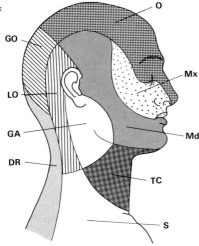

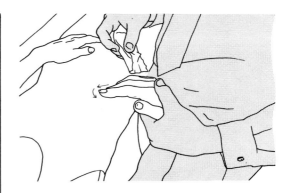

Fig. 6.4 Compare sensation between the digits and along each digit

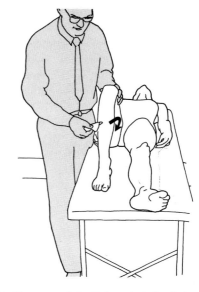

Fig. 6.5 Test around the limb to include all dermatomes and cutaneous fields

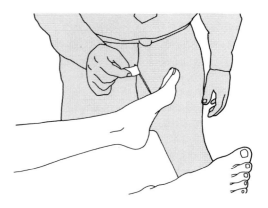

Fig. 6.6 Use of the flagged pin to test the sensation of superficial pain

Fig. 6.3 Cutaneous innervation fields. **A** upper limb posterior view, **B** upper limb anterior view. SC supraclavicular C3,4; ULC upper lateral cutaneous C5,6; I intercostobrachial T2; PCA posterior cutaneous of the arm C5,6,7,8; MCA medial cutaneous of the arm C8,T1, MCF medial cutaneous of the forearm C8,T1; M median C6,7,8; SBR superficial branch of the radial C6,7,8; LCF lateral cutaneous of the forearm C5,6; LLC lower lateral cutaneous of the arm; U ulnar C8,T1; PCF posterior cutaneous of the forearm. **C** lower limb posterior view, **D** lower limb anterior view. Su subcostal T12; II ilio-inguinal L1; DRL dorsal rami lumbar L1,2,3; DRS dorsal rami sacral S1,2,3, LCT lateral cutaneous of the thigh L2,3; O obturator L2,3,4; MCT medial cutaneous of the thigh L2,3; PCT posterior cutaneous of the thigh S1,2,3; LC lateral cutaneous of the calf L4,5,S1; SA saphenous L3,4; S sural L5,S1,2; MC medial calcaneal S1,2; DP deep peroneal; SP superficial peroneal L4,5,S1; M & I medial and intermediate cutaneous of the thigh L2,3; FG femoral branch of the genito-femoral L1,2; IH iliohypogastric L1, **E** sole of the foot. T tibial S1,2; MP medial plantar L4,5; LP lateral plantar S1,2; S sural L5,S1,2; Sa saphenous L3,4
F the scalp and face. DR dorsal rami C3,4,5; GA greater auricular C2,3; LO lesser occipital C2; GO greater occipital C2,3; O ophthalmic; Mx maxillary, Md mandibular, TC transverse cutaneous C2,3; S supraclavicular C3,4. From: Williams P L, Warwick R, Dyson M, Bannister L H (eds) 1989 Gray's anatomy, 37th edn. Churchill Livingstone, Edinburgh, with permission

via axoplasmic flow alterations rather than altered impulse conduction. Sensation changes in the trunk can be detected by light touch and pinprick applied in the longitudinal axis to include all fields of innervation.

Some patients may complain of itching. This may also be worth mapping out. The physiological mechanisms behind itching are probably similar to those of pain.

Vibration

Vibration sensation (pallesthesia) will be diminished or lost with disease and/or injury in the peripheral nerves and in the dorsal columns. The sense of vibration is not regularly tested by physiotherapists, although some hand therapists use it. Plenty of recent evidence exists suggesting that vibration is the first sensation to diminish with failing nerve conduction (Szabo et al 1984, Beatty et al 1987, Phillips et al 1987). In peripheral nerve, vibration sensation is carried in large group A fibres and these are more susceptible to a depletion of blood than the small fibres.

A tuning fork with a frequency of 256 Hz is best, not the higher frequency fork used for tests of hearing (Phillips et al 1987). The best areas to test are bony surfaces such as the medial epicondyle and the clavicle. Bony surfaces along the whole limb should be tested. A prong of the fork is struck and the single pronged end placed onto a distal bony surface (Fig. 6.7). As with all testing, the patient must

be made to understand the sensation that the physiotherapist wants him/her to feel. Initially placing the vibrating fork on the forehead or sternum may help the patient understand the sensation about to be applied. A clear verbal relationship must exist. For example the patient must say 'yes' or 'no' or 'buzzing' or 'not buzzing' during the test. Vibration testing is compared inter-limb and intra-limb. Once the prongs are struck, the fork slowly loses amplitude, hence double testing is required to allow for this (i.e., test left side first and then test the right side first).

The Mayo Clinic (1981) suggests that a sharp gradient of vibration loss with a deficit distally but not proximally in a limb indicates a peripheral nerve disorder. A central nervous system disorder is more likely when there is little change in the vibration gradient from limbs to the girdles.

Vibration sense should never be absent on the shins or fingers in normal, healthy people (van Allen & Rodnitsky 1976). It is known, however, that in older people, (say over 60) that vibration sense may be absent in the toes. Vibration sense is closely allied with position sense. If vibration sense is intact, then position sense will rarely be altered (van Allen & Rodnitzky 1976).

Proprioception

This is not routinely tested but is worthwhile, especially in the more severe nerve injuries. Loss of proprioception is evident in disorders such as sprained ankles, where not only the non-neural structures are damaged but almost inevitably the nervous system is as well. Subjects can usually identify 1–2 mm of movement in an extremity joint. It can be tested by asking the patient to mimic the position of one digit on the opposing limb or by asking them what you are doing to a particular digit. The patient can say 'up' or 'down' in response to the physiotherapist's movement. Make sure that the patient's eyes are closed.

Tests of balance, such as standing on one foot and hopping, could be relevant tests of altered conduction.

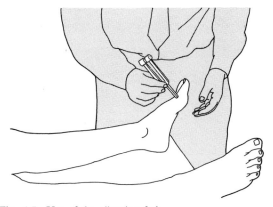

Fig. 6.7 Use of the vibration fork

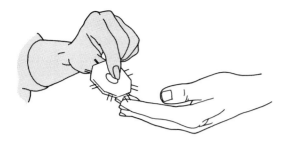

Fig. 6.8 The two point discrimator as suggested by Mackinnon & Dellon (1988)

Two point discrimination

With further loss of conduction the normal appreciation of static and two point discrimination may begin to diminish. Mackinnon & Dellon (1989) suggest use of their discriminator (Fig. 6.8). It certainly looks more convenient, scientific, and a far better reassessment tool, than opened out paper clips. Szabo et al (1984) showed that, while changes in the vibration threshhold were noted with amplitude changes of 12%, two point discrimination was normal until the amplitude had decreased by 70%. A normal subject should be able to distinguish between points 3 mm apart on the pulps of the fingers and 2–3 cm apart on the soles of the foot.

Age and sensory testing

With increasing age, a slow decline in the senses of pain, vibration, and touch occurs. Some possible causes are changes in skin properties, diminished blood flow in the nervous system and a reduction in the number of Meissner's corpuscles (Bolton et al 1966). Perhaps there may also be increased communication difficulties with some of the more aged patients.

EXAMINATION OF MOTOR FUNCTION

Wasting

Wasting can sometimes be observed in the undressed patient. This is an objective change which the patient can relate to and be willing to try to alter. Patients will often be unaware of wasting, especially in the calf and gluteals and may be quite shocked when you point

it out. Some clarification will be needed to ensure that wasting or muscle weakness is due to the presenting disorder. The wasting may be due to a previous injury (either muscular or neurological) that has left a degree of permanent muscle weakness. Swelling and oedema can sometimes mask the extent of wasting.

By palpating the texture of the muscle and comparing it to the contralateral muscle a change in texture may be evident. It can be useful to observe wasting in different positions such as standing and lying and also with the relevant muscles contracted and relaxed.

Reflex testing

Reflex testing utilises the fact that a sudden stretch of a skeletal muscle will result in a reflex contraction of that muscle. The results will be dependant on the state of the reflex arc. Central influences can modify the responsiveness of the motor unit. Testing requires:

1. Complete relaxation of the patient
2. The tendon to be tested placed in a position of slight stretch. The limb could be moved passively before the reflex is tested
3. An adequate stimulus
4. Reinforcement if needed.

There is an art to reflex testing. The tendon should be struck a few times, letting the tendon hammer drop onto the tendon. In this way, an even amplitude of force can be applied, i.e., just the weight of the hammer. The physiotherapist will require some experience regarding the ranges of normality. Minor differences in responses between sides can be neglected. If a response is hard to elicit, reinforcement via muscular exertion elsewhere (e.g., clench jaw, make a fist) can be used. Make sure that reinforcement does not directly influence the muscles being tested, i.e., clench the jaw for testing lower limbs.

A reflex will be decreased in a lower motor neurone injury and may be exaggerated with upper motor neurone disease or injury. A spread of reflexes may also be indicative of an upper motor neurone lesion. Here, testing the biceps

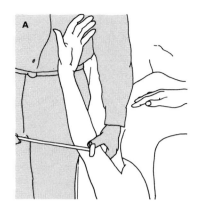

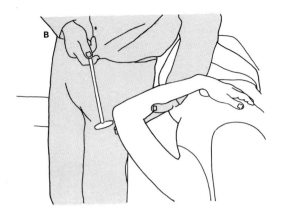

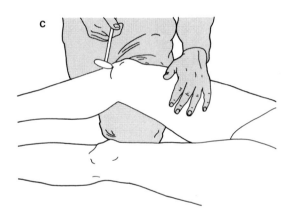

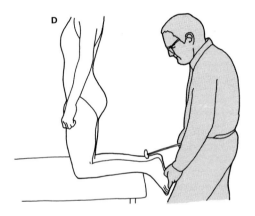

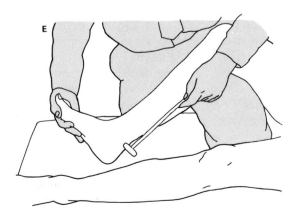

Fig. 6.9 Reflex testing. A biceps (C6), B triceps (C7),
C quadriceps (L3,4), D calf (S1,2), E alternative method
for the calf

jerk may elicit the triceps jerk or testing the brachioradialis jerk may elicit both biceps and triceps jerks. Reflexes can also appear brisker after exercise or if the patient is anxious. Interpretation of results should be done in relation to other conduction tests. For example, with a diminished knee jerk (L3,4) it is likely that the strength of the quadriceps would be diminished. In Figures 6.9 A,B,C,D,E the most commonly tested reflexes of the upper and lower limbs are illustrated.

Some clinical observations made by physiotherapists indicate that reflexes may be more quickly changed than previously thought. For example, lower limb reflexes can change while a patient is on lumbar traction. They can also change after the nervous system has been mobilised. The mechanisms behind these anecdotal observations are not clear.

Muscle power testing

Muscle testing is also an art requiring concise handling, a knowledge of neuroanatomy and patient communication. There are many systems of grading (Daniels & Worthingham 1972, Mayo Clinic 1981). The standard 0–5 grading as taught in Australian physiotherapy schools is shown in Table 6.1.

Within this classification, there will, by necessity, be subgroups, especially within the grade 5 category. For example, the extensor hallucis longus muscle may move the underlying joints of the great toe through full range against resistance, but the tendon of the contracted muscle could be a little 'soft' to palpate, compared with the other side. I prefer to add 5+ for full strength, use 5 for slightly decreased strength and 5− for a more moderate decrease

Table 6.1 Grades of muscle power

0 = no flicker
1 = perceptible flicker
2 = some movement if gravity eliminated
3 = full range of movement against gravity
4 = full range of movement against some resistance
5 = full range against full resistance

in strength. These strength tests are made in comparison with the other limb, or to what is considered normal. Included in testing and discussed later in this chapter are some quick tests which may be more relevant to the patient as a measure of his/her improvement than to the physiotherapist. These are discussed and illustrated below. The results of muscle testing will need interpretation. For example, pain may inhibit the strength of contraction available. After a period of denervation, compensatory mechanisms in affected muscle groups occur, such as collateral axon sprouting, increased frequency of motor unit firing and hypertrophy of existing muscle fibres. Bohannon & Gajdosik (1987) have reviewed these mechanisms. Consideration must also be given to the possible occult strength deficit. The amount of innervation loss necessary before manual tests can detect the loss is not known. Wohlfart (1959) suggested that, with the partial denervation caused by amyotrophic lateral sclerosis, up to a third of the motor fibres may disappear without any appreciable loss of strength.

Like a dermatome, a myotome is a muscle or group of muscles supplied by a given cranial or spinal nerve. Due to fascicular splitting in the area of plexuses especially, the muscles innervated by a spinal nerve may be widely dispersed. However, some muscle groups can be isolated and tested for a single spinal nerve or peripheral nerve. For example, the extensor hallucis longus receives innervation primarily via the L5 spinal nerve.

Muscle testing upper limb

As a general guide, a maximal contraction is required, then the physiotherapist gently breaks the contraction. Some muscles can be too strong to test such as the calf and the biceps muscles. Here, techniques may need to be varied. For example, calf strength can be tested in standing and the biceps can be tested in its outer range.

There are a number of effective methods of testing. I prefer testing in supine as this offers better stabilisation of the rest of the body. Others may prefer to do some of the tests in sitting. In

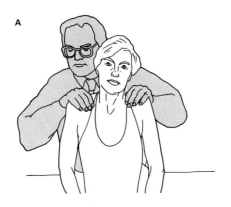

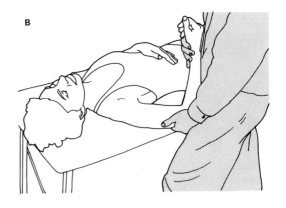

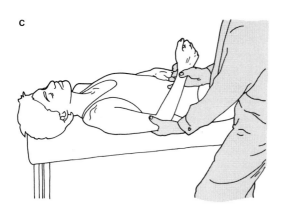

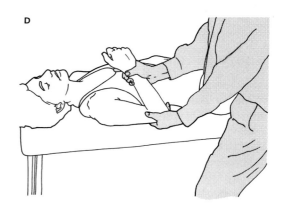

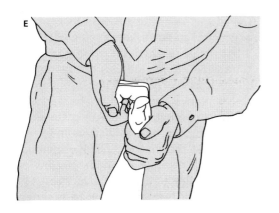

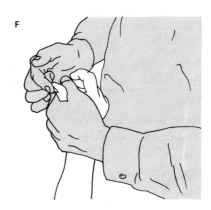

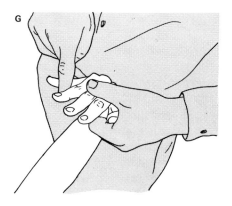

Fig. 6.10 Muscle tests of segmental levels. A shoulder elevators, B deltoids, C biceps, D triceps, E long flexors of the fingers, F flexor pollicus longus, G interrossei and lumbricals

descriptions of tests, the patient is referred to in the feminine and the physiotherapist in the masculine.

Tests for segmental levels

C4 *The scapular elevators*. This is best done in sitting. The physiotherapist stands behind and places his hands on the patient's shoulder girdles. He asks the patient to shrug her shoulders as high as possible, then he gradually increases downward pressure on the shoulders (Fig. 6.10.A).

C5 *Deltoids*. The physiotherapist stands by the patients side with her shoulder in thirty degrees of abduction. Using his body weight, he asks the patient to 'hold against me' (Fig. 6.10B).

C6 *Biceps*. Biceps strength is best tested with the elbow in greater than 90° of extension. It is often too strong in its inner ranges to be tested accurately. On retesting, the same starting range should be used (Fig. 6.10C).

C7 *Triceps*. Triceps is best tested with the elbow more flexed (Fig. 6.10D). Note, in both biceps and triceps testing, the physiotherapist's body weight is strategically placed to assist with testing.

C8 *Long finger flexors*. Care is required with testing muscle power in the hand. It is easy for the patient to cheat. The patient is asked to fold her fingers in while the physiotherapist holds the fingertips. He then tries to straighten the

fingers out (Fig. 6.10E). Extension of the interphalangeal joint of the thumb can also be used. The physiotherapist places his hand and thumb around the patient's thumb and thenar eminence, thus blocking the carpometacarpal and metacarpophalangeal movements. With one finger on the patients nail, he asks her to push her thumb tip towards her head (Fig. 6.10F). I feel this is a more sensitive test than the test using all the fingers.

T1 *Interrossei and lumbricals*. These are best observed by asking the patient to fully spread her fingers. For stronger grades, the patient is asked to 'make a platform' by flexing the metacarpophalangeal joints to ninety degrees with the interphalangeal joints extended. This position is supported as in Figure 6.10G and the examiner then places a finger between each of her fingers and asks her to 'hold my finger as hard as you can' while he tries to pull it from her grip.

Tests for individual nerve trunks

Any muscle or muscle group can be tested and the results used as part of the overall process of determining the source of the weakness. Greater detail is given in muscle testing manuals such as Kendall et al (1971) and Daniels & Worthingham (1972).

Radial nerve. The patient's wrist is extended and this position held resisted. The tendons of extensor carpi radialis and extensor carpi ulnaris can be palpated for firmness while the wrist is extended.

Median nerve. The patient flexes the distal interphalangeal joint of the index finger. The physiotherapist supports this position with one hand and then resists the movement with his own index finger.

Ulnar nerve. This can be examined by testing resisted abduction of the index finger or by observing the contraction of the first dorsal interrosseus muscle. Wasting in the hypothenar eminence may be evident.

Other nerves. The rhomboids (dorsal scapular nerve) and serratus anterior (long thoracic nerve) can also be tested. A winged scapula may be the result of a nerve injury to muscle rather than a muscle injury.

Quick tests and tests for the patient

For the median nerve, the patient tries to make an 'O' with the thumb and index finger. With weakness of the flexor digitorum longus, the patient can only manage a pear shape (Fig. 6.11). If there is an obvious movement that the patient cannot perform, this should be pointed out to the patient and improving it made a goal for the patient. The lateral key pinch test (Fig. 6.12) is a useful test of the ulnar innervated first dorsal interosseus muscle.

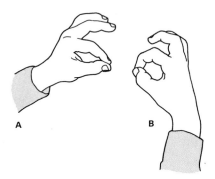

Fig. 6.11 'Pears and oranges'

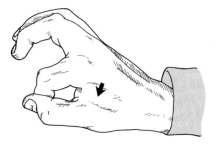

Fig. 6.12 Lateral key pinch test

Muscle testing lower limb

L2 Hip flexors. The physiotherapist holds his hands around the patient's thigh and then asks her to start holding against his increasing pressure until she is using all her strength. He then assesses the strength (Fig. 6.13A) As in all tests a comparison is made with the other side.

L3 Knee extensors. The physiotherapist places the patient's knee over his knee and then encourages her to straighten her knee as hard as

possible. The physiotherapist then tries to break the hold (Fig. 6.13B). The muscle can also be tested through the last 30° of knee extension where the knee can generate more power.

L4 Ankle dorsiflexors. The patient is asked to dorsiflex her ankles. The tendon of tibialis anterior can be palpated for firmness. The patient is then asked to hold the dorsiflexion position while the physiotherapist tries to pull her feet towards plantarflexion. This is best achieved by putting his hands between her feet and pulling down and out (Fig. 6.13C).

L5,S1 Extensors of the distal phalanx of the great toe. The patient maximally dorsiflexes her ankles and then her great toes. The physiotherapist places the tips of his index fingers on the great toenails and asks the patient to 'hold against me'. It is then advisable to change hands and perform the test using the opposite hand to eliminate any left or right side bias in strength of the physiotherapist. (Fig. 6.13D). Like the tendon of tibialis anterior, the tendon of extensor hallucis longus can be palpated for alterations in tension. Extension of the toes (L5, S1) can also be tested (Fig. 6.13E).

S1 Everters of the ankle. The patient places her heels together. The physiotherapist places his hands on the outside of her feet and asks her to turn her feet out. Hand placing will be necessary to stop any plantarflexion.

S1,2 Ankle plantarflexors. This is best done in standing as the calf muscles are normally too strong to test in lying. The organised physiotherapist will have done this test before asking the patient to lie down for other tests or treatment. The patient stands on one foot, the physiotherapist assists with balance and the patient goes up onto her toes as far as she can. This should be repeated for both feet at least six times. Lots of verbal encouragement is needed to ensure that the patient goes to the full plantar flexion position. Watch for signs of fatigue. If there is suspicion that the muscle is only slightly weak, ask the patient to go up on her toes more times.

S2 Toe flexors. The physiotherapist places the tips of his fingers on the pads of the patient's toes and asks her to 'bend your toes under'. He then tries to put the toes into dorsiflexion while the patient resists (Fig. 6.13F).

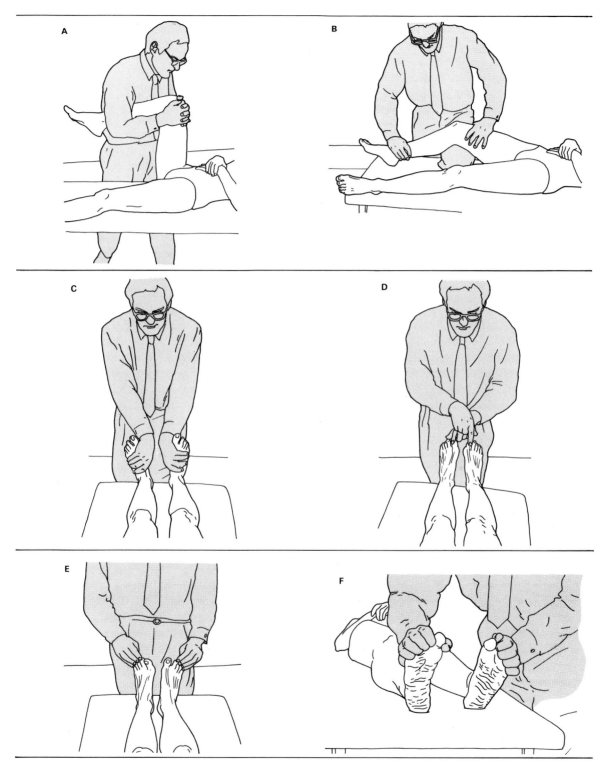

Fig. 6.13 Muscle testing in the lower limb. A hip flexors, B quadriceps, C ankle dorsiflexion, D the great toe extensors, E toe extension, F toe flexion

Quick tests and tests for the patient

Walking on the heels is a good test of the strength of the dorsiflexors whereas walking on the toes tests the calf strength. These are good functional tests that the patient can use as a self reassessment. In cases of severer paralysis there may be other functional signs useful for the patient and physiotherapist. For example, with weakness of the hip flexors, lifting the thigh in sitting is a useful test and is easily repeatable each time the patient attends for treatment. Patients can be taught to measure their own quadriceps lag in sitting and compare it with the opposite limb.

FURTHER TESTING AND ANALYSIS

Tests of the autonomic nervous system

Physiotherapists can only test a very small part of the functions of the autonomic nervous system. Detailed testing requires specialised equipment.

In the early stages of sympathetic involvement, vasomotor instability results from sympathetic hyperactivity. Redness, warmth and sweating may be noted. In later stages there may be pain on movement although the oedema and vasomotor changes may have settled (Mackinnon & Dellon 1988). Complete sympathetic lesions result in the absence of sweating, however, partial changes will result in excess sweating (Bickerstaff & Spillane 1989)

Horner's syndrome results from a lack of sympathetic input to the eye. On the affected side, the pupil is constricted, the eyelid droops and sweating is lost. Possible sites of sympathetic interference are in the brainstem, the cord and the cervical sympathetic trunk. Lesions in the thoracic spine can cause Horner's syndrome (Mathers 1985).

Tinel's sign

Tinel (1915) described this simple test whereby a peripheral nerve is tapped. 'Tingling' so emitted was indicative of axonal regeneration. The test is a useful reassessment sign but care needs to be taken in interpretation. Its use is limited to where nerves are superficial (see Ch. 9) and it is quite frequently positive in normal subjects (Dellon 1984). Phalen (1966) promoted use of the test as part of the diagnosis of carpal tunnel syndrome. Seror (1987) reviewed the literature on the use of the test in carpal tunnel syndrome and found that it was positive in 58% of the total tested (although expressing some doubts about what various authors considered a positive test). Dellon (1984) pointed out that in many cases of carpal tunnel syndrome, there are no regenerating axons either because the injury is too severe or, quite possibly, because degenerative axons are not the source.

Staging the disorder

The neurological examination findings can be interpreted further than just the assignment of an involved segmental level. The stage of the disorder may be ascertained. Weakness is the first finding in motor nerve conduction alteration. Wasting due to loss of innervation may be at a later stage and implies a loss or degeneration of nerve fibres. Mackinnon & Dellon (1988) make the analogies in the sensory system. Early on in nerve compression, a hypersensitive response may be present. Later, with increasing nerve compression, sensation is decreased. The first sensation to alter is the appreciation of vibration.

TESTS OF CORD FUNCTION

Subjective examination

Severe upper motor neurone disorders are easily evident by spasticity, gross altered movement patterns and paralysis. For the less severe cord disorders there are clues that can alert the physiotherapist to the presence of 'cord signs' or raise the index of suspicion about possible spinal cord involvement.

1. Bilateral pins and needles in the extremities. This is not a definite indicator of cord dysfunction as it is possible to have bilateral nerve root compression or bilateral lower limb entrapment. Pins and needles in all four extremities would raise the index of suspicion. Some patients with cord injuries may report a feeling of walking on cotton wool.

2. In cervical spondylotic myelopathy, Clark (1988) has described loss of dexterity in the upper extremity, abnormal sensations in the hand and diffuse non-specific weakness. He also notes a broad based, jerky gait.

3. Lhermitte sign may be present. With flexion and extension of the neck, the patient may complain of a generalised electric shock in the body.

Physical tests of cord function

Some confusion can arise because a patient may have upper as well as lower motor neurone involvement. There are two essential tests, ankle clonus and the Babinski test.

1. Ankle clonus. To test for clonus, the physiotherapist bends the patient's knee a little and then rapidly dorsiflexes the ankle (Fig. 6.14). If positive, a strong 'cogwheel type' rigidity is elicited.

2. Babinski test. The Babinski sign is part of the primitive flexion reflex. If present after 12–16 months it indicates some form of dysfunction of the motor area of the brain or the corticospinal tracts and thus loss of suppression of the flexion reflex. It is an important test and if normal, provides good evidence that the corticospinal system is functioning normally (Van Allen & Rodnitzky 1981). An applicator stick, the blunt end of a pen, or the end of a reflex hammer can be used (Fig. 6.15). The Mayo Clinic (1981) suggests that if an abnormal response is not achieved, and if cord involvement is sus-

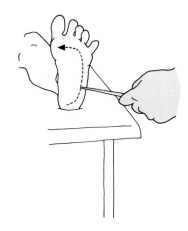

Fig. 6.15 The Babinski test

pected, the technique can be done using a sharp and unpleasant stimulus such as a nail file. The normal response is flexion and adduction of the toes. An abnormal response is dorsiflexion of the great toe and fanning of the others. This test is also rather ticklish, and there are people who will not allow adequate testing. Stroking the lateral aspect of the foot below the malleolus (Chaddock reflex), squeezing the calf, or running the examiner's fingers down the shin (Oppenheim reflex) may evoke a response (Mayo clinic 1981, Van Allen & Rodnitzky 1981).

The sign of Babinski is reported as present or absent.

ELECTRODIAGNOSIS

This is a brief introduction to the uses and pitfalls of the main forms of electrodiagnosis. References giving further details of these tests are given.

Uses, advantages and disadvantages of electrodiagnosis

Some authors have questioned the value of electrodiagnosis in peripheral nerve injuries (Sunderland 1978, Mackinnon & Dellon 1988). There is the problem that exists where a patient has a normal nerve conduction test (NCT), yet symptoms persist, and doubts creep in as to the organic basis of the patient' complaints. Electrodiagnosis cannot be taken a true indicator of the underlying disorder. If used, results must be taken

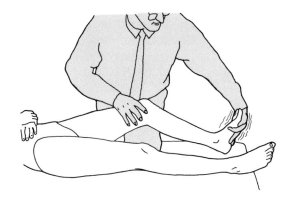

Fig. 6.14 Testing for clonus

along with clinical findings. Further details on testing procedures and analysis may be found in Haldeman (1983), Kimura (1983), Robertson (1985), Peterson & Will (1988), Lieberman & Taylor (1989), Taylor & Lieberman (1989). Electrodiagnosis may be useful for:

1. Deciding whether a neuropathy is from a peripheral nerve or is actually a myopathy
2. Diagnosis of systemic conditions such as alcoholic or diabetic neuropathy
3. Guidance in possible recovery of a severe nerve injury and assisting with the timing of surgical intervention. Tests may help in staging of nerve compression hence prognosis of decompression operations
4. Providing an objective measurement by which treatment results can be compared and thus may form part of clinical research. Difficulties will be encountered with the more minor nerve injuries that physiotherapists encounter
5. Identification of some anomalies in neuroanatomy.

There are some difficulties and pitfalls with electrodiagnosis, which are discussed below.

1. Technical. NCT requires that one electrode can be placed proximal to the compression site. With compression close to the neuraxis this may not be possible. There are also technical problems such as deep nerves (e.g., ulnar nerve in the forearm) for surface stimulation, and difficulties stimulating one nerve without stimulating an adjacent nerve. Variations in technique and interpretation occur and normal values vary between laboratories (Kimura 1984).

2. Anatomical and physiological. There are variations in skin thicknesses overlying nerves that may interfere with results. Measurable alteration may not occur for some weeks following a partial nerve injury. The temperature of a nerve effects conduction. Cooling causes slowing of conduction velocities and a prolongation of latencies (Kimura 1983). Latencies are longer and conduction slows past the age of 60 (Peterson & Will, 1988). Anomalies in neuroanatomy are very common and may lead to confusing results.

3. Problems associated with pathology.

The tests are not sensitive enough to pick up early and minor alterations in nerve conduction. Of course, the tests do not measure the extent of any neural connective tissue pathology. Proximal nerve injuries may appear to be more distal lesions on the basis of EMG and nerve conduction studies. With multiple nerve injuries such as from trauma, disease such as diabetes, or a double or multiple crush syndrome, testing for a mononeuropathy can clearly be misleading (Peterson & Will 1988).

The 'normal' electrodiagnostic test result on a patient with pain associated with tension tests and a history that infers neural involvement presents a clinical paradox not uncommonly encountered by physiotherapists. Mackinnon & Dellon (1988) take up this issue and urge clinical correlation and consideration of more minor entrapments when examining the results of electrodiagnosis. In support, they cite two studies. First, Louis & Hankin (1987) found that patients with carpal tunnel syndrome and normal electrodiagnostic studies but abnormal clinical findings do well with surgery decompressing the carpal tunnel. A second study (Spindler & Dellon 1982) correlated detailed electrodiagnostic studies with a neurosensory evaluation for the carpal tunnel syndrome. The electrical and clinical evaluations were in disagreement in 70% of the cases of early carpal tunnel syndrome, 64% in moderate and 30% in severe nerve compression. The likely basis for this situation is uneven fascicular pathology. There may be a pathological fascicle yet the tests are testing a normal fascicle. Tests cannot be fascicle specific (Mackinnon & Dellon 1988). This suggestion is supported by clinical findings of variable manifestations of median nerve compression such as severe sensory loss but no motor loss (Mackinnon et al 1987). Similarly, an EMG test can only sample a few muscle fibres around the tip of the needle. There does not have to be a particular site of entrapment. Multiple constraints on axoplasmic flow along the entire nerve could be responsible for changes in a measured target tissue such as muscle.

One interesting thought that arises is the position of the patient during the test. Theoretically, in a normal person, conduction should be the same;

the desired afferent and efferent impulses should be available no matter what physiological position the body is in. The advice given in the nerve conduction manuals on positioning the patient is often confusing and contradictory. Bielawski & Hallett (1989) measured motor conduction velocities in the ulnar nerve across the elbow in patients selected for possible ulnar nerve abnor-malities unrelated to motor conduction. They found no major differences in velocities from flexion to extension. This is not surprising as the nerves could have been normal. However, if the nervous system was abnormal with a mechani-cally sensitive abnormal impulse generating site, which was put on stretch, then it may show up electrodiagnostically.

REFERENCES

Beatty S E, Phillips J E, Mackinnon et al 1987 Vibratory sensory testing in acute compartment syndrome: a clinical and experimental study. Plastic and Reconstructive Surgery 79: 796–801

Bickerstaff E R, Spillane J A 1989 Neurological examination in clinical practice, 5th edn. Blackwell, Oxford

Bielawski M, Hallet M 1989 Position of the elbow in determination of abnormal motor conduction of the ulnar nerve across the elbow. Muscle & Nerve 12: 803–809

Bohannon R W, Gajdosik R L 1987 Spinal nerve root compression: some clinical implications. Physical Therapy 67: 376–382

Bolton C F, Winkelmann R K, Dyck P J 1966 A quantitative study of Meissner's corpuscles in man. Neurology (Minneap) 16: 1–9

Clark C R 1988 Cervical spondylotic myelopathy: history and physical findings. Spine 13: 847–849

Daniels L, Worthingham C 1972 Muscle testing, 3rd edn. Saunders, Philadelphia

Dellon A L 1984 Tinel or not Tinel? Journal of Hand Surgery 9B: 216

Haldeman S 1983 The electrodiagnostic evaluation of nerve root function. Spine 9: 42–48

Kendall H O, Kendall F P, Wadsworth G E 1971 Muscle testing and function. Baltimore, Williams & Wilkins

Kerr A T 1918 The brachial plexus of nerves in man: the variations in its formations and its branches. American Journal of Anatomy 23: 285

Kimura J 1983 Electrodiagnosis in diseases of nerves and muscles. Davis, Philadelphia

Kimura J 1984 Principles and pitfalls of nerve conduction studies. Annals of Neurology 16: 415–429

Lieberman J S, Taylor R G 1989 Electrodiagnosis in upper extremity nerve compression. In: Szabo R M (ed) Nerve compression syndromes. Slack, Thorofare

Louis D S, Hankin F M 1987 Symptomatic relief following carpal tunnel decompression with normal electroneuromyographic studies. Orthopaedics 10: 434–436

Mackinnon S E et al 1987 Chronic human nerve compression: a histological assessment. Neuropathology and Applied Neurobiology 12: 547–565

Mackinnon S E, Dellon A L 1988 Surgery of the peripheral nerve. Thieme, New York

Maitland G D 1986 Vertebral manipulation, 5th ed. Butterworths, London

Mathers L H 1985 The peripheral nervous system. Butterworths, Boston Mayo Clinic 1981 Clinical examinations in neurology, 5th ed. Saunders, Philadelphia

McLeod J C, Lance J W 1989 Introductory neurology, 2nd ed. Blackwell, Melbourne

Peterson G W, Will A D 1988 Newer electrodiagnostic techniques in peripheral nerve injuries. Orthopaedic Clinics of North America 19: 13–25

Phalen G S 1966 The carpal tunnel syndrome: seventeen years experience in diagnosis and treatment of 654 hands. The Journal of Bone and Joint Surgery 48A: 211–228

Phillips J H, Mackinnon S E, Dellon A L et al 1987 Vibratory sensory testing in acute compartment syndromes: a clinical and experimental study. Plastic and Reconstructive Surgery 79: 796–801

Robertson K B 1985 Electrodiagnosis in neurological rehabilitation. In: Umphred D A (ed) Neurological rehabilitation. Mosby, St. Louis

Seddon H 1972 Surgical disorders of the peripheral nerve. Williams & Wilkins, Baltimore.

Seror P 1987 Tinel's sign in the diagnosis of carpal tunnel syndrome. The Journal of Hand Surgery 12B: 364–365

Spindler H A, Dellon A L 1982 Nerve conduction studies and sensibility testing in carpal tunnel syndrome. Journal of Hand Surgery 7: 260–263

Sunderland S 1978 Nerves and nerve injuries, 2nd ed. Churchill Livingstone, Edinburgh

Szabo R M, Gelberman R H, Williamson R V et al 1984 Vibratory sensory testing in acute peripheral nerve compression. Journal of Hand Surgery 9A: 104–108

Taylor R G, Lieberman J S, 1989 Electrodiagnosis in upper extremity nerve compression. In: Szabo R M (ed) Nerve compression syndromes. Slack, Thorofare

Tinel J 1915 Le signe du fourmillement dans les lesions des nerfs peripheriques. La Presse Medicale 47: 388–389

Torg J S, Pavlov H, Genuario S E et al 1986 Neuropraxia of the cervical spinal cord with transient quadriplegia. Journal of Bone and Joint Surgery 68A: 1354–1370

Van Allen M W, Rodnitzky 1981 Pictorial manual of neurological tests: a guide to the performance and interpretation of the neurological examination, 2nd edn. Year book, Chicago

Wohlfart G 1959 Clinical considerations on innervation of skeletal muscle. Americal Journal of Physical Medicine 38: 223–230

7. Tension testing — the lower limbs and trunk

THE CONCEPT OF BASE TENSION TESTS

Tension tests such as the Straight Leg Raise (SLR), Prone Knee Bend (PKB) and Passive Neck Flexion (PNF) are familiar and established components of a neuro-orthopaedic examination. These traditional tests and some relatively new tension tests are suggested as base tests. Because the nervous system forms a complex mesh throughout the body, a system of easily repeatable base tests, with known normative responses, is needed for routine examination, and as a starting point to examine further. Examination and treatment will often involve derivations of these tests, for example, hip adduction and medial rotation may be added to the base test of the SLR. The base tests are:

- Passive Neck Flexion (PNF)
- Straight Leg Raise (SLR)
- Slump Test
- Prone Knee Bend (PKB)
- Upper Limb Tension Tests (ULTT) 1, 2 and 3.

It would be useful to have a tension test for each of the major nerves in the body such as 'the median nerve tension test', but this is not possible. In addition to the complexity of the nervous system mesh, anomalies and interconnections are very common and with the addition of pathologies to such a complex system, enormous variations in the clinical presentations are possible. Hence, while the base tests may have a bias towards a particular nerve trunk, in most situations it is difficult to say they are a definite test for that particular segment of nervous system. This is especially so in the upper limb where the neuroanatomy is more complex than in the lower limb.

The base tests have been kept as simple as possible. This not only allows ease of handling and accurate repetition of the test, it also makes research involving the tests easier.

Handling mastery of the base tests is essential before a physiotherapist can adequately examine, using derivations of the tests. As well as the descriptions of the tests in the next two chapters, there is a section in Chapter 9 entitled 'keys to better tension testing'.

The notation used to describe combinations of movement is the 'IN: DID:' system. For example, if dorsiflexion of the ankle was performed with the leg in hip adduction and Straight Leg Raise, this would read 'IN: SLR/H Ad DID: DF'. This method allows recording of the sequence of additional sensitising tests. In the example, dorsiflexion was added last. Recording is discussed in greater detail in Chapter 9.

Each base test is described under the headings of:

1. History of the test
2. Method. The method described is for a non-irritable condition where examination can be taken to the end of range and is not limited by the severity or irritability of the presenting disorder. Tension testing the irritable disorder and aspects of analysis of tension testing are discussed in Chapter 9. That chapter is essential associated reading

3. Normal responses to the test
4. Indications for performing the test
5. Commonly used variations and sensitising tests
6. Pertinent biomechanics of the nervous system involved in the test.

In the descriptions of tests, the patient is 'she' and the physiotherapist 'he' for convenience of description.

Information needed from all tension tests

The following information should be elicited from all tension tests:

1. The symptom response. Useful information is the range at which symptoms start (P1), what those symptoms are (eg., pain, paraesthesia), whether the symptoms are the ones that the patient complains of, and what the symptoms are at the limit of range (P2).

2. The resistance encountered. Useful information is when range resistance is first encountered (R1) and when resistance stops any further movement (R2). The behaviour of resistance (eg., abrupt increase or gradual increase) during the movement should also be noted.

3. An assessment of both the symptom responses and the resistance must be made after each component of a tension test is added or subtracted. These issues are discussed in detail in Chapter 9.

PASSIVE NECK FLEXION

History

O'Connell (1946) lists the Passive Neck Flexion sign of Brudzinski (1909) as one of the clinical signs of meningitis. Troup (1986) described Passive Neck Flexion in sitting and in combination with the Straight Leg Raise. PNF is an important base test and should always be considered as a test that stands alone as well as in combination with other tests.

Method

A standard position is employed for all tests and

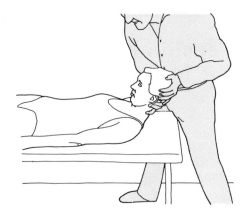

Fig. 7.1 Passive neck flexion

retests. The patient's arms are by her sides and her legs together.

The patient lies supine, preferably without a pillow. The physiotherapist asks the patient to lift her head off the bed a little and then he takes over, passively flexing the neck in a 'chin on chest' direction. One hand may be used to stabilise the chest or both hands can hold her head (Fig. 7.1). As in all tension tests, the symptom responses, range of movement and resistance encountered through movement are noted and analysed.

Normal responses

PNF should be a painless test, although asymptomatic individuals may feel a pulling at the cervico-thoracic junction. This is probably related to joint or muscle rather than the neuraxis or the meningeal tissues. However, differentiation is easy, by maintaining the Passive Neck Flexion and adding a manoeuvre such as a Straight Leg Raise. The basis of structural differentiation was discussed in Chapter 5 and is discussed further in Chapter 9.

Indications

PNF is indicated for all possible spinal disorders. It may also be indicated for headache symptoms and for arm and leg pain of possible spinal origin. I feel it can be an easily forgotten tension test and, in many situations, it is not 'cleared' for lumbar disorders when the SLR may well be. It is often forgotten as a test for thoracic symptoms.

A study by Troup (1981) has clearly shown its importance. Troup (1981) reported PNF to be positive in 22% of all cases of back and sciatic pain seen in an industrial survey and in 35% who were referred to hospital. These figures come from testing neck flexion in sitting. However, a positive PNF for lumbar/sciatic pain is regularly seen when carried out in supine, and I would think that the figures are comparable to the test being carried out in supine. An advantage of performing a PNF in supine is that other spinal components are neutralised, thus allowing better interpretation of test results. It is also easier to reproduce the same test on different treatment days because the rest of the spine is automatically placed in the same position. Neck flexion in sitting is an integral part of the Slump Tests and, in many patients, the two tests should be carried out separately. The possible differences encountered in testing PNF in sitting and in supine should be apparent after reading Part I of this text.

Variations and sensitising additions

Any neck movement will mechanically influence the nervous system and could be considered a tension test. For example, passive neck extension and neck lateral flexion, or a combination of lateral flexion, and rotation, may well be useful tests of adverse tension. Once a desired response is found, the most common additional sensitising manoeuvres are the addition of Straight Leg Raise or an Upper Limb Tension Test. Alternatively, PNF is also a sensitising component of the ULTTs and SLR. Less commonly, PNF can be added to the PKB. The patient needs to be in sidelying for this particular technique, described later in the chapter.

The flexion component can be taken further by adding upper thoracic flexion to the PNF. The physiotherapist needs to slide his hand down to the thoracic level that needs flexing (Fig. 7.2). With this test, it is still possible to move only the neuraxis and meninges in the lumbar spine with negligible effect on the non-neural structures.

In some patients, the flexion component can

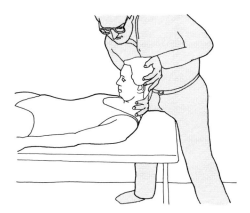

Fig. 7.2 Passive neck/upper thoracic flexion

be broken down into upper cervical flexion or lower cervical flexion. The responses may be different depending on the site of the adverse tension.

Passive neck movements should not be/limited to flexion. Passive Neck Extension (PNE), while not performed routinely, is a useful test. This is especially so if there is a high level of suspicion of adverse tension in a disorder, or the subjective complaints of the patient indicate that cervical extension is an involved movement in the disorder. The nervous system still has to adapt to shortening of the spinal canal and this adaptation to extension may be symptomatic. The patient is asked to move to the end of the bed, and with

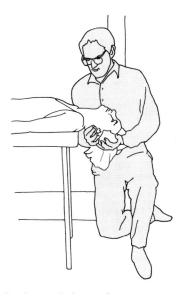

Fig. 7.3 Passive cervical extension

the examiner supporting the head, the patient is asked to carefully wriggle so the cervico-thoracic junction is over the end of the bed. Cervical extension is then occiput to thoracic spine (Fig. 7.3). This is also a good position to examine upper and lower cervical extension plus neck retraction. The effect of cervical extension on any other tension test, such as the SLR or the Upper Limb Tension Test, may be tested if required.

Biomechanics

The effects of passively flexing the neck are not limited to the cervical and upper thoracic spine. There is some experimental support for Troup's (1981) clinical study, and our common finding that PNF can alter lumbar symptoms. It has been shown in cadaver studies that, by passively flexing the neck, the neuraxis and the meninges in the lumbar spine and in part of the sciatic tract are moved and tensioned also (Breig & Marions 1963, Breig 1978, Tencer et al 1985). Since there is no tension on the nervous system at the 'other end', i.e., the sciatic tract and lumbosacral nerve roots are relatively slack, movement of the neuro-meningeal tissues is allowed. Less movement is likely, but more tension will be developed, if the PNF is performed with the leg or legs in a SLR position. This feature has been discussed and illustrated in Chapter 2. Extension creates less tension throughout the tract, but surely, will allow some migration of the tract. This migration may be symptomatic, for example, if a sensitive segment of dural sleeve moves onto a osteophyte or disc bulge.

As PNF and its variations allow some alteration in the nervous system in the lumbar spine without moving other lumbar structures such as zygapophyseal joints, sacroiliac joints and erector spinae muscles, this is a diagnostic bonus. If PNF reproduces lumbar pain, it can be inferred that the source of that pain lies within the nervous system (for example, arachnoiditis or scarred dura) or in a pathological relationship with the structures to which it is attached.

STRAIGHT LEG RAISE

History

The origins of the SLR are somewhat unclear and disputed. Dyck (1984) has given an interesting historical overview. According to Dyck's interpretation of the literature, the first person to recognise that pain produced on straight leg raising was due to the sciatic nerve was a Serbian, Lazar Lazarevic, in 1880. Most textbooks refer to the initiator of the test as Leseague in 1864, with the test brought into prominence by his pupil, Forst. Leseague, however, referred to the pain from a SLR as coming from compression of the sciatic nerve by the hamstrings. Lazarevic also demonstrated that dorsiflexion of the foot intensified patients' sciatica and that the same manoeuvre would increase the tension in the sciatic tract in a cadaver. If the mechanics of the SLR are interfered with, the resultant inability to extend the leg is so obvious in many activities that it must have been noticed by laymen as well as doctors throughout the centuries. Indeed, there are reports around the year 2800 BC suggesting that extension of the legs should be used to examine sprained vertebrae (Beasley 1982).

The term 'Straight Leg Raise' has far wider use and merit than 'Leseague's test' or even 'Lazarevic's test'. The test, such as Forst described and named 'Leseague's test', whereby the extended leg is lifted to a pain response and then the knee flexed to see if the pain ceased, is probably one of the first described methods of differentiation, in this case between the hip joint and sciatica. If pain ceased, sciatica was the diagnosis (Fig. 7.4 A,B).

Method

The patient lies supine, relaxed and comfortable on the examination bed, towards the side of the examiner. The trunk and hips should be in a neutral position. The examiner places one hand under the Achilles tendon and the other above the knee. The leg is lifted perpendicular to the bed, with the hand above the knee preventing any knee flexion. The leg should be lifted as a solid lever moving at a fixed point in the hip joint. (Fig. 7.5). This simple, easily reproducible straight lift is the protocol suggested by Breig & Troup (1979). The leg is then taken to a predetermined symptom response or range of movement. As in all tension testing, range, symptom response and resistance encountered through the

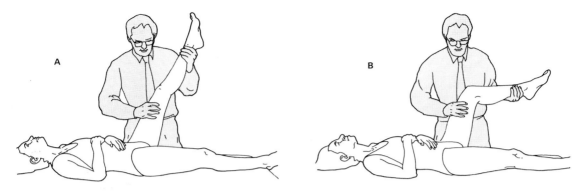

Fig. 7.4 The Leseague sign according to Forst. In A, hip area pain provoked by the SLR could be from the hip joint or the sciatic nerve. In B, if knee flexion decreased the pain, the sciatic nerve is culpable because the hip joint structures have not been altered

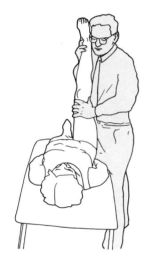

Fig. 7.5 The SLR test

movement are noted. These responses are then compared to the SLR of the other leg, and to what is considered normal (see below). If possible, a pillow should not be used under the head, but if a pillow is necessary, the same pillow should be used in later retesting. Given the difference that cervical position can make on the SLR range and pain response (Lew & Peuntedura 1985), this is essential for accurate reassessment. Some examples of situations where a pillow or two might be used are fixed flexion deformities, and severe pain in extension.

Normal responses

The normal responses to a SLR vary widely. Troup (1986) suggested that the normal range of

SLR in healthy individuals is between 50°–120°. Sweetman et al (1974) examined the SLR in 500 post office workers aged between 22 and 63 years, finding a minimum of 56°, a maximum of 115° and a mean of 83.4°. There is also a group of hypermobile individuals whose SLR would exceed this range, but still must be considered normal. A degree measurement by itself is of little clinical use as Troup (1986) acknowledges. It must be interpreted along with the symptom response, the SLR range of the contralateral limb and the overall patient presentation. The range of SLR may also show a diurnal variation (Gifford 1987). Miller (1987) and Slater (1989) examined the SLR in 100 and 49 'normal' individuals respectively. The results were similar. The three main symptom areas in normals were posterior thigh, posterior knee, and posterior calf into the foot.

There may be some postural responses during the SLR worth assessing. Some patients, even those asymptomatic to the SLR, may extend, flex, or laterally flex their neck. The hip of the contralateral leg may extend. These responses should be noted.

Indications

The SLR is probably the key tension test. So much information can be gleaned from it; and it is far more than a mere test to assess whether a low lumbar discogenic problem is interfering with the biomechanics of the nervous system. The SLR is routine for all spinal and leg symptoms as it tests aspects of nervous system mechanics from the toes to the brain, including the sympathetic trunk. This includes headache and foot symptoms, although further sensitising tests will probably be needed in these cases. Where there has been severe trauma or where a disorder is deemed irritable, a SLR, or components of it such as dorsiflexion, or knee extension in some hip flexion, should also be performed for upper limb symptoms. The nervous system link between the upper and lower limb has been discussed in Part I.

Variations and sensitising additions

Although the SLR is usually performed in supine, there may be situations which require testing in side lying. It should be noted that the normal responses will be slightly different in sidelying, perhaps due to the side flexion of the lumbar spine (Miller 1987). It is also possible to do a form of SLR in prone, this being a useful position to palpate the sciatic nerve in the buttock while the sciatic tract is on tension (see Ch. 9). In this technique, the patient moves to the side of the bed and the leg is lowered.

All variations to the test can be named by the movements and the sequence of addition of the movements such as HF/KE (IN: hip flexion DID: knee extension).

The most commonly used and useful sensitising additions are:

- ankle dorsiflexion
- ankle plantar flexion inversion
- hip adduction
- hip medial rotation
- passive neck flexion.

There are two ways of including a sensitising addition into a tension test. The movement could be included first (DF/SLR), or at a certain range of the SLR, the sensitising addition could be included (SLR/DF). The differences between these two ways is discussed in Chapter 3 and Chapter 9. Essentially, the best response will be gained if movements at the site of tension are taken up first.

Combinations of sensitising additions may be useful. For example the SLR could be performed with hip adduction and medial rotation.

Ankle dorsiflexion (DF)

The addition of dorsiflexion will add further tension along the tibial tract (Lazarevic 1884, MacNab 1971, Breig & Troup 1979). Dorsiflexion can be added first and then the limb lifted, or it can be added at the limit of SLR. I find that placing the limb on my shoulder, using one hand to maintain extension and then using the other hand to dorsiflex the foot as in Figure 7.6, is the most useful. Another suggested method, perhaps more useful for the patient with a small leg, is shown in Figure 7.7. Note that the knee extension is maintained by the examiner's forearm down the shaft of the tibia. When performing a SLR, dorsiflexion added first would be useful if dorsiflexion with the leg in neutral caused a relevant symptom, say in the Achilles tendon region. If this

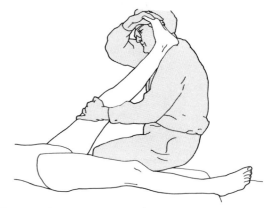

Fig. 7.6 SLR/Dorsiflexion

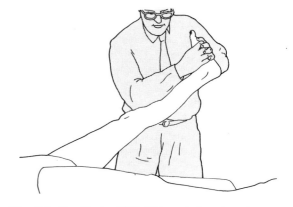

Fig. 7.7 Dorsiflexion/SLR. This technique lets the examiner keep two hands on the foot and maintain the knee extension by their forearm

position was maintained and the addition of SLR made this symptom worse, then a nervous system component to the disorder would be apparent. The Achilles tendon had not been moved, only the hip. Dorsiflexion added to the SLR would be a useful sensitiser if it could alter a spinal symptom provoked by the SLR.

SLR/DF can be further sensitised by everting the foot, extending the toes and stretching the plantar fascia. This will place more tension along the tibial tract. Eversion of the ankle when in SLR/DF is a powerful yet unreported sensitising movement. Logically, it places more tension along the tibial tract. Another useful combination using dorsiflexion is to place the foot in SLR/DF and then to add inversion (SLR/DF/INV). This places tension along the sural nerve and is probably localised enough to call it the 'sural nerve tension test'. I feel that the sural nerve is a forgotten nerve and is responsible for far more symptoms than it is given credit for (see Ch. 12).

Ankle plantarflexion/inversion (PF/I)

PF/I will add tension along the common peroneal tract (Nobel 1966, Sunderland 1978, Borges et al 1981, Styf 1988, Slater 1989). Like dorsiflexion, PF/I may be added before the SLR or at the completion of the SLR. If PF/I is taken up first, the technique shown in Figure 7.8 is effective. Here, the foot position can be stabilised with two hands while the examiner's forearm maintains the knee extension. In Figure 7.9, the addition of PF/I to a SLR using the shoulder lift technique is shown.

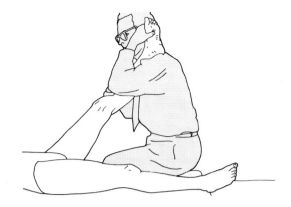

Fig. 7.9 SLR/Plantarflexion/Inversion

The leg is taken to the desired range of SLR and then the PF/I is added. The addition of plantarflexion and inversion to the SLR is of great clinical value in the examination of disorders such as shin splints and chronic ankle sprains.

Hip adduction

This is a powerful sensitising addition to the SLR (Sutton 1979, Breig & Troup 1979). The sciatic tract is lateral to the ischial tuberosity and the addition of adduction to a SLR (or simply adduction in neutral) will add further tension to the nervous system (Fig. 7.10). If a considerable range of adduction has to be examined, the physio-

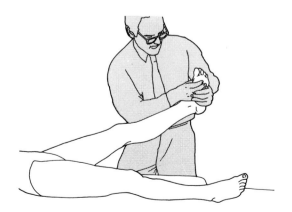

Fig. 7.8 Plantarflexion/Inversion/SLR

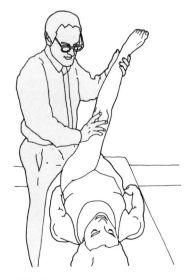

Fig. 7.10 SLR/Hip adduction

therapist may have better control of the test when they stand on the opposite side of the leg being tested. The same range of SLR must be maintained when the hip adduction is added.

Hip medial rotation

The addition of hip medial rotation (Fig. 7.11) will further sensitise the sciatic tract (Breig & Troup 1979). Note in Figure 7.12 that, during the addition of medial rotation with the leg in a neutral position, the nerve root moves cephalad in relation to the interfacing structures rather than the expected caudad, yet the increased tension in the nerve is obvious. This emphasises the elasticity and movement reversibility of the nervous system. It may well be the opposite if the medial rotation is added when the leg is in Straight Leg Raise. What is important is that, clinically, the addition of medial hip rotation to a SLR will often worsen spinal/leg symptoms. It probably sensitises the common peroneal division more than the tibial division of the sciatic nerve.

Cervical flexion/extension

This is a useful addition at 'the other end' (Fig. 7.13). Cyriax (1978) suggested it, and Lew's (1979) normative study and followup study (Lew

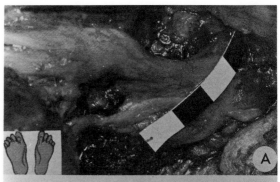
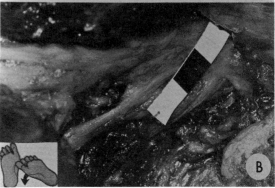

Fig. 7.12 The effect of medial hip rotation on the left sacral plexus. A 4 cm marker has been stitched to the S2 and S3 roots, lying obliquely across the sacral plexus with one end into the greater sciatic foramen. The position of the feet show the leg movement. In B, the slack has been taken up and the end pulled up into the greater sciatic foramen. From: Breig A, Troup J D G 1979 Biomechanical considerations in the straight-leg-raising test. Spine 4: 242–250, with permission from the publishers and authors

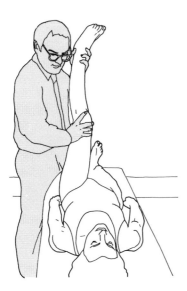

Fig. 7.11 SLR/Hip medial rotation

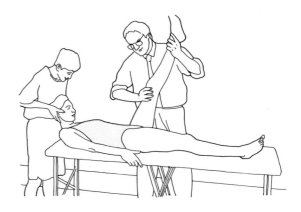

Fig. 7.13 SLR/Cervical flexion with an assistant

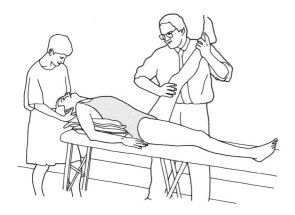

Fig. 7.14 SLR in spinal extension with an assistant

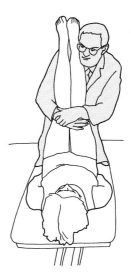

Fig. 7.15 Bilateral Straight Leg Raise

& Peuntedura 1985) showed that the addition of cervical flexion to a SLR would change the symptom response and range of movement of the SLR. Equally, passive neck extension and passive lateral flexions could be useful additions in suitable patients. The SLR responses to the test will be different depending on whether the CF is added before or after the SLR. There is a difficulty with handling here which becomes more obvious as the extent and complexity of tension testing increases, that is, the physical limitations of the physiotherapist. Few physiotherapists have the luxury of an assistant to hold and take up other components of a tension test. With the addition of cervical movement to the SLR, only the largest and most flexible physiotherapist with a small patient will be able to perform Passive Neck Flexion. The alternatives are to get the patient to do it actively, place the patient's head on a pillow first, or seek help.

Cervical extension can also be examined. In Figure 7.14, with the help of an assistant, the effect of cervical extension on the SLR response has been measured. Note also in this figure that the spine has been placed in extension over pillows. With the neuraxis and meninges slack in this position, the SLR responses may be different.

Other Straight Leg Raises

The bowstring test (Macnab 1977) is used by some clinicians. The SLR is taken up to the point of symptom response and then back to a point just short of this response. In this position, the tibial nerve at the knee crease is palpated. If pressure on the nerve at this point makes the symptoms worse, then the test is positive. In a situation where palpation at the posterior aspect of the knee was painful, the bowstring test could be used to see if there was a nervous system component to the symptoms. In a SLR, with the nervous system tightened, these symptoms are likely to be worse.

To perform a Bilateral Straight Leg Raise (BSLR), the examiner kneels on the bed and places the patient's legs on his shoulders and then lifts them perpendicular from the bed (Fig. 7.15). Smaller patients' legs can perhaps be lifted with the examiner standing by the side of the bed, but the physiotherapist should be careful as it can be a heavy and cumbersome test. Once in the BSLR, if the need arises, either of the legs can be further raised.

The crossed SLR is regarded as positive if, in patients with unilateral leg pain, the SLR on the opposite side of their symptoms reproduces the symptoms. The test is also known as 'the well-leg-raising test' This test has been shown to be the best indicator of a disc prolapse (Hudgins 1979, Urban 1985, Khuffash & Porter 1989), presumably because the irritated or adhered dural theca is moved across the bulge or extruded disc material.

Biomechanics

There are many structures moved when a SLR is performed. These include the hamstring muscles, the lumbar spine, hip and sacroiliac joints and fascia, as well as the nervous system. The biomechanics of all these structures are important and pathology involving any of these structures may affect the SLR. This text concentrates on the nervous system.

A SLR moves and tensions the nervous system from the foot and along the neuraxis to the brain (Breig 1978). This includes the lumbar sympathetic trunk (Breig 1978) and, from extrapolation of clinical observations and its anatomy, the sympathetic chain. It also includes the nervous system in the upper limb (Ch. 2). In Chapter 2, the biomechanics of the SLR have been discussed in greater detail, including the concept of tension points and the effects of the sequence of addition of components.

Clinically, the response to a BSLR is usually different to a unilateral SLR. In the unilateral SLR, the dural theca and nerve roots are drawn across the spinal canal, whereas in BSLR such movement will not be allowed because the contralateral leg is already in SLR. BSLR will also flex the lumbar spine more than the unilateral SLR.

PRONE KNEE BEND

History

Upper lumbar radiculopathy is less common than in the lower lumbar spine. Hence the PKB exists as a poor, often forgotten, cousin to the SLR. Credit can be given to Wasserman in 1919, according to Estridge et al (1982), for first suggesting the manoeuvre as a tension test after searching for physical signs to match complaints of anterior thigh and shin pain in soldiers. To further increase tension in the PKB, O'Connell (1946) recommended the inclusion of hip extension. Recently Davidson (1987) performed normative studies of the PKB in varying spinal positions. A PKB may be the same, or not dissimilar, to a quadriceps stretch. The question should arise during all tension testing' 'Just what are the structures being stretched?'

Method

The patient lies prone, towards the side of the physiotherapist, with the head turned towards the physiotherapist. If this position is maintained each time the PKB is tested, the retest will be more valid. The examiner grasps the lower leg and flexes the knee to a predetermined symptom response. As with all testing, range, symptom response and resistance through the movement are noted (Fig. 7.16). The response must be compared to the contralateral PKB.

Normal responses

The responses to the PKB in a large group of asymptomatic volunteers have not been documented. However, from clinical observations, it is possible to flex the knees of most people so that their heel touches their buttocks. The normal symptom response is a pulling or pain in the area of the quadriceps muscle. There are postural responses worth evaluating also. The buttocks may lift or the patient may try to rotate their hips. Of course, the source of this pain and resultant antalgic posture may not necessarily be directly from the nervous system — it could also be from muscle, fascia or from the extension forced

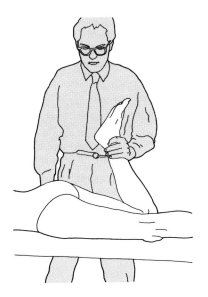

Fig. 7.16 Routine Prone Knee Bend

upon the lumbar spine. Differentiation is not quite as easy as in the SLR. The technique of PKB in the slump position, as described below, is one method of differentiation between structures, as is the use of the 'saphenous nerve tension test'. The physiotherapist will need to rely on subjective clues as well, to allow structural localisation of the source of the limitation.

Indications

The PKB is a recommended routine test for any patient with knee, anterior thigh and hip and upper lumbar symptoms. The variation described below to test the saphenous nerve should be used for symptoms in the saphenous nerve distribution. A PKB is worthwhile testing when SLR is markedly positive. It follows that, if there is marked involvement of the lower lumbar and the sacral nerve roots, then the upper lumbar roots may be secondarily involved. It should also be tested if the patient gives the clue that a similar manoeuvre is responsible for their symptoms. Pain from kneeling and hurdling would be two such examples.

Variations and sensitising additions

Authors such as O'Connell (1943) Macnab (1977), Grieve (1981) and Corrigan and Maitland (1983) have suggested extending the hip with the knee flexed to further sensitise the PKB. However, Davidson (1987) showed in 100 normal asymptomatic volunteers that PKB in neutral was a more sensitive test for the reproduction of symptoms than the PKB with the hip in extension. Clinically, in patients with a 'meralgia paraesthetica' (lateral femoral cutaneous nerve entrapment, see Ch.12), reproduction of their symptoms is often better, using the PKB/HE. It can also be made even more sensitive if the test is done in some hip adduction. Hip extension can be added by placing the flexed knee on a pillow or over the examiner's knee (Fig. 7.17). This variation is probably localised enough to call it the 'lateral femoral cutaneous nerve tension test'.

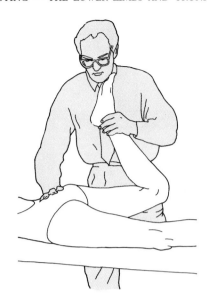

Fig. 7.17 Hip extension/Prone Knee Bend

The PKB can also be performed in hip abduction or adduction and medial or lateral rotation. These manoeuvres appear to cause only minor alterations in tension and movement in normals, but with the addition of pathology, any of these tests may be relevant. The best clues come from the aggravating positions of which the patient complains.

Adding the Slump Test to the PKB (Davidson 1987) is useful and may be a way to allow differentiation of nervous system involvement from non-nervous system structures. Side lying is the best position (Fig. 7.18) and an assistant (preferably experienced) is required. The less ex-

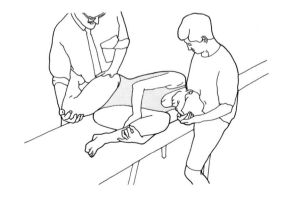

Fig. 7.18 Slump/Prone Knee Bend

perienced operator should take the head end. The patient's trunk and neck must be held in flexion, yet the operator must be in a position to allow neck extension when required. The other examiner then places the foot of the side to be tested on his hip and then flexes the knee. Further hip extension can be added if required. In this position, once the desired response has been achieved, then the 'head end' operator can extend the neck while keeping the spine and leg positions constant. Any alteration in leg symptoms will implicate some involvement of the nervous system. While in this position, confirmation of the response can be made by adding on the cervical flexion again. Davidson (1987) recorded that, in the PKB/Slump position in 40 volunteers, cervical flexion increased the response in 62.5% of asymptomatic volunteers and decreased it in 12.5%. Cervical extension decreased the responses in 20% and increased the responses in 30%.

The femoral nerve continues medial to the knee as the saphenous nerve with a cutaneous supply at about the instep. This makes it evident that the PKB is really a tension test on the upper parts of the femoral nerve by its connections in the quadriceps group of muscles, as Dyck (1976) has suggested. The test probably lessens tension on the saphenous nerve. A femoral/saphenous test can be performed in prone. The extended leg is abducted, the knee is extended and then the hip extended and laterally rotated. In this position, a neat differentiation can be performed by using the ankle. Eversion and dorsiflexion appear to be the most sensitive additions, although the saphenous nerve does have a wayward distribution and plantarflexion may well mechanically sensitise the saphenous tract (Fig. 7.19).

The addition of ankle dorsiflexion and ankle plantar flexion/inversion to the PKB position will often alter the traditional PKB response, especially when there is some pathology along the tract. It is difficult to analyse why this happens since, anatomically, the nervous system connections cannot be tightened. Perhaps further tension is placed on the femoral nerve in the thigh via fascial tracts.

Like the SLR, it may be useful to perform a bilateral PKB. The ranges of knee flexion can

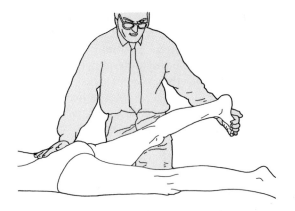

Fig. 7.19   The saphenous nerve tension test

be easily compared. The pain responses are likely to be different from the unilateral PKB.

Biomechanics

The saphenous nerve runs behind the axis of knee flexion and extension and hence, in PKB, it will be lax. Thus, as stated above, the PKB is probably a tension test via the attachments of the femoral nerve in the quadriceps muscle and surrounding fascia. Tension is transmitted via the femoral nerve to the L2,3,4 nerve roots placing some tension and causing some movement of the neuraxis and meninges (Dyck 1976, Davidson 1987). The spread of tension and movement along the neuraxis is probably less than the spread with a SLR. Christodoulides (1989) presented myelographic support for the PKB to be used as a test for a L4,5 disc protrusion. Here, movement of the L4 root pulls on an already tense and inflamed L5 root.

If the PKB is performed in hip extension, more tension is placed along the lateral femoral cutaneous nerve, since the nerve is anterior to the hip axis of flexion and extension, and the main femoral nerve trunk. However, hip extension inevitably forces the lumbar spine into extension, hence lessening tension along the neuraxis. Davidson (1987) tested the PKB in neutral and in hip extension in 100 young, normal, male and female subjects and found that the test was more sensitive with the hip in neutral. However, if the test is done in hip extension, this would presumably allow more migration of the femoral nerve in relation to interfacing structures. This may be the symptomatic movement if the nervous system touches a pathological interface.

THE SLUMP TEST

History

The Slump Test is one of the newer tension tests, although performing knee extension in the sitting position has been suggested for many years. According to Woodhall & Hayes (1950), Petren in 1909 was the first to employ knee extension in sitting as a tension test. In 1942, Cyriax used combinations of knee extension in sitting with cervical flexion to diagnose 'sciatic perineuritis'. Inman & Saunders (1942) also suggested using combinations of spinal flexion and Straight Leg Raise to try and localise the source of lumbar pain. An increase in symptoms with an increase in the range of SLR was indicative of lower lumbar pathology, whereas an increase in symptoms with trunk flexion was indicative of upper lumbar pathology. Maitland (1979) carried out a normative study naming the test the 'Slump Test' and has been primarily responsible for its now increasing use in manual therapy (1986). In retrospect, the test is a logical progression, utilising the continuum of the nervous system and the established tests of PNF and SLR.

Method

It must be stressed that the sequence described is for a patient with a non-irritable disorder. Examination of the irritable disorder is discussed in Chapter 9.

1. The patient sits well back on the end of a plinth with thighs fully supported and knees together. The knee creases should be at the very edge of the plinth. This starting position allows a repeatable hip position. The patient's hands are linked gently behind her back. The examiner stands beside and close to the patient, perhaps with one leg up on the couch (Fig. 7.20A). Resting symptoms are noted as are the symptoms or alteration in the symptoms after each stage listed below. The range of movement of components after each stage is visually estimated.

2. The patient is asked to 'slump' or 'sag' (a gentle push in the abdomen may facilitate this) while the examiner maintains the cervical spine in a neutral position (Fig. 7.20B). Overpressure is applied to the lumbar and thoracic flexion, in an attempt to 'bow' the spine, rather than flex the hips. The sacrum must remain vertical. I find it easier to have one knee up on the bed and my axilla on the patients cervico-thoracic junction area. This means that I can use my ribs and my forearm to bow the spine and, at the same time, keep an even pressure on either side. Remember to assess responses after each component.

3. With the spinal flexion position maintained, the patient is asked to bend her neck 'chin to chest' and then an overpressure in the same direction is added. The response is assessed after neck flexion and after overpressure. If the 'axilla on C7' technique is used, then both hands will be free to control the patient's head (Fig. 7.20C).

4. The patient is asked to extend her knee actively, and the response assessed (Fig. 7.20D). Always make it a habit to extend the left knee first as it makes it easier to recall the responses to record them. If there is a side with a pain dominance, then examine the good side first. This gives a better idea about what to expect from the painful side. 'Straighten your knee' is probably the best command.

5. The patient is asked to dorsiflex her ankle (Fig. 7.20E). More patients will understand 'bend your ankle up' rather than 'dorsiflex your foot'. Sometimes patients will try to straighten the whole leg. It may be better to say 'bend your ankle up, only the ankle'.

6. Neck flexion is slowly released (Fig. 7.20F), and the response carefully assessed. Some subjects will feel an instant ease or alteration in symptoms, others will have an alteration further back in a cervical extension position, a few will have no alteration. It is

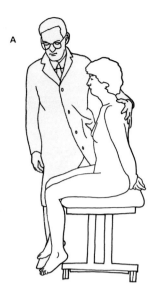

Fig. 7.20A Slump stage 1

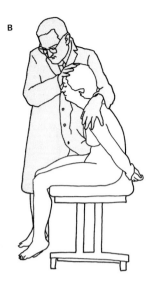

Fig. 7.20B Slump stage 2

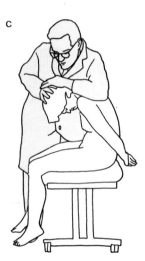

Fig. 7.20C Slump stage 3

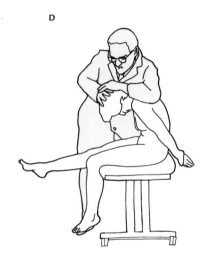

Fig. 7.20D Slump stage 4

important to know where in the range of cervical extension the alteration, if any, occurs.

7. The same procedure is repeated for the other leg. The range of movement and the pain responses are compared.

8. In the slump position, both knees are extended and the effect of the release of neck flexion noted (Fig. 7.20G). Any asymmetry in ranges of knee extension is noted.

This is a description of the test for a non-symptomatic subject. Once the test has been completed, if, say in Slump/Neck Flexion the left knee extension was restricted by pain in the hamstring region, this position could be held and the neck flexion slowly released. If there was a change in symptoms in the hamstring area, it could be inferred that these symptoms are neurogenic in origin.

Some clinicians use slight variations of the above method, such as the greater hip flexion used by Maitland (1986). The above method was used in the normative studies by Massey (1982), Leung (1983), Grant (1983) and Butler (1985).

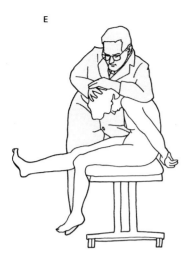

Fig. 7.20E Slump stage 5

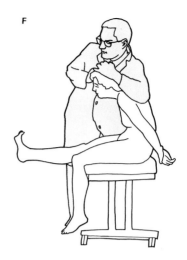

Fig. 7.20F Slump stage 6

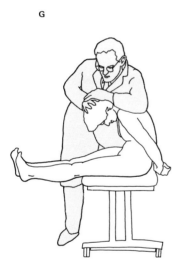

Fig. 7.20G Testing bilateral knee extension in Slump

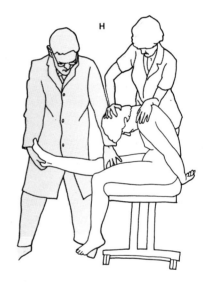

Fig. 7.20H The Slump Test with an assistant

Hip flexion can be added later as a sensitising movement (by flexing the trunk as well as flexing the thigh).

The Slump Test is a powerful test of many structures, and careful handling is required to accurately assess and thus interpret the responses. If the sacrum can be kept vertical, accurate reassessments will be easier. Note too that the base test does not use full hip flexion. There is, therefore, a nervous system tensioning component not used unless needed. This makes testing a little safer.

If an experienced assistant is available, he/she can be used to maintain the trunk position while the physiotherapist examines the leg movements (Fig. 7.20H).

Precautions related to the Slump Test

The Slump Test is a complex test requiring skilled handling and interpretation. The general precautions and contraindications listed in Chapter 5 must be considered, especially those involving the central nervous system.

1. The whole test does not have to be performed. If a disorder is deemed irritable, part of the Slump Test can be examined. For example, the patient's lumbar symptoms may be reproduced on Slump without overpressure and then made worse with slight cervical flexion. This might be all that is needed in that particular patient. It may not be necessary or wise to perform a Slump Test in some patients or at a particular stage of their disorder.

2. The flexion component of the Slump may place an unstable discogenic disorder at risk. Flexion often worsens the symptoms of an apparent disc injury by increasing the pressure in the disc or bulging the disc onto the posterior longitudinal ligament or the dura mater. If there is any possibility of an unstable discogenic disorder, the test should either not be performed or performed short of the onset of symptoms. All physiotherapists who perform a Slump Test should have had it performed on themselves. It can be quite an uncomfortable, even claustrophobic test.

Normal responses

In nearly all subjects, the Slump Test is associated with some discomfort, even pain. These responses require analysis to determine whether they are normal or not (see Ch. 9). The responses listed below are the suggested normal responses to the method above. They come from studies of approximately 250 asymptomatic subjects (Maitland 1979, Leung 1982, Grant 1983, Butler 1985). The normal responses from these studies are:

- Stage 2. (Fig. 7.20B) On Slump — nil
- Stage 3. (Fig. 7.20C) On Slump/Neck Flexion — pain in the area of T8 and T9 in approximately 50% of normals. This response is less common in older subjects (Butler 1985).
- Stage 4. (Fig. 7.20E) On Slump/Neck Flexion/Knee Extension — pain behind the extended knee and in the hamstring area plus some restriction of knee extension. This restriction should be symmetrical.

- Stage 5. (Fig. 7.20F) On Slump/Neck Flexion/Knee Extension\Ankle Dorsiflexion — some restriction of ankle dorsiflexion.
- Stage 6. (Fig. 7.20G) On release of neck flexion — a decrease of symptoms in all areas and an increase in the range of knee extension and range of ankle dorsiflexion.

Indications

The Slump Test should be a routine test (though not necessarily on the first examination) when:

1. There are spinal symptoms.
2. There are indications from the subjective examination that a positive Slump Test may be possible. For example, the patient may complain that symptoms are worse getting into a car or kicking a football.
3. Treatment is going to be nerve mobilisation, say by SLR or PKB. It is useful to have another tension test to reassess the responses and possibly progress to.
4. To ensure that the nervous system moves and stretches properly in a patient ready for discharge.

Variations

Once the base test has been performed, the test will need varying to accommodate the various disorders. The irritable disorder (Ch. 9) and the hypermobile patient are two such examples.

To examine the nervous system fully in the hypermobile patient, the Slump Test will need to be taken further. Greater hip flexion will be needed as will hip adduction and medial rotation. Some lateral flexion of the spine may be required to get the desired response. Any of the sensitising additions used for the SLR (hip adduction, medial rotation, varying foot positions) can be easily added to the Slump Test.

The Slump Test also offers a good position to examine the nerve role (most likely the obturator nerve) in groin sprain. If the patient

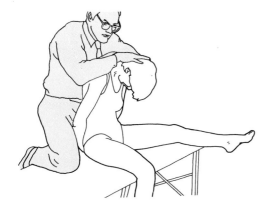

Fig. 7.21 The obturator nerve can be examined as a variation of the Slump Test

were to abduct the leg to the onset of symptoms, then the trunk could be flexed and neck position altered (Fig. 7.21). The leg could be supported on a chair. Where neck flexion/extension alters the groin pain response, there is likely to be a neurogenic component to that disorder.

The Upper Limb Tension Tests and variations (ULTT), either bilaterally or unilaterally can be added to the Slump Test position. McLaughlin (1989) examined combined Slump/Bilateral ULTT positions in 50 asymptomatic subjects and found that responses were reasonably similar to the standard Slump Test in a sitting position. The addition of the bilateral ULTT could induce fixation of the nervous system at the C8,T1 level and be useful in the examination and treatment of adverse tension upper disorders originating in the spine and upper limb.

Slump Test in Longsitting (Slump LS)

The Slump Test can be conveniently performed in Longsitting both as an assessment and a treatment technique. It is also a useful test to observe how the patient performs the test by themselves; this can provide evidence as to the site of the restriction. The restriction is not necessarily nervous system. This hypothesis will have to be proven or disproven by moving distal components, for example, further extending the knee or dorsiflexing the ankles.

The Slump LS test is essentially performing a Slump 'from the other end'. That is, the tension in the nervous system from the legs and lower trunk has been taken up first. This means different tensions and nervous system/interface relationships are examined. Clinically, the responses are often different to the Slump Test in a sitting position.

Method

1. The patient sits in longsitting (Fig. 7.22A). If needed, ankle dorsiflexion can be added by placing her feet against a wall.
2. Trunk flexion is added. Overpressure to the movement can be given to bow the spine (Fig. 7.22B).
3. With this position maintained, neck flexion is added (Fig. 7.22C). If the examiner kneels behind the patient, good control of the head and maintenance of trunk position is possible.
4. In this position, it is easy to examine cervical and upper thoracic movements in Slump. In Figure 7.22D, cervical rotation to the right is being examined. It is also useful, as a variation, to examine the effect of allowing one knee to flex over the side of the bed and then to move the patient to the other side of the bed and compare the same manoeuvre on the other leg. Variations on the Upper Limb Tension Test could also be added. As in many of the more complex tension tests, an assistant is extremely useful. Straps could also be used to maintain knee extension.

Indications

The Slump LS Test is especially indicated for the patient who complains of symptoms in the Slump Longsitting position. Some positional examples are reading in bed or rowing. It is also a convenient position to examine cervical and thoracic movements in sitting and an effective way to give the patient a home exercise that involves the Slump Test (see Ch. 11).

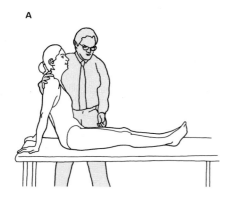

Fig. 7.22A Slump Longsitting stage 1

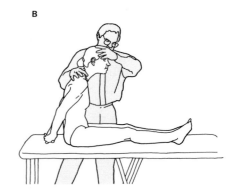

Fig. 7.22B Slump Longsitting stage 2

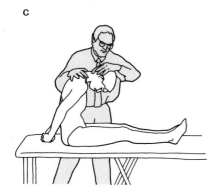

Fig. 7.22C Slump Longsitting/Cervical flexion

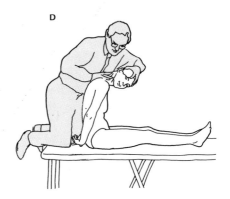

Fig. 7.22D Slump Longsitting/Cervical flexion and Rotation

Biomechanics

What actually occurs to the neuromeningeal tissues during the Slump Test can only be postulated and extrapolated from the few cadaver studies available and the in-vivo studies (these are discussed in Ch. 2).

It appears that in the complete Slump Test position, the limitation to any further neck flexion, knee extension and dorsiflexion is due to the peripheral and central nervous systems being on full stretch and physically restricting any further movement. Evidence of this is found in the normal response of an increased range of knee extension and ankle dorsiflexion when the cervical flexion is released. The nervous system is the most direct structural connection.

Because all the body components are tightened up, the Slump Test must create maximal tension in the nervous system. This correlates well with

Massey's study (1985) of 50 patients with low back pain. She examined PNF, PKB, SLR and Slump in these patients. The Slump Test was the most sensitive for reproducing the symptoms.

It is possible to interpret the Slump test responses further. Some patients have a SLR and/or PNF reproducing symptoms and yet a negative Slump. This may be due to the Slump not allowing as much movement of the nervous system as the PNF or SLR allow. This may be because tension and movement have been taken up at one end, therefore, not as much movement is allowed at the other. In the case of irritative pathology or a 'strategic adhesion', because tension has been taken up at the other end, it may not allow the nerve/interface relationship necessary for symptom reproduction.

Another important consideration is that, although the Slump may well be testing tension in the nervous system, it is also testing the antero-posterior movement of the dural sac in the spinal canal or perhaps antero/lateral movement if combined movements are used. Structures like the dorsomedian plica (Ch. 1) may be stretched. PNF and SLR may not be adequate tests to test these tissues.

Many authors have, over the years, noted that a SLR result was different in sitting compared with the traditional supine position. Some clinicians still use this to conclude that a patient's symptoms may not be valid. However, sitting dramatically changes interfacing tissues and the spine will not be in the same position for the test as in supine. The patient will be in more spinal flexion in the sitting test. In the light of what is already known about spinal canal biomechanics and pathology, this test as evidence of the existence or not of organic pathology should be disregarded. With what is known about the biomechanics of the nervous system including the potential of little movements and slight postural adjustments to alter symptoms, these tests appear very gross, and it seems unfair that such a weighty emphasis is often placed upon them.

REFERENCES

Beasley A W 1982 The origin of orthopaedics. The Journal of the Royal Society of Medicine 75: 648–655

Borges L F, Hallett M, Selkoe D J, Welch K 1981 The anterior tarsal tunnel syndrome. Journal of Neurosurgery 54: 89–92

Breig A, Marions O 1963 Biomechanics of the lumbosacral nerve roots. Acta Radiologica 4: 602–604

Breig A, Troup J D G 1979 Biomechanical considerations in the straight-leg-raising test. Spine 4: 242–250

Breig A 1978 Adverse mechanical tension in the central nervous system. Almqvist & Wiksell, Stockholm

Butler D S 1985 The effects of age and gender on the slump test. Unpublished thesis, South Australian Institute of Technology, Adelaide

Christodoulides A N 1989 Ipsilateral sciatica on femoral nerve stretch test is pathognomic of an L4/5 disc protrusion. Journal of Bone and Joint Surgery 71B: 81–89

Corrigan B, Maitland G D 1983 Practical orthopaedic medicine. Butterworths, London

Cyriax J 1942 Perineuritis. British Medical Journal 578–580

Cyriax J 1978 Textbook of orthopaedic medicine, 7th edn. Baillierre Tindall, London, vol 1

Davidson S 1987 Prone knee bend: an investigation into the effect of cervical flexion and extension. In: Dalziell B A, Snowsill J C (eds) Proceedings of the Manipulative Therapists Association of Australia, 5th Biennial Conference, Melbourne

Dyck P 1976 The femoral nerve traction test with lumbar disc protrusion. Surgical Neurology 6: 163–166

Dyck P 1984 Lumbar nerve root: the enigmatic eponyms. Spine 9: 3–6

Estridge M N, Rouhe S A, Johnson N G 1982 The femoral stretching test. Journal of Neurosurgery 57: 813–817

Gifford L 1987 Circadian variation in human flexibility and grip strength. In: Dalziel B A, Snowsill J C (eds) Fifth biennial conference proceedings, Manipulative Therapists Association of Australia, Melbourne

Grant A 1983 The slump test. Unpublished thesis, South Australian Institute of Technology, Adelaide

Greive G P 1981 Common vertebral joint problems. Churchill Livingstone, Edinburgh

Hudgins W R 1979 The crossed straight leg raising test: a diagnostic sign of herniated disc. Journal of Occupational Medicine. 21: 407–408

Inman V T, Saunders J B 1942 The clinico-anatomical aspects of the lumbosacral region. Radiology 38: 669–678

Khuffash B, Porter R W 1989 Cross leg pain and trunk list. Spine 602–603

Leung A L 1983 Effects of cervical lateral flexion on the slump test in normal young subjects. Unpublished thesis, South Australian Institute of Technology, Adelaide

Lew P C 1979 The straight leg raise and lumbar stiffness. Unpublished thesis, South Australian Institute of Technology, Adelaide

Lew P C, Puentedura E J 1985 The straight-leg-raise test and spinal posture. In: Proceedings Fourth Biennial Conference, Manipulative Therapists Association of Australia, Brisbane

Macnab I 1971 Negative disc exploration. Journal of Bone and Joint Surgery 53A: 891–903

Macnab I 1977 Backache. Williams & Williams, Baltimore

Maitland G D 1979 Negative disc exploration: positive canal signs. Australian Journal of Physiotherapy 25: 129–134

Maitland G D 1986 Vertebral manipulation, 5th edn. Butterworths, London

Massey A E 1985 Movement of pain sensitive structures in the neural canal. In: Grieve G P (ed) Modern manual therapy of the vertebral column. Churchill Livingstone, Edinburgh

McLaughlin A 1989 Combined slump tests. Unpublished thesis, South Australian Institute of Technology, Adelaide

Miller A M 1987 Neuro-meningeal limitation of straight leg raising. In: Dalziel B A, Snowsill J C (eds) Fifth biennial conference, Manipulative Therapists Association of Australia, Melbourne

Nobel W 1966 Peroneal palsy due to haematoma in the common peroneal nerve sheath after distal torsional fractures and inversion ankle sprains. The Journal of Bone and Joint Surgery 48A: 1484–1495

O'Connell J E A 1946 The clinical signs of meningeal irritation. Brain LXIX: 9–21

O'Connell J E A 1943 Sciatica and the mechanism of the production of the clinical syndrome in protrusions of the lumbar intervertebral discs. British Journal of Surgery 30: 315–327

Slater H 1989 The effect of foot position on the SLR responses. In: Jones H, Jones M A, Milde M (eds) Sixth biennial conference, Manipulative Therapists Association of Australia, Adelaide

Styf J R 1988 Diagnosis of exercise induced pain in the anterior aspect of the lower leg. American Journal of Sports Medicine 16: 165–169

Sunderland S 1978 Nerves and nerve injuries, 2nd edn. Churchill Livingstone, Edinburgh

Sutton J L 1979 The straight leg raising test, unpublished thesis, South Australian Institute of Technology, Adelaide, Australia

Sweetham B J, Anderson J A, Dalton E R 1974 The relationships between little finger mobility, lumbar mobility, straight leg raising and low back pain. Rheumatology and Rehabilitation 13: 161–166

Tencer A F, Allen B L, Ferguson R L 1985 A biomechanical study of thoracolumbar spine fractures with bone in the canal, Part III. Spine 10: 741–749

Troup J D G 1981 Straight-leg-raising (SLR) and the qualifying tests for increased root tension. Spine 6: 526–527

Troup J D G 1986 Biomechanics of the lumbar spinal canal. Clinical Biomechanics 1: 31–43

Urban L M 1985 The straight leg raising test: a review. In: Grieve G P (ed) Modern manual therapy of the vertebral column. Churchill Livingstone, Edinburgh

Woodhall B, Hayes G J 1950 The well leg raising test of Fajersztajn in the diagnosis of ruptured intervertebral disc. The Journal of Bone and Joint Surgery 32A: 786–792

8. Tension testing — the upper limbs

The tests of neural tension proposed for the upper limb (Upper Limb Tension Tests (ULTTs)) have been developed much more recently than those used for the lower limb and trunk. They are used, almost exclusively, by physiotherapists. More time and research will be needed before they become an accepted part of a neuro-orthopaedic examination by professions other than physiotherapy. There is, however, no reason why they cannot be incorporated into the assessment and treatment approach of Maitland. I will describe four base tension tests for the left upper limb and a non-irritable disorder.

- ULTT1. median nerve dominant utilising shoulder abduction
- ULTT2 a. median nerve dominant utilising shoulder girdle depression and external rotation of the shoulder
- ULTT2 b. radial nerve dominant utilising shoulder girdle depression plus internal rotation of the shoulder
- ULTT3. ulnar nerve dominant utilising shoulder abduction and elbow flexion.

UPPER LIMB TENSION TEST 1

History

The Upper Limb Tension Test (also known as the 'Brachial Plexus Tension Test' and 'Elvey's test') is the most recent of the tension tests. The test was developed by Elvey in 1979 and further developed and popularised in recent years. (Elvey, 1983, 1986, Elvey et al 1986, Kenneally et al 1988). Kenneally et al (1988) have called the Upper Limb Tension Test the 'straight leg raise of the arm'. This is a useful and helpful analogue, for the test is every bit as useful for examining upper limb and neck disorders as the SLR is in assessment and treatment of patients with lower limb and spinal disorders.

For many years, clinicians and researchers have hinted that there could be useful tension tests of the arm. Chavany (1934) suggested a test using traction applied along the extended, abducted and elevated arm. Frykolm (1951) also described a similar test. However, it differed in that the nervous system was tightened up by adding cervical lateral flexion to the opposite side of the test. In 1956, Smith did cadaver studies (human and monkey) involving arm movements, similar to those described in this text, for the ULTT1. Resultant movements on the cervical cord were duly noted in these studies. Pechan (1973) devised a test known as the 'ulnar nerve tension test'; it is rather similar to the Upper Limb Tension Test 3 described later in this chapter. Cyriax (1978), who clearly was very aware of the importance of neurobiomechanics, suggested the addition of elbow extension to symptomatic wrist positions.

Surgeons have been aware for many years, that if the arms of anaesthetised patients were placed in certain positions, there existed a risk of a stretch neuropathy. Abduction of the shoulder and depression of the shoulder girdle have been identified as the positions posing the most danger.

Since Elvey's initial reports and cadaver studies, many undergraduate and postgraduate studies in Australian tertiary institutions have examined the test and its variants. Over 500 subjects have participated in normative studies at the South Australian Institute of Technology alone (Kenneally 1985, Rubenach 1985, Fardy 1985, Bell 1987, Landers 1987). Cadaver studies have also been utilised to investigate the Upper Limb Tension Test (Elvey 1983, 1988, Ginn 1989, Selvaratnam et al 1989). Recently, the test has been applied and its strong relevance noted in various disorders including Colles' fracture (Young 1989), whiplash (Quintner 1989), and post-surgical hypersensitivity of the hand (Sweeney & Harms 1990). Still, the test needs greater exposure in the mainstream medical literature.

The possibility of tension tests for the various nerves of the upper limb has been suggested (Kenneally et al 1988). By examining the location of nerves in relation to the joint axes of movement, Kenneally et al (1988) suggested it should be possible to develop techniques that selectively stress individual nerves. Clinical experience shows this is not always possible, especially when considering the complex neuroanatomy of the arm. I suggest that, for the upper limb, four base tests be used. These tests are based on powerful nervous system tensioning manoeuvres, each individual test allowing a bias to a particular nerve trunk.

Method

The technique described is for a left ULTT1 in a non-irritable disorder where full range of finger, wrist, elbow, shoulder and neck movements are present. As in the previous chapter the patient is described as 'she' and the physiotherapist as 'he' for convenience.

1. The patient is positioned in neutral supine, towards the left hand side of the couch. A pillow is not normally required, however, if used, it should become a standard feature of later re-testing. The examiner faces the patient in stride standing, his right hand holding her left hand ensuring control right down to the thumb and finger tips. Her upper arm rests on the examiner's left thigh (Fig. 8.1A).

2. A constant depression force is placed on the shoulder girdle during the movement. This is best achieved by the examiner's fist being pushed down vertically into the bed such that the neutral shoulder girdle position can be maintained. Consequently, elevation of the shoulder girdle is prevented during abduction.

Note that a convenient alternative position is preferred by some physiotherapists and is discussed below. The patient's arm is subsequently abducted in the coronal plane to approximately 110°. Greater control and support of the arm can be achieved if the abduction component is performed with the patient's arm resting on the physiotherapist's thigh. In this way, the physiotherapist can walk the arm up into abduction whilst maintaining complete support and control of the movement (Fig. 8.1B).

3. With this position maintained, the forearm is supinated and the wrist and fingers extended (Fig. 8.1C).

4. The shoulder is laterally rotated (Fig. 8.1D.

5. The elbow is extended (Fig. 8.1E). Earlier component positions must be strictly maintained.

6. With this position held, cervical lateral flexion to the left and then to the right are added (Fig. 8.1F). If asked to turn her head to the side, the patient will inevitably rotate rather than laterally flex the neck. Before performing the test, it is best to explain to the patient what is expected. 'Keep looking at the ceiling and take your ear to your shoulder' is a useful command.

The most important part of the test, and indeed of any tension test, is that once part of the test has been taken up, these positions must be firmly maintained before the addition of the next component. Symptoms and symptom changes must be identified and interpreted after each step.

An alternative method of handling

In Figure 8.2 an alternative method of handling, preferred by some physiotherapists, is illustrated. In the second stage, rather than maintaining the shoulder girdle depression by the examiner's fist on the bed, the physiotherapist can place his left elbow on the patient's shoulder girdle with his forearm along her upper arm. In some patient/physiotherapist combinations this may provide more support. Note also that supination is performed early in the test. Some clinicians prefer to add supination after the lateral rotation.

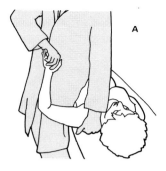

Fig. 8.1A ULTT1 stage 1

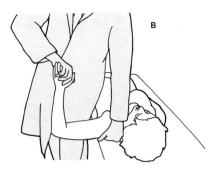

Fig. 8.1B ULTT1 stage 2

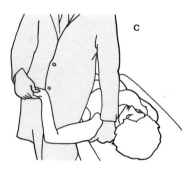

Fig. 8.1C ULTT1 stage 3

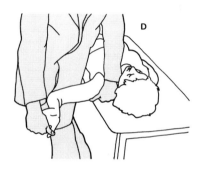

Fig. 8.1D ULTT1 stage 4

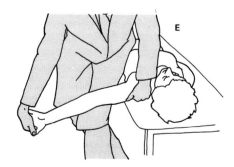

Fig. 8.1E ULTT1 stage 5

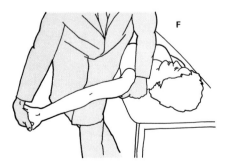

Fig. 8.1F ULTT1 stage 6

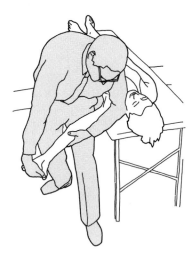

Fig. 8.2 ULTT1 alternative method of handling

Clinically this is not of great consequence, as long as the same base test is used each time and the physiotherapist is aware that altering the sequence of additions may have an effect on the reproduction of symptoms.

Comment on the test procedure

The test method proposed by Kenneally et al (1988) utilises wrist and finger extension last. However, I suggest that elbow extension should be the last component added. It is easier to visually measure the range of elbow extension than it is to measure the range of wrist extension. Another important factor is that it is probably safer to have elbow extension as the last component. Simply, nerves are stronger at the elbow than at the wrist and the heavy handed or inexperienced clinician is less likely to aggravate an upper quadrant disorder. Kenneally et al (1988) also stress the addition of shoulder girdle depression to the test. As the ULTT2 test described below is strongly dependent on shoulder girdle depression, I feel that, in the ULTT1, it is sufficient just to maintain the depression component. This, therefore, allows better examination of abduction.

There may be a temptation to pre-stress the nervous system by placing the patient in contralateral lateral flexion first, thus avoiding the potentially messy business of having to ask the patient to flex the neck laterally. Although this is sometimes required, I feel the test should be performed initially with the neck in neutral; it will nearly always be adequately sensitive in this position. This makes it easier to repeat the test accurately and is safer for the patient since there remains some slack in the nervous system within the cervical spine. It also means that lateral flexion away and towards the test side can be used to differentiate the structural source of symptoms in the limb, rather than use only of lateral flexion towards the side being tested.

Precautions

Great care is needed with this test. The precautions and contraindications listed in Chapter 5 should be reviewed, as should the 'Guide to better tension testing' in the next chapter (see page 168). Other than the general precautions, there are two particular precautions for the ULTT:

1. Physiotherapists should remember that it is much easier to aggravate upper limb symptoms than those in the lower limbs. Nerves are weaker and run more complex courses in the arm. With the repetitive activities that many jobs demand of the upper limb, there is also the greater possibility of confronting the irritated and inflamed nervous system.
2. The test is complex and involves many joints and muscles. It can be easy to forget that one of these structures (for example, a strained zygapophyseal joint) could be irritated during testing.

Providing the subjective examination is as comprehensive as possible and the physiotherapist is able to link this information with a knowledge of pathology; with adequate handling skills, unintentional aggravations of disorders will be extremely rare.

Indications

ULTT1 is a recommended test for all patients with symptoms anywhere in the arm, head, neck and thoracic spine. It should be performed on the first examination if indications in the subjective and physical examination imply that impaired nervous system mechanics are a component of the patient's disorder (Chs 4 & 5). In severe and irritable disorders the test could be omitted initially or, more likely, would be examined as for an irritable disorder (see Ch. 9). For physiotherapists unaccustomed to examining the nervous system, it is a good idea to examine the ULTTs in all non-irritable disorders to gain some idea of the tests' relevance.

Normal responses

Kenneally et al (1988) listed the normal responses to the ULTT as seen in 400 'normal' volunteers:

1. A deep stretch or ache in the cubital fossa, (99% of volunteers) extending down the anterior and radial aspects of the forearm and into the radial hand (80%)
2. A definite tingling sensation in the thumb and first three fingers
3. A small percentage of subjects may feel stretch in the anterior shoulder area
4. Cervical lateral flexion away from the side tested increases the response in approximately 90% of normals
5. Cervical lateral flexion towards the tested side decreases the test response in 70% of normals.

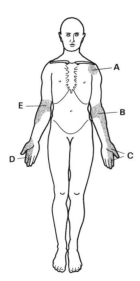

Fig. 8.3 The normal responses to the ULTT1 (adapted from Kenneally et al 1988)

These responses are summarised in Figure 8.3. Pullos (1986) applied the test to 100 normal subjects and reported that the normal deficit in range of elbow extension during the test was 16.5–53.2°.

Sensitising additions and variations

There are many components to this test and perhaps 'variations' is a better word than 'sensitising'. The same clear sensitising additions that occur in the lower limb are not as evident in the upper quarter. In the arm, due to the complexity of nerve anatomy, a small movement which acts to sensitise one nerve will rapidly take tension off another. Any of the components can be changed, and, while an increase in the range of most of the components will increase the sensitivity of the test, this is not always so.

Once the base test responses have been confirmed, there are many variations and directions that further examination could take, for example, pronation instead of supination, wrist radial/lateral deviation, varying degrees of shoulder extension or flexion to name a few. The possible combinations are endless, provided the examiner is guided by a knowledge of neurobiomechanics and the complaints of the patient regarding aggravating activities. In Chapter 9 the issues of further developing the base tests are discussed.

The ULTT can be performed from 'the other end', that is, from the hand first. This is useful for symptoms which may have their source in the hand or the wrist and forearm. Here, a painful position can be reproduced, say wrist extension and radial deviation. Tension can then be added by tightening the proximal components. Tensioning other limbs can also be added. Two very useful additions to the test are the the ULTT of the contralateral arm and the SLR (Fig 8.4)

Some of the normative studies performed at the South Australian Institute of Technology have examined variations to the ULTT1. These give an indication of the widespread effects of the test and the need for a comprehensive examination in patients with adverse ternsion syndromes. Rubenach (1985) examined the implications of adding a contralateral ULTT1 to an existing ULTT1. Most of the symptoms in the initial test

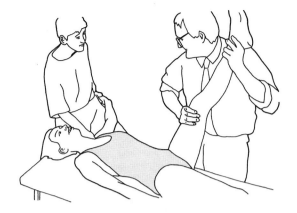

Fig. 8.4 Adding the SLR to the ULTT1

arm decreased. A similar alteration in symptoms was reported with the addition of Bilateral Straight Leg Raise to the test (Bell 1987). Fardy (1985) investigated the effect of neck position on the ULTT1 and confirmed that cervical lateral flexion away from the test side maximally increased the ULTT response in young asymptomatic subjects. Landers (1987) performed the ULTT1 in different positions of shoulder abduction (70°, 110°, 130°, and 150°) and concluded that 110° was the optimal position for symptoms related to the fifth, sixth and seventh cervical nerve roots. McLaughlin (1989) examined the effects of bilateral ULTT1 on the Slump Test. This test had only a minimal effect on the response to the Slump, although enough to support the use of the test in patients with arm and trunk symptoms.

Biomechanics

The test is certainly complex in nature. Every structure in the arm and many structures in the neck and thorax are moved during testing. By the anatomy and the evidence of symptomatic responses in normals, it can be deduced that the nervous system structure maximally tested is the median nerve; including the anterior interosseus nerve. It is possible, however, to ascertain further what happens to the nervous system during movement. See Chapter 2 for some of the studies outlining the amount of movement and tension occurring during arm movements.

During shoulder abduction, the C5,6, and 7

nerve roots are tensioned and pulled out of their individual foramina. Maintenance of depression will also keep the nerve roots and brachial plexus on some tension. Lord and Rosati (1971) describe a 'pulley effect' on the brachial plexus during shoulder abduction as it wraps around the coracoid process. All cords of the plexus would be tensioned in this position, with no bias to a particular nerve trunk. With regard to abduction, it has been noted clinically (Maitland 1977, Davidson et al 1981) that patients with fifth cervical nerve root pain obtain relief by scapular elevation and glenohumeral abduction. Some patients rest the hand of the painful limb on their head. The maintenance of depression and the pulley effect therefore seem essential to the symptom reproduction.

The effect of shoulder lateral rotation on the nervous system is not as clear. Reid (1987), conducted buckle transducer studies on two cadavers; one embalmed, one un-embalmed. Her studies revealed that lateral rotation decreased tension in the cords of the plexus and it was concluded that the movement should be left out of the test. Reid (1987) also noted clinically that lateral rotation often decreased the symptoms created by shoulder abduction. This finding is common. I feel that anything which makes the tests simpler will be useful. However, it is important to consider that, although tension may be reduced during lateral rotation in this small study, movement of the nervous system may be the sensitive feature. Lateral rotation, especially towards the end of the range is often painful, commonly thought of as a glenohumeral capsular restriction. It is not difficult, via structural differentiation, to analyse whether the limitation is from the nervous system or from the glenohumeral capsule. In the ultimate treatment selected in some patient presentations, the lateral rotation component may not be required.

Elbow extension will clearly tension the radial and median nerves together with slackening the ulnar nerve at the elbow. Wrist and finger extension tighten the median and ulnar nerves and slacken the radial nerve.

Remember that the pattern of tension distribution and hence the symptomatic responses can be completely different with the addition of a pathological process. Once sensitised, there is repeated clinical evidence that the ULTT1 can effect headache and spinal symptoms (occasionally even in the lumbar spine).

UPPER LIMB TENSION TEST 2

History

It rapidly became obvious to physiotherapists who were clinically reasoning, and using the ULTT1, that patients with symptoms, suspected to be neurogenic in origin, did not necessarily alter them in the elevated arm position. A difficulty was further encountered with the ULTT1 because, during the shoulder abduction component, shoulder girdle depression could not be adequately maintained. New tests and varieties of the ULTT1 were clearly needed. The ULTT2, which is derived from a number of sources, was subsequently developed, as a result of these circumstances. Initially, a test was required to match the positions used by keyboard operators and typists, particularly the shoulder girdle depression and protraction positions (Butler 1987). Disections by Smith (1956) revealed the significant effect that depression of the shoulder girdle had on the brachial plexus and cervical cord in monkeys and a human cadaver. Indeed, a cursory investigation of the neuroanatomy of the upper limb shows the obvious effect that shoulder depression has on the neural structures. Elvey (1986) has suggested using shoulder depression as part of a mobilisation treatment for cervical nerve roots. Sunderland (pers. comm. 1988, 1989) has often urged the incorporation of more shoulder girdle depression in upper limb tension testing techniques.

The methodology suggested here is that which I, personally, have found to be the best. Depression of the shoulder girdle places potent tension forces upon the nervous system and I feel it is worthwhile including two base tension tests with depression as the key position; one is biased towards the median nerve and one biased towards the radial nerve.

Method (median nerve bias)

The test is described for the left arm

1. The patient lies slightly diagonally across the bed with her head towards the left hand side of the bed and her scapula free of the bed. The examiner's right thigh rests against the patients left shoulder. His right hand holds the patient's elbow and his left hand holds her wrist (Fig. 8.5A). This crossed-arms starting position means that the position of the physiotherapist's hands will require minimal changes during the manoeuvre, and the technique will be smoother and better controlled.

2. Using his thigh, the examiner carefully depresses the patient's shoulder girdle (Fig. 8.5B). In this position and indeed, throughout the test, it is possible to look at the patient's face from under the examiner's arm to pick up any non-verbal information. Quite a sensitive feel can be developed with the thigh and the obvious advantage is that the depression can be maintained, leaving two hands free for movement combinations of the rest of the arm. The test will have to be performed in approximately 10° of shoulder abduction so that the arm is clear and parallel to the side of the bed.

3. The shoulder depression is maintained and then the examiner subsequently extends the patient's elbow (Fig. 8.5C).

4. The shoulder girdle depression/elbow extension position is maintained and the examiner, using both arms, laterally rotates the patient's whole arm (Fig. 8.5D).

5. With this position maintained, the examiner's left forearm is pronated and slides down to the patient's hand. The examiner's thumb is slipped in the web space between the patient's thumb and index finger. The examiner then extends the patient's wrist, fingers and thumb. This position provides good control over the arm, including the tips of the fingers (Fig. 8.5E).

6. The most common sensitising addition is abduction of the shoulder (Fig. 8.5F). Other variations and sensitising positions which can be added to the ULTT2 are discussed following the description of the ULTT2 for the radial nerve.

Once a symptom has been reproduced, if more distal, then shoulder depression can be released and the effects assessed. If more proximal, the

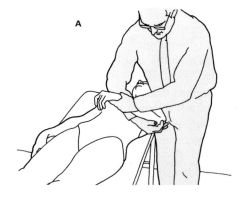

Fig. 8.5A ULTT2 (median nerve bias) stage 1

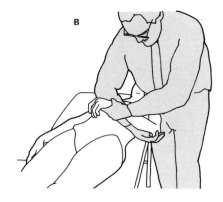

Fig. 8.5B ULTT2 (median nerve bias) stage 2

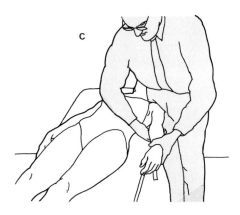

Fig. 8.5C ULTT2 (median nerve bias) stage 3

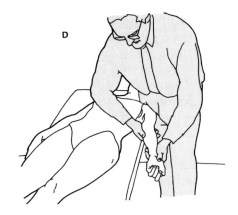

Fig. 8.5D ULTT2 (median nerve bias) stage 4

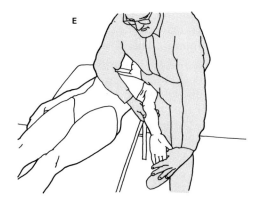

Fig. 8.5E ULTT2 (median nerve bias) stage 5

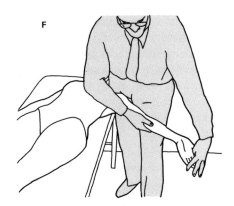

Fig. 8.5F ULTT2 (median nerve bias) stage 6

wrist can be moved to assess if there are any alterations in the reproduced symptoms. It is worth noting the sensitivity of shoulder girdle depression. Once a forearm symptom response is obtained, if of neurogenic origin, then the slightest release of the depression will usually ease this symptom response.

Method (radial nerve bias)

1. The starting position, shoulder girdle movements and the elbow extension are the same as for the test with a median nerve bias.

2. With this position maintained, the shoulder is then medially rotated. This is the key factor to the test. The examiner must reach under the patient's arm as far as possible with his left arm and grasp her wrist (Fig. 8.6A). The patient's whole arm is then guided into medial rotation at the shoulder,

inevitably with pronation of the forearm. With the medial rotation taken up, it should be possible for the examiner's left elbow to 'lock' against the patient's left elbow, thus keeping it in extension and maintaining the medial rotation (Fig. 8.6B). The examiner will know if the position is held securely enough because his right arm will be relatively free to guide the patient's arm. This free arm will ultimately be invaluable for treatment techniques, for example, techniques such as mobilising the radial head or deep frictioning at the elbow for the common involvement of the nervous system in tennis elbow (Ch. 14).

3. The patient's wrist is then flexed, either actively or passively using the examiner's left hand (Fig. 8.6C). Flexion of the thumb joints and ulnar deviation of the wrist will further sensitise the radial nerve via the superficial sensory branch. Alternatively, the examiner

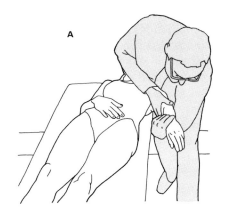

Fig. 8.6A ULTT2 (radial nerve bias) stage 1

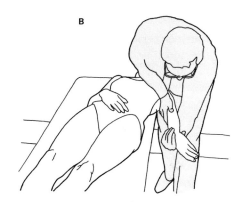

Fig. 8.6B ULTT2 (radial nerve bias) stage 2

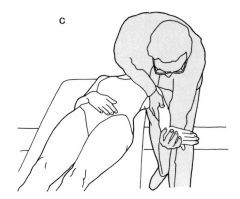

Fig. 8.6C ULTT2 (radial nerve bias) stage 3

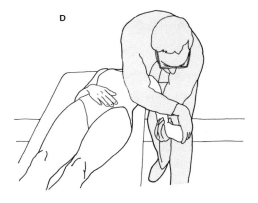

Fig. 8.6D ULTT2 (radial nerve bias) stage 4

can slide his right hand down the patient's arm a little to control the wrist, thumb and finger flexion (Fig. 8.6D.

Indications

Like the ULTT1, the ULTT2 should be examined in all cervical, thoracic and upper limb disorders. High priority (meaning that the test is essential on the initial examination) would be given if there are subjective indications of an adverse tension component; especially if these symptoms appear to be related to activities which involve shoulder depression. Symptoms in the radial nerve distribution would clearly indicate the need for the test with the radial nerve bias. Disorders presenting with diagnoses such as 'tennis elbow' and de Quervain's disease would also make the ULTT2 radial nerve bias test a priority.

Normal responses

No studies have been undertaken which indicate the normal responses to the ULTT2 tests. Comparison must be made with the other arm. Symptoms should be expected in the innervation fields of either the radial or median nerves, depending on the bias of the test, or along the nerves. In any of these tests it is quite normal to feel some symptoms. The ULTT2 manoeuvres provide a method of testing tension and movement of the nervous system with the interfacing structures positioned relatively in mid range. In some situations, this may allow better examination and ultimately better treatment of the nervous system in contrast with the ULTT1 where the shoulder non-neural structures are on considerable stretch as well.

Common variations

1. During shoulder girdle depression, the physiotherapist can add either shoulder girdle protraction or retraction. Squatting a little and 'picking up' the shoulder girdle (Fig. 8.7) adds protraction. If the patient is moved to the side of the bed a little more, the examiner can come up onto his toes and retract the shoulder girdle using his thigh. Protraction will tighten up the suprascapular nerve.

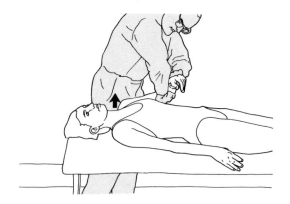

Fig. 8.7 Picking the shoulder girdle up in the ULTT2 positions

2. In the ULTT2 position, useful further sensitising procedures are to add cervical lateral flexion away and/or some abduction or extension of the shoulder. Shoulder abduction is usually possible up to 40° or 50° before the shoulder depression component is lost.

3. Rather than elbow extension, elbow flexion and/or combinations of supination and protraction can be added if required.

4. Wrist radial and ulnar deviations together with supination and pronation can be added. In some of these more complex positions, help from an assistant can be very welcome.

5. As in all tests, the sequence of additions can be altered. For example, in the median nerve bias test, the shoulder lateral rotation could be added before the elbow extension. In the radial nerve bias test, the distal components of thumb and wrist flexion could be the first movements taken up.

6. The ULTT2 (both radial and median nerve bias tests) can also be performed with the patient in prone. This is convenient if a technique such as unilateral pressures on the cervical spine, or a thoracic spine technique is being performed. The physiotherapist is able to reassess the effect of treatment on the ULTT2 quickly without moving the patient. This is a good position to examine the effect of shoulder retraction on the test (Fig. 8.8).

UPPER LIMB TENSION TEST 3

The tests previously described rely on shoulder girdle depression or glenohumeral abduction as

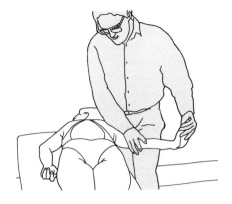

Fig. 8.8 ULTT2 in prone

base positions to move and tension the nervous system. Because the tests all involve elbow extension, the ulnar nerve and its origins may miss out on effective examination. Hence, I feel it is necessary to add a test that includes elbow flexion as part of a base test.

History

Perhaps due to its more obvious anatomy, compared with other nerves at the elbow, and the common occurrence of 'funny bone' symptoms, there are a number of reported tests designed to stretch the ulnar nerve. Pechan (1973) seems to have been the first person to devise a test to stress the ulnar nerve. In a recent journal, the 'elbow flexion test', as in Figure 8.9 was presented (Buehler & Thayer 1988). Clearly, in their test, more tension could have been added by using

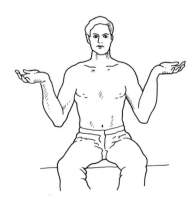

Fig. 8.9 The elbow flexion test. From: Buehler M J, Thayer D T 1988 The elbow flexion test: a clinical test for the cubital tunnel syndrome. Clinical Orthopaedics and Related Research 233: 213–216, with permission

shoulder girdle abduction and depression. The test I describe below is derived to some extent from those tests. Handling convenience and clinical analysis of the best way to reproduce symptoms related to the ulnar nerve and its origins also contribute.

Method

1. The patient and the physiotherapist are in the same starting position as for ULTT1. Note the stride standing position of the physiotherapist, such that the body can be used to make the test a smooth flowing action with minimal foot movements. The patient's elbow is rested just below the anterior superior iliac spine, in the examiner's left groin (Fig. 8.10A), although some may find the right side easier.

2. The patient's wrist is extended and the forearm supinated (Fig. 8.10B).

3. With the above position maintained, the elbow is fully flexed (Fig. 8.10C).

4. Shoulder depression is then taken up by the examiner's right arm pushing into the bed, taking up the depression and then 'punching' down into the bed to block and hold the depression. In this position, shoulder lateral rotation can be added (Fig. 8.10D).

5. With this position maintained, shoulder abduction is added as though it were a matter of placing the patient's hand over her ear. To do this in a smooth action, the physiotherapist's body should be placed so that a pivot around the arm pushed into the bed is achieved. The initial stride standing position is essential (Fig. 8.10E).

6. The test can be done with the neck initially in a position of lateral flexion (or any other desired position) or the patient's head can be pushed across into lateral flexion during the course of the test (Fig. 8.10F).

There are many components of this test and it is easy to lose them during the procedure. All components must be held and kept stable before the addition of a subsequent movement. This tension test takes a little practice. Like all tension tests, once the base test has been performed, the components can be added in any desired order.

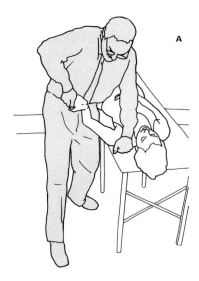

Fig. 8.10A ULTT3 stage 1

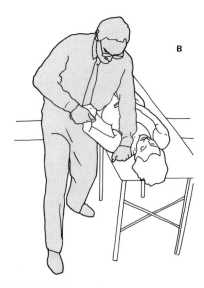

Fig. 8.10B ULTT3 stage 2

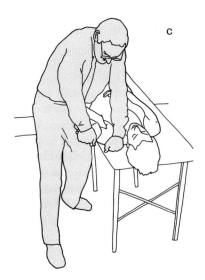

Fig. 8.10C ULTT3 stage 3

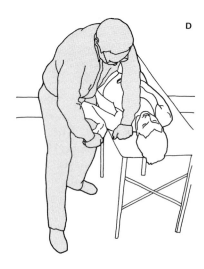

Fig. 8.10D ULTT3 stage 4

Indications

ULTT3 is clearly an ulnar nerve biased tension test. I feel it should be regarded as a base test because the ULTT1 and 2 do not routinely use elbow flexion and hence may not place enough tension on the ulnar nerve and its continuations. Nerve root lesions at C8 and T1 are well known for being obstinate to manual therapy, and hunting out ways to get at all the structures involved

in such a disorder has prompted my regular clinical usage of this test. In doing so, the role of the ulnar nerve in other disorders of the upper limb, such as 'golfers elbow', came to light. The test should be done where any suspicion of ulnar nerve involvement exists in the disorder. An example of a clue which the patient may offer is, at the top of a golf swing, they have wrist pain along the ulnar border. Such a position is similar to ULTT3.

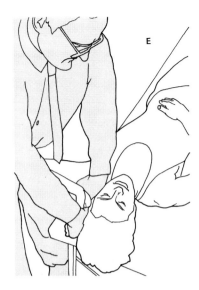

Fig. 8.10E ULTT3 stage 5

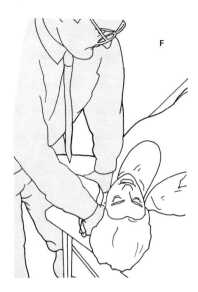

Fig. 8.10F ULTT3 stage 6

If a patient presented with a restricted ULTT1 and with symptoms in a median nerve distribution, an ULTT3 could still be worthwhile, especially if a site of tension is in the brachial plexus. The best possible movements of the plexus connections of the ulnar nerve are needed for the best movement and tension of those of the median nerve. Hence, treatment via the ulnar nerve tension test could be part of a treatment for carpal tunnel syndrome.

Normal responses

No normative studies have been undertaken on the ULTT3. Responses should be compared with those obtained from the other arm. In asymptomatic young people, a common response is a degree of burning and tingling in the ulnar nerve distribution in the hand or in the medial aspect of the elbow. Apparently, the test is not as sensitive in normal subjects as the ULTT1 and ULTT2. In some, there may be no symptoms provoked or resistance reached. These are my quick observations from testing many participants on adverse neural tension courses.

OTHER UPPER LIMB TENSION TESTS

These base tests and variations should apply tension and move all neural structures in the arm and neck. However, the musculocutaneous nerve, the long thoracic nerve, the axillary nerve and the suprascapular nerve may need a little more stress placed upon them during testing. Certainly, the examiner should be aware of these nerves during the test procedure. The long thoracic nerve will be tensioned by shoulder depression and lateral flexion away of the cervical and thoracic spine. Protraction of the arm will tension the suprascapular nerve. Both the musculocutaneous nerve and its terminal branch, the lateral antebrachial cutaneous nerve of the forearm, will be tensioned by shoulder girdle depression, elbow extension and lateral rotation; more so with some concomitant shoulder abduction. Abduction and lateral rotation of the shoulder will stretch the axillary nerve.

Further refinements and analysis of tension tests are discussed in the next chapter.

REFERENCES

Bell A 1987 The upper limb tension test and straight leg raising. In: Dalziell B A, Snowsill J C (eds) Manipulative Therapists Association of Australia, Proceedings 5th biennial conference, Melbourne

Buehler M J, Thayer D T 1988 The elbow flexion test: a clinical test for the cubital tunnel syndrome. Clinical Orthopaedics and Related Research 233: 213–216

Butler D S 1987 The concept and treatment of adverse mechanical tension in the nervous system — application to repetition strain injury. In: Dalziel B A, Snowsill J C (eds) Manipulative Therapists Association of Australia, Fifth biennial conference, Melbourne

Chavany J A 1934 A propos des neuralgies cervico-brachiales. Bulletin Medical (Paris) 48: 335–339

Cyriax J 1978 Textbook of orthopaedic medicine, 7th edn. Baillierre Tindall, London, vol 1

Davidson R I, Dunn E J, Metzmaker J N 1981 The shoulder abduction test in the diagnosis or radicular pain in cervical extradural compressive monoradiculopathies. Spine 6: 441–445

Elvey R L 1979 Painful restriction of shoulder movement: a clinical observational study. In: Proceedings, Disorders of the knee, ankle and shoulder. Western Australian Institute of Technology, Perth

Elvey R L 1986 Treatment of arm pain associated with abnormal brachial plexus tension. Australian Journal of Physiotherapy 32: 224–229

Elvey R L, Quintner J L, Thomas A N 1986 A clinical study of RSI. Australian Family Physician 15: 1314–1322

Fardy E 1985 The upper limb tension test: an investigation of responses to the upper limb tension test and the effect of passive movement of the head in sagittal and coronal planes in young asymptomatic subjects. Unpublished thesis, South Australian Institute of Technology, Adelaide

Frykolm R 1951 Cervical nerve root compression resulting from disc degeneration and root-sleeve fibrosis: a clinical investigation. Acta Chirurgica Scandinavica (Suppl) 160: 1–149

Ginn K 1989 An investigation of tension development in upper limb soft tissues during the upper limb tension test. In: Proceedings, International Federation of Orthopaedic Manipulative Therapists, Congress, Cambridge

Kenneally M, Rubenach H, Elvey R 1988 The upper limb tension test: the SLR test of the arm. In: Grant R (ed) Physical therapy of the cervical and thoracic spine, Clinics in physical therapy 17. Churchill Livingstone, Edinburgh

Kenneally M 1985 The upper limb tension test. In: Proceedings, Manipulative Therapists Association of Australia, 4th biennial conference, Brisbane

Landers J 1987 The upper limb tension test. In: Dalziell B A, Snowsill J C (eds) Manipulative Therapists Association of Australia, Proceedings 5th biennial conference, Melbourne

Lord J W, Roseti L M 1971 Thoracic outlet syndromes. In: CIBA Clinical Symposia 23: 20–23

Maitland G D 1977 Vertebral manipulation, 4th edn. Butterworths, London

McLaughlin A 1989 Combined slump tests. Unpublished thesis, South Australian Institute of Technology, Adelaide

Pechan 1973 Ulnar nerve manoeuvre as a diagnostic aid in its pressure lesions in the cubital region. Ceskoslovenska Neurologie 36: 13–19

Pullos J 1986 The upper limb tension test. Australian Journal of Physiotherapy 32: 258–259

Quintner J L 1989 A study of upper limb pain and paraesthesiae following neck injury in motor vehicle accidents: assessment of the brachial plexus tension test of Elvey. British Journal of Rheumatology 28: 528–533

Rubenach H 1985 The upper limb tension test: the effect of the position and movement of the contralateral arm. In: Proceedings, Manipulative Therapists Association of Australia, 4th biennial conference, Brisbane

Selvaratnam P J, Glasgow E F, Matyas T 1989 Differential strain produced by the brachial plexus tension test on C5 to T1 nerve roots. In: Jones H M, Jones M A, Milde M R (eds) Manipulative Therapists Association of Australia, Sixth biennial conference proceedings

Smith C G 1956 Changes in length and posture of the segments of the spinal cord with changes in posture in the monkey. Radiology 66: 259–265

Sweeney J E, Harms A D 1990 Hand hypersensitivity and the upper limb tension test: another angle. Pain (Suppl) 5, S466

Young L 1989 The upper limb tension test response in a group of post Colle's fracture patients. Unpublished thesis, South Australian Institute of Technology, Adelaide

9. Application, analysis and further testing

ESSENTIALS OF TESTING

The physical examination methods described in the previous three chapters may have to be altered slightly to suit all physiotherapists. Physiotherapists come in different shapes and sizes, so do patients, plinths and physiotherapy departments. There are different hand placements, examiner's stances, and adaptations to particular patients that will make a test fit one physiotherapist/patient combination better than others. What is important is that the physical examination procedure accurately tests the desired movement, allows interpretation of that movement and that the technique is safe for both the physiotherapist and the patient. Most physiotherapists should have no trouble with the examination procedures described. It is important that the base tests are learnt and that the physiotherapist acquires a feel for tension testing. Handling skills for new tension tests and variations on the old should progress rapidly once the base tests are mastered. There are, however, a few essentials with testing.

When performing a tension test the examiner must:

1. Know details of all the patient's symptoms
2. Know details of the symptoms in the starting position
3. Carefully monitor symptoms throughout the procedure and make the patient clear about the symptoms complained of in comparison to any pain or discomfort caused by the test. Symptoms should be reassessed after each component of the test. (It is essential that the patient concentrates, and knows that any changes in symptoms must be reported to the physiotherapist.)
4. Note and record if necessary:

(a) The range of movement at which symptoms first start (P1)
(b) Whether the disorder is non-irritable. If so take the test to the predetermined symptom response or range of movement and note the responses
(c) The type and area of symptoms
(e) The resistance to movement encountered during the test, especially when in range, resistance begins
(f) The above findings compared to the test of the contralateral limb and to what is known to be normal

5. Take the test far enough to establish if adverse tension is a relevant component of the disorder and if a claim of symptoms being adverse tension related can be made. This may require the addition of sensitising or desensitising manoeuvres. From the information gained during the subjective examination, the physiotherapist should be aware of how far into range, how much of the symptoms and which symptoms can be reproduced.

THE RELEVANCE OF EXAMINATION FINDINGS

The tension test examination findings can be analysed in three broad ways. Firstly, whether the findings indicate that the mechanics of the nervous system are abnormal. Secondly, whether these findings are relevant to the particular patient

161

being examined. Thirdly, can further analysis of the test findings assist in locating the site or sites of the altered mechanics, hence providing assistance in treatment.

Normal responses to tension tests

In most people, tension testing causes some discomfort (Kenneally et al 1988). There will be normal responses, either a resistance from tight tissues, a pain response, or both, to any combination of movements in the body. For tension tests such as the Slump Test and the ULTT1, the normal responses have been documented (see Chs 7 & 8). Normal responses are useful but are not essential. If a base test system, as suggested, is used, then it is very useful to have normal responses for these tests. Otherwise, using the points from the 'essentials of testing' listed earlier in this chapter, will allow adequate testing. It is worth remembering that some of the tests are complex and the exact replication of a test will be very difficult, although Philip et al (1989) have shown a high inter-therapist reliability when the patient's symptoms are the criterion for a positive or negative Slump Test. After some experience with tension tests, normal responses to a particular disorder, such as a positive ULTT2 with radial bias in tennis elbow, may become evident. As well as the need to compare with expected normal responses, it is important to consider whether the responses are relevant to the particular patient being examined.

Positivity/relevance

Usually the term 'positive' is applied to a tension test if the test reproduces relevant symptoms or is limited at a particular range. I urge examiners to consider relevance of the test as well as positivity. Rather than merely assigning a range of movement, say 90° of knee flexion for a positive Prone Knee Bend, the findings need to take features of the presenting disorder, other than the pain response and the range of movement, into account. The whole patient perspective needs analysis. These two examples emphasise the importance of such thinking:

1. A long distance runner complains of mild but annoying right anterior thigh pain after running for one hour. On physical examination of all relevant possible contributing structures, there is little evidence of any injury. However, the right PKB, though full range, is slightly tighter than the left and causes a slight pulling in the anterior thigh and low back, more so on the right than the left. In this patient, such symptoms and the sign are relevant and probably need improving before the annoying pain is alleviated. This patient may also be better examined if the disorder is sensitised. That is, the patient is examined after running for an hour.

2. A patient complains of severe debilitating right anterior thigh pain that is easily aggravated, difficult to ease and limits him to walking 50 yards before he has to stop and rest. On physical examination, active spinal movements are limited by pain at approximately half range and hip flexion is limited at 40°. The PKB causes some pain at 80° of knee flexion. Although, in this case, the PKB is more 'positive' than in the first example it is far less relevant at this stage of examination. The hip and the lumbar spine deserve greater attention, at least in the above presenting stage of the disorder.

Definition — a positive tension test

The term 'positive' has been retained, although it must include relevance if it is to be of great clinical use. A tension test can be considered positive if:

1. It reproduces the patient's symptoms. Note that this may not yet implicate the nervous system and further testing may be required.

2. The test responses can be altered by movement of distant body parts. For example, if a Passive Neck Flexion test alters a Straight Leg Raise response of posterior thigh pain, then the SLR is instantly made a more relevant test of nervous system mechanics.

3. There are differences in the test from the left side to the right side and from what is

known to be normal. These differences may be in ranges of movement, resistance encountered during movement and in symptom responses during movement. Be wary that the good side, if used for comparison, could also be affected by the same disorder.

To enable further analysis of the tension tests and ultimately, to ascertain the sites of adverse tension, some features of examination require discussion.

ESSENTIAL FEATURES OF TENSION TEST ANALYSIS

1. A positive tension test does not necessarily indicate a mechanical disorder of the nervous system. There may be a physiological disorder, such as irritation, existing alone, without structural changes such as tethering or intraneural scarring (pathomechanics).

Alterations in microcirculation and tissue pressures around the nervous system are likely to be present well before any structural changes are evident. Symptoms related to target tissue hypersensitivity could perhaps be reproduced by tension testing. A pathophysiological situation may occur alone or in combination with pathomechanics. It is difficult to envisage a pathomechanical situation existing without any pathophysiological changes.

Another important consideration is that the test could be placing a force on a surrounding symptomatic interfacing structure, yet the nervous system itself is normal. For example, a SLR could be pulling on dural ligaments which, in turn, could be placing a force on an irritated posterior longitudinal ligament.

2. A positive tension test gives the examiner a valid reason to examine away from the symptom area and known sources capable of referring pain to that area. For example, if Passive Neck Flexion reproduces lumbar pain, then a site of adverse tension may be anywhere between, and including, the neck and lumbar spine (and possibly beyond). Similarly, in an Upper Limb Tension Test, if wrist extension alters neck symptoms, then a

site anywhere along the nerve trunks, roots and neuraxis may be responsible. There could be a number of sites of tension with a marked additive effect. Even if a site of adverse tension contributes only a few percent to the 'main site', alleviation of tension at this location could have a marked symptomatic alterations at the main site. For example, I have often noted clinically that treatment at the T6 tension point area can alter symptoms and signs related to a known disc injury at the L4 area. This is an important issue. It takes time to get used to handling the nervous system and most physiotherapists are not used to the idea of examining well away from the symptom area, or of sites that can refer into the symptom area.

Where examination away from the symptom area and referral sites is undertaken, the vulnerable areas are best examined first. For example with a positive Straight Leg Raise reproducing a relevant hamstring area pain, possible sites for early examination would be the T6 tension point area and the area around the superior tibio-fibula joint.

3. The examination techniques must be part of an overall concept of examination (Elvey 1986). The base tension tests, by themselves, are quite crude and limited. For example, in a patient with left buttock pain, it is not enough to examine a SLR, find it negative and from that amount of examination, declare that adverse tension has no part in the patient's symptoms. Neurogenic symptoms may not be reproduced in the pure SLR position. They may be reproduced in a combination of the SLR with hip adduction and medial rotation together with a spinal lateral flexion position. In the upper limb, examination of one tension test, such as ULTT1, is not enough. The patient's symptoms may not be reproduced in the elevated arm position, yet they could be in a behind the back position. Subjective clues about positions that cause the symptoms and a knowledge of biomechanics must be used to make up new tension positions that fit with the patient's complaints and with nervous system biomechanics. This is discussed later in this chapter. The base tests can be used as

tests from which to explore and as reassessments to come back to after a treatment which may be in a completely different position.

Physiotherapists adept in joint examination will examine joint movement in many directions and combinations of movements. The nervous system needs such detailed assessment also.

4. Sensitising or desensitising additions are a great help in proving a nervous system component of a disorder. This is especially so if the addition is some distance away from the symptom site. For example, if a SLR reproduces thoracic pain the nervous system as a source is immediately suspect. Then, if ankle dorsiflexion further increases that pain, altered mechanics of the nervous system is even more strongly suspected. The only structure that has been altered in these examples is the nervous system. Desensitising additions are useful too. For example, in standing spinal forward flexion, if cervical extension decreases symptoms in the lumbar spine (presuming the physiotherapist has carefully stabilised the lumbar spine) a nervous system disorder must be strongly suspected. We can infer that the symptoms are at least part neurogenic in origin (see section on 'Quick tests' later in this chapter).

5. Relevant nerve trunks should always be palpated along their length. This helps to identify sites of tension, entrapment and also gives some indication about the pathology present. For example, irritated epineurial tissue can be tender to palpate, and tapping the nerve (Tinel's sign) may produce paraesthesia in the nerve distribution — an indication that nerve fibres are affected in the disorder. Techniques of palpation are discussed later in this chapter.

6. Sometimes with tension testing, 'the' pain or symptoms cannot be completely reproduced, and the physiotherapist may have to be content with reproduction of similar symptoms or symptoms that are different from the contralateral limb. This again underlines the crudity of testing. It may take half an hour or more to find the desired symptomatic

relationship of tension, movement and the interfacing tissue. This is not usually necessary and the time taken may be unproductive. An examining physiotherapist may feel that a comparable symptom could be a familiar symptom. It should also fit the examination. Those patients who report more vague pains or occasional catches are unlikely to have such symptoms completely reproduced.

7. A neurological examination for all patients treated via tension tests is mandatory (Ch. 6). This includes subjective and objective tests of upper and lower motor neurone conduction. This is not only for safety, but also for diagnosis and prognosis. Neurological signs make excellent reassessments. It is often surprising how neurological changes can occur with normalising of nervous system mechanics.

8. The examining physiotherapist should remember that it is possible to examine the mechanics of the nervous system in three ways (Figure 9.1A,B,C & D). Firstly, the elasticity can be examined (Fig. 9.1B), for example by the Slump Test or the ULTT1 including cervical lateral flexion away from the test side. Secondly, the ability to move in relation to an interface (Fig. 9.1C), as in any movement out of tension, for example shoulder depression with the elbow flexed and the cervical spine in neutral may be examined. Thirdly, in some areas such as the dorsum of the foot, by palpation, the transverse movements of the nervous system can be examined. Some physiological movements, such as elbow flexion, also move the nervous system in a perpendicular direction to the interfacing structures (Fig. 9.1D).

9. Analysis of the sources of adverse tension signs and symptoms can be difficult especially with a widespread distribution of symptoms, the possibility of multiple sites along the nervous system and the contributions of non-neural structures. However, any analysis can only be an hypothesis that is proven or disproven by the clinical reasoning process. An hypothesis may not be proven but strengthened or weakened. It is the making of the hypothesis, the 'having a go' at the site and origin of symptoms, and the collection of

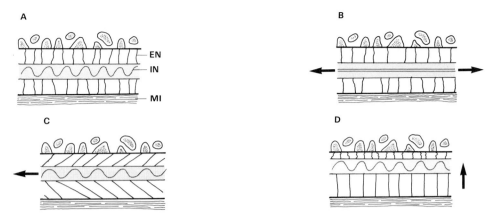

Fig. 9.1 The mechanics of the nervous system available to examination, A. Representation of a segment of nervous system surrounded by a mechanical interface, The lines represent the intraneural and extraneural connective tissues. MI mechanical interface, IN intraneural EN extraneural, B. examination of the intraneural component or the elasticity of the system (e.g., Slump test), C. examination of the extraneural component or the movement of the system in relation to the interface (e.g., knee extension in hip flexion) D. examination of the movement of the nervous system perpendicular to the interface (e.g., palpation)

information to support or reject the hypothesis that will enable progress in this area of physiotherapy.

ESTABLISHING SITES OF ADVERSE TENSION

The importance of accurate symptom localisation

It is crucial to an accurate assessment that the patient is questioned about the site of symptoms, not only before testing but during testing. The SLR provides a good example. If the patient complains of pain at a tension point, i.e., at a point behind the knee or at the head of the fibula during a SLR, then this is regarded as a possible 'tension point pain'. A hamstring limitation is un-likely to cause a limitation at this area. This symptom response may be an indication that something is wrong with the mechanics of the nervous system, even though the symptoms are not what the patient complains of. In the case of the SLR, sites of adverse tension could be in the foot or the lumbar spine, or even higher in the thoracic spine. Further proof and interpretation will be needed to decide whether the site is ex-traneural or intraneural. The common peroneal tension point pain or 'burn' is quite common. It

follows that the physiotherapist who is clinically reasoning as he/she assesses will then look for contributing sites of tension below in the calf or foot or higher in the thigh or spine.

The symptoms evoked on tension testing can be categorised:

1. Physiological symptoms, i.e, normal symptomatic responses to the stretch of structures

2. Clinical physiological symptoms, i.e., abnormal symptoms provoked by the test but in areas where there is nothing wrong with the underlying structures. For example, testing a SLR in a patient with low back pain may produce a pain posterior to the knee at 60° while, in the other leg, it reproduces a pain in the hamstring area at 80°. There may be nothing wrong with the structures posterior to the knee, but this area is showing up as symptomatic, whereas the source of the symptoms could be elsewhere, such as in the lumbar spine. Sometimes altered patterns of clinical physiological symptoms are evident. For example, in a patient with a right 'Achilles tendonitis', the response to right knee extension during the Slump Test could be calf pain then hamstring pain, whereas to left knee extension during the Slump Test, the response is hamstring area pain, then calf. Such a

response can only indicate that something is wrong, maybe involving the nervous system. It is up to the skilled examiner to prove or disprove the hypothesis that the pain is from the nervous system and to find out where the sources of adverse tension are. With sensitising and desensitising manoeuvres, physiological and clinical physiological symptoms could be analysed further to prove whether they are neurogenic in origin

3. Neurogenic/Neuropathic symptoms. Here, the symptoms are presumed to originate from some pathology involving the nervous system, as far as can possibly be ascertained by examination. All available information must be used to make this inference, including structural differentiation, information gained from the subjective examination and investigative tests. I have used the term broadly to include all symptoms from the nervous system. Absolute proof is difficult with the more minor injuries.

Site(s) along the nervous system

Clinicians are reminded that there is nearly always likely to be more than one segment of nervous system and more than one structure involved. The site(s) of adverse tension along the nervous system may be ascertained from various sources:

1. The subjective examination. The area of symptoms (e.g., dermatomal, along a nerve, known vulnerable point) will assist in source identification. Clearly, the history could be particularly helpful especially with isolated trauma.

2. The neurological examination. Sensory and motor deficits could indicate involvement at nerve trunk, nerve root or cord level. The level of nerve root and the sites along the nerve trunk could also be identified (see Ch. 6).

3. Palpation of the nervous system (see page 172).

4. In some situations, if the patient's symptoms are evoked by tension testing, the area of symptoms is likely to be the source of symptoms. For example, with medial knee pain and especially with a history of injury to

the area, if the saphenous nerve tension test reproduces that pain, the major site is logically the saphenous nerve and interfacing structures at the knee. In other situations, clinical physiological symptoms and referral of symptoms will make such an analysis difficult.

5. Order of component addition. It is expected that the best reproduction of symptoms will come if the source of symptoms is tensioned first and then tension is added via other components. For example, if the sensory radial nerve is injured at the wrist, the ULTT2 (radial bias) should be more sensitive if the wrist ulnar deviation and pronation components are taken up first, instead of last as proposed in the base test (Ch. 8).

6. Examination of interfacing structures. Because the effects of pathology will not be limited to the nervous system, examination of the interfacing structures is one of the best ways to localise sites of tension. Physiotherapists have become specialised in the examination of joint and muscle, but the physical findings from testing these structures may not always be due to that structure. For example, the pain and resistance encountered on palpating a symptomatic costo-transverse joint could be due to an intercostal nerve or the sympathetic trunk. Likewise, an iliopsoas muscle may be tight because the genito-femoral nerve is painful if stretched. The known vulnerable sites should also be accorded preferential examination.

Intraneural and extraneural sites

The sites of pathology that create positive tension tests can be extraneural, intraneural or both. These processes have been discussed in Chapter 3 and related to neurobiomechanics in Chapter 2. In many situations the site(s) or the predominant site(s) can be identified and then treated accordingly. For example, if the source of a positive tension test is extraneural, i.e, in the nerve bed or the interfacing structure, then the interfacing structure requires treatment or the nerve needs to be moved in the nerve bed. If a process is inside the nervous system then some tension

Table 9.1 Some signs and symptoms that may indicate intraneural and extraneural sites of adverse neural tension — A hypothesis. (adapted from Asbury and Fields, 1984, Butler 1989)

	Extraneural	Intraneural	
		Conducting tissues	Connective tissues
Description and distribution	Catches, twinges around vulnerable areas	'Burning, tingling, electric' in innervation field	Lines of pain, along trunks, nondermatomal
Constancy	Intermittant → constant short symptom duration	More constant, longer symptom duration	Intermittent → constant
Recognition	Familiar	Unfamiliar, 'bizarre', 'nervey'	More familiar
Aggravating/easing factors	↑ With movement of interface	↑With tension of nervous system Activity specific	↑With tension ↓↑ With movement
Physical signs	Comparable signs in interfacing structures	Neurological signs & symptoms Palpation → symptoms elsewhere	Palpation → local pain
Tension test symptom response	↑ or ↓ With movement	↑ With tension	↑ With movement ↑ With tension
Examples	Tight scalenei → irritation of nervous system	Neuroma and immature axons in scarred endoneurium	Irritated epineurium

generation during the treatment will be needed. Where both processes are involved, the best treatment response will be from treating both extraneurally and intraneurally. If a disorder is intraneural, further localisation of the site is possible. The disorder may involve the conducting tissues and/or the connective tissues. Table 9.1 is a hypothesis that provides further examples of clues to either extraneural or intraneural sites of tension. These are derived from my clinical analysis, logic and the hypothesis of Asbury & Fields (1984) (see Ch. 4). Equally, in the central nervous system, where possible, cord signs and symptoms should be differentiated from those from the connective tissues.

Consideration of symptoms from non-neural tissues

The non-neural structures can be a source of symptoms from direct injury to their tissues. Be aware that the patient's expression of these symptoms may be impaired by injury to the primary neurones involved either in the peripheral or central nervous system. A patent nervous system is vital,

especially for approaches that are heavily dependent on symptomatology.

The non-neural tissues could also be directly affected by a site of adverse tension in the form of trophic changes due to impaired axonal transport mechanisms, or even disuse or misuse. If there are suggestions that altered axoplasmic flow is an element in the disorder, then treatment of the tension signs may become more of a priority. Unaccountable maintenance of symptoms and signs, observable changes in skin such as reddening, shininess, and puffiness are examples of clues. Further to this would be changes on X-ray such as osteoporosis and whether, in the history, there was enough evidence to implicate the non-neural structure, i.e., 'Did features fit?'. In more severe nerve injuries that have led to paralysis, maintenance of the extensibility of the soft tissues by passive movement may be needed.

TAKING TENSION TESTING FURTHER

The base tests alone are not enough to examine a patient's disorder. It would be a rare situation where one of the base tests was the best possible way of reproducing symptoms. Already in the last two chapters, sensitising tests and variations to the tests have been discussed. New tests can be devised, and this can be done using expanded clinical reasoning skills. The reasoning will be primarily determined by the use of anatomical knowledge and by listening to the patient.

1. Use of anatomical knowledge. For example, it is clear that the addition of plantar-flexion and inversion to a SLR will place tension and movement along the common peroneal tract. Equally, it should be evident that passive neck extension will lessen tension and allow movement of the nervous system. An awareness of common anomalies is also needed.

2. Listening to the patient. For example, if a patient says she gets her symptoms on doing up a bra strap, then this position can be turned into a tension test. By placing the arm into the pain reproductive position, other components such as cervical flexion and wrist movements may be added and subtracted. If a patient said that, during walking, there was left hip pain when turning to the left, hip medial rotation as a known nervous system sensitiser would be a logical component to add into examination. In supine, the hip could be medially rotated and then hip flexion, knee extension and cervical movements added. Hip medial rotation could also be examined as part of the Slump Test. If the patient said a fast movement or a sustained position was symptomatic then these features could be included in the test.

As well as adding physiological movements, accessory movements of joints, muscle contractions or fascial stretches could be added. For example, a postero-anterior pressure could be placed on the head of the humerus in an ULTT1 position in prone, the hamstrings could be contracted in a SLR position or the plantar fascia could be stretched in a position of SLR/ankle dorsiflexion.

This also raises the idea of 'hunting out' symptoms or, as Maitland (1986) says, 'Find the pain and hurt it'. In this regard, all information possible from the subjective examination, a knowledge of anatomy and some trial and error movements will be required.

Tension testing the irritable disorder

The tension tests in the previous chapter have been described for the non-irritable disorder where a complete examination is possible. However, they can also be used as part of the examination of severe and irritable disorders. With the nervous system being a continuum throughout the entire body, the ability to move just one structure gently in remote parts without touching that structure is invaluable both diagnostically and for treatment purposes. For example, in a severe lumbar area injury, a PNF can move the nervous system in the lumbar spine but not other structures. In some nasty whiplash injuries to the cervical spine, just ankle dorsiflexion alone may increase the neck symptoms.

With the more irritable disorders, it is unlikely that the whole test will need to be performed. For example, in an ULTT1 if shoulder abduction of 50° makes symptoms that are deemed irritable, worse, and wrist extension worsens them again, that may be the extent of the examination. Enough information has been obtained at that stage. More information (perhaps from the contralateral ULTT or the SLR) may be required if the nervous system is going to be mobilised. However, if an interfacing structure is to be mobilised, then the amended test can be used as a reassessment. The nervous system has already been implicated as part of that disorder. In a Slump Test, if sitting with a few degrees of spinal flexion causes a lumbar pain and a few degrees of neck flexion makes this pain worse, that is enough examination to establish the nervous system as part of the disorder. With the ULTT2 positions, the use of the physiotherapist's thigh to depress the shoulder girdle is probably not needed. Better support can be given by leaving the arm on the bed and then gently depressing the shoulder using the physiotherapist's arms. Further guides to better tension testing are given below.

Guide to better tension testing

1. There is a skill in handling that some people pick up very quickly and others have to

learn. The base tests must be performed adequately and practised before any derivatives are added. The Slump Test and the Upper Limb Tension Tests are the most difficult tests to master. They need to be practised on asymptomatic subjects before they are attempted on patients.

2. As in the examination of any structure, it is best to begin knowing what to expect. The subjective examination should allow this. That is, the physical findings should match the patient's complaints. For example, if the patient says he/she can kick a football, then a good range of SLR should be expected. During the physical examination if the physiotherapist tests the good limb first then he/she should have a better idea about what to expect from the affected limb. This is particularly important where the disorder is irritable or the physiotherapist is unsure of the level of irritability.

Patients should also know what to expect from the test. They must be told about the test and any likely symptoms. They need to know that all responses, especially those relating to their symptoms, are of interest. The most common handling difficulty with the ULTT1 is when the patient is asked to flex his/her head laterally away from the test side. Nearly all patients will rotate their heads away. The lateral flexion manoeuvre you want them to perform must be demonstrated at the start of the test.

3. A clearer interpretation will be possible if a component of the tension test is taken just to the onset of symptoms (P1) and then taken back to just off P1, into a symptom-free range, before the next movement is added on. The patient may then relax more and will find it easier to describe aspects of symptoms if they are not superimposed on a pre-existing symptom. Similarly, if a component to the tension test is added on or taken off, the most minimal movement possible to get an alteration in responses is desirable. The more movement, the more structures are involved. These handling suggestions ultimately make it easier to make the inference of a symptom

being neurogenic in origin. They also assist with handling the patient with an irritable or potentially irritable disorder. In some non-irritable disorders, especially where symptoms are hunted out, the position reproducing the symptom may need to be maintained while other components are added.

4. Some assistance with these tests can be extremely valuable. Other physiotherapists skilled in tension testing are obviously the best. However, any of the staff in a physiotherapy department could be trained to assist. Combinations, such as adding cervical positions to the SLR or adding in the contralateral ULTT, are so much easier with help. Make sure, if possible, the assistant holds the non-moving part so that the physiotherapist can move one component and feel the resistance to the movement and thus interpret this in relation to the symptoms provoked.

5. Remember to feel for resistance to the movement and not just 'symptom hunt'. Resistance related to altered nervous system mechanics is often felt earlier in range than the reproduction of symptoms. A treatment may be defined by the amount of resistance encountered rather than the symptom response. The importance of symptom localisation has been discussed in an earlier section.

Sustained tests

Some authors have suggested and demonstrated the value of sustained positions as tests for the nervous system. For example, Mackinnon & Dellon (1988) suggested holding the forearm in hyperpronation to test for entrapment of the superficial radial nerve, with symptoms expected within a minute. Buehler & Thayer (1988) suggested a sustained elbow flexion position (illustrated in Ch. 8) for entrapment of the ulnar nerve in the cubital tunnel. Clare (1989) described a 'free arm hanging test' of up to 60 seconds to assist in the assessment of the responses of upper limb neural tissue to tension in the longitudinal axis. Patients diagnosed as suffering from repetition strain injury (Ch. 14) reported symptoms earlier in the test than a group of asymptomatic normals.

I feel that the symptoms provoked by these sustained tests could also be reproduced by the appropriate tension test as described in the last chapter. However, they can provide an accurate reassessment following treatment. The time taken to reproduce symptoms gives an objective measure and the tests are easily reproducable and accurate because there is no movement.

These sustained tests would also be appropriate if a patient complained of symptoms after a period of time in a sustained position.

Quick tests

During the physical examination of a patient, it is possible to incorporate quick tension tests. A good example of this is when the patient stands and forward flexes his/her spine and complains of a pain, say around L4. Diagnostically, this pain could come from a number of sources with joints, muscles and nerves of the lumbar spine being the most likely culprits. But, if the patient can be held at that pain provoking position and then the cervical spine flexed and extended to see if there is any change in the pain response, this may point to an adverse tension component to the disorder (Fig. 9.2). This will help to prioritise the examination. For example, if in the patient mentioned, neck movements could alter the lumbar pain, then it would mean the Slump Test should be performed on the first visit.

Some other examples are:

1. If a patient complains of pain in the shoulder quadrant position it is an easy matter to perform the same technique and alter elbow extension, wrist and hand movements (Fig. 9.3). The patient could make these alterations actively. Other joints which could be altered to give similar information would be the cervical spine, and those involved in the contralateral arm or the SLR.

2. If the length of the upper trapezius muscle is tested, the contribution of the

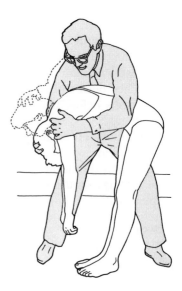

Fig. 9.2 Flexion and extension of the cervical spine in a position which provokes symptoms in the lumbar spine. A quick test for the nervous system

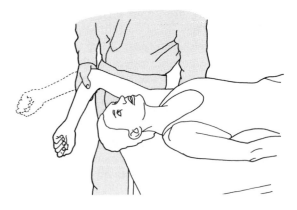

Fig. 9.3 Quick testing for the nervous system in the quadrant position

nervous system to its length and any symptoms provoked can be tested by performing the technique with the elbow flexed and then comparing the same movement with the elbow extended (Fig. 9.4).

The crucial part of all these examinations is that a technique is performed in differing nervous system tensions and nerve/interface relationships, yet the non-neural structures underlying are not, or only negligibly, altered.

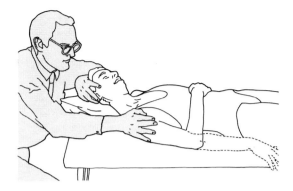

Fig. 9.4 Testing for the role of the nervous system during examination of trapezius length

Table 9.3 Recording a treatment

IN: WE	GHAb 90 into mod p	DID: EE 2 × IV + into p, S.O. p + n

RECORDING

Accurate records must be kept and updated with each attendance or contact. It is particularly important that, on the first assessment, a base is made from which to treat. For example, an initial examination of ULTT1 in a patient with a pain in her upper arm and pins and needles in her thumb may be recorded as in Table 9.2. Table 9.2 is read as:

At glenohumeral abduction of 85°, the patient's arm pain and pins and needles were reproduced. Wrist extension was full range, symptoms from the shoulder abduction did not change although the movement produced a wrist pain. Supination was full range and did not alter any of the symptoms. Lateral rotation was limited to 45°, the pain increased, the pins and needles were the same. Elbow extension was limited to 120°, all symptoms increased dramatically and the patient complained of a sensation of headache. Cervical lateral flexion towards the test side reduced all symptoms except those in the wrist. At 5°, cervical lateral flexion away from the test side, all symptoms increased except those in the wrist.

Recording is a rather personal thing. No one physiotherapist's recording will be the same as

the next, though hopefully recording will be similar and easily transferable from one physiotherapist to another. Note my personal preferences in the above example. If the patient's symptoms are reproduced, then they are underlined (compare the symptoms reproduced on shoulder abduction compared to wrist extension). If a component has a dramatic effect on the test, then this is emphasised by a number of pluses. Note too that a range of movement has been added where possible and this has been qualified by a symptom response. This symptom response does not have to be pain, it could be a headache or even a feeling of nausea.

To record a particular treatment, along the same line as the assessment, I use the 'IN: DID:' system. An example of a treatment could be as shown in Table 9.3.

In this example, wrist extension was taken up first, followed by shoulder abduction to 90°, which was in the area of moderate symptoms for this patient. The technique performed was elbow extension, two repetitions at a grade IV+ into the patient's pain, but short of reproducing the pins and needles. Note another piece of personal recording, if two repetitions are carried out, then the number is underlined. If a series of oscillatory movements of 20 seconds duration is carried out, then this is not underlined.

If the patient has been treated for some time, a shorthand version will probably be all that is necessary, although full responses will need to be recorded from time to time. e.g., 'IN: ULTT2 (radial with wrist in neutral)/DID: Sh Dep 2 ×

Table 9.2 Recording on initial ULTT1 test.

GHAb	WE	SUP	LR	EE	CxLF	CxLF
85 p arm	√	√	45 P ↑	120	to	away
S1 p + n	ISQ	ISQ	p + n ISQ	all p ↑ ++	↓ all	5°
thumb	+ SI W			H	exc W.	↑ all
	pain					exc W.

IV sl pain.' This reads as: 'IN: ULTT 2 position with the radial nerve bias, DID: shoulder depression 2 lots of 20 secs at grade IV which reproduced a slight amount of pain.'

PALPATION OF THE NERVOUS SYSTEM

Tension testing and the examination of conduction form two parts of the examination of the nervous system. The third way in which the nervous system can be examined is by palpation. Palpation of the nervous system is a new idea to many physiotherapists. Perhaps the dominance of joint and muscle thinking has made it rather redundant. Yet, the peripheral nervous system is readily available to palpation and much valuable information can be gleaned. Some revision may be required to recall the location of nerves in the body. I have always been surprised at the amazement of postgraduate course participants when they find how accessible the branches of the superficial peroneal nerve in the dorsum of the foot are and that it is so visually obvious. Most seem to think that the nerve is a tendon.

The uses of palpation

1. There is no better way to learn (or re-learn) the clinical anatomy of the peripheral nervous system than by palpating it. Palpation opens up an awareness and appreciation of the anatomy of the nervous system, especially for the physiotherapist whose treatment and thinking is joint dominant. It also creates an awareness of the great differences in individual nerves. Nerves are not homogeneous structures. For example, palpation of the ulnar nerve at the elbow or in the upper arm easily creates a paraesthesia, whereas palpation of the radial nerve creates more of a local pain and less commonly, a paraesthesia. While the innervated connective tissues of nerve could be in part responsible for the radial nerve symptoms, it seems more likely that the contained primary neurones are responsible for those of the ulnar nerve. Where nerve has more fascicles and more connective tissue, it will be harder to get a neural response from palpation Fascicular arrangement was discussed in Chapter 1.

I also feel that, when physiotherapists reproduce a pain by palpation around a joint or muscle, they could well have their palpating fingers on a nerve. An example is the posterior primary ramus in the lumbar spine. It would seem that pressure on this nerve is unavoidable when performing a unilateral postero-anterior pressure as described by Maitland (1986). When an antero-posterior pressure is placed on the head of the radius, the palpating thumb invariably palpates the radial nerve. Similarly, with an antero-posterior pressure on the talus, the peroneal nerves are palpated. Palpation could elicit pain from a nerve of any size. One only has to remember toothache. Nerves to the teeth are small, yet who can deny the pain of toothache.

2. Injury to nerve may be assessed by palpation. A normal nerve, where accessible, should feel hard and round. It should be able to be moved from side to side. This transverse range of movement will be lessened if the nerve is in tension. Part of the transverse range of movement can be lost if the nerve is adhered to surrounding interface structures. The nerve could be swollen. It may also feel hard and thickened, usually above the site of entrapment. Some peripheral neuropathies, such as leprosy and hereditary motor and sensory neuropathies, can present with long segments of thickened nerve. Entrapment sites are likely to have only small areas thickened. Localised nerve enlargement could also indicate the presence of a peripheral nerve tumour, such as a schwannoma. These can be rolled over the nerve transversely but not axially along the nerve (Thomas 1984).

3. The symptom response from palpation can assist in the localisation of a site of adverse tension. Palpation is likely to evoke local pain from irritated and/or scarred connective tissue sheaths of nerve, or from mechanosensitive sites of abnormal impulse generation. Identification of sites of abnormal impulse generation can be made if a nerve is 'twanged' as is described below and a symptom is felt elsewhere along the nerve track. The site could be the source of symptoms. Palpation can also assist in structural differentiation. For example, if the

superficial radial nerve is twanged on the radius and this reproduces a symptom further distal in the wrist or hand, then this symptom is likely to be related to a neurogenic source. The non-neural structures have not been touched. Where the nervous system is particularly mechanically or chemically sensitised, palpation of a nerve in the extremities, say the superficial radial nerve in the forearm, could reproduce proximal symptoms such as neck pain. There appears to be a spinal canal equivalent here. The patient who complains of lumbar pain while his/her neck is being palpated or vice versa, is often one who has a positive Slump Test.

The nervous system can be further implicated if a site palpated is found to be painful and the pain is increased when the nervous system is tightened. For example, if the saphenous nerve medial to the knee is tenderer to palpation and is tenderer if the saphenous nerve is tightened up via ankle movements, then the tenderness elicited on palpation can be inferred as neurogenic (see Ch. 7). If a spot pain in the arch of the foot is worse when palpated with the leg in SLR, a similar inference may be made.

Nerve tenderness is very common at the site of entrapment (Saal et al 1988). Many clinicians find nerve tenderness the most helpful physical sign for a diagnosis of entrapment. In general, nerves are more sensitive to palpate if there is a source of adverse tension somewhere along the track.

4. Palpation may turn into a local massage or friction treatment. Oscillatory pressures can be placed on the nerve or the surrounding fascia can be frictioned. In retrospect, some of the transverse friction techniques suggested by Cyriax & Russell (1977) must also have included some nerve trunks. Perhaps some of the benefit of the frictions could be attributed to the forces placed through the nerve or effects on nerve from alterations of the interface.

5. Palpation may pick up anomalies. For example, in the foot, if the sural nerve is unusually large, it may be carrying some of the axons that normally would be in the branches of the superficial peroneal nerve. In this case, the branches of the superficial peroneal nerve would be smaller or perhaps even absent.

Techniques of palpation and treatment

Nerves can be directly palpated; they can be 'twanged' and they can be 'tapped', as in Tinel's test. Twanging means gently pulling a finger or thumb nail across the nerve. This may reproduce symptoms under, above or below the site of application. The sural nerve and branches of the common peroneal nerve in the foot, the superficial radial nerve in the forearm, and the median and ulnar nerves in the arm are some good examples where this technique can be applied. Tinel's test of tapping the nerve with the intent of reproducing symptoms in the distribution of the nerve has been discussed in Chapter 6.

It is useful to palpate nerves when the nerve trunk is in tension. If they are tighter then it will be easier to reproduce symptoms, especially if symptoms are related to an intraneural process. An appreciation of common nervous system anomalies is needed. Some are discussed in Chapter 3. Anomalies is probably not the best word, normal variations is better; the nervous system often runs a wayward course. It is recommended that a copy of a good anatomical text book is kept by one's side.

Areas easily palpable

Nerves can be palpated where superficial or, in the cases of large nerves, through some soft tissue. All major nerve trunks have at least two areas where they can be palpated. Like any manual skill, it may take some practice. Listed below are some of the easier areas to palpate.

Lower limb

At approximately one third of the distance between the ischial tuberosity and the greater trochanter, the sciatic nerve can be palpated. The nerve is easier to palpate if the patient is put in prone and the nerve tightened up using a SLR over the side of the bed (Fig. 9.5). The tibial nerve can be palpated centrally and posteriorly at the knee crease where it lies lateral to the popliteal artery

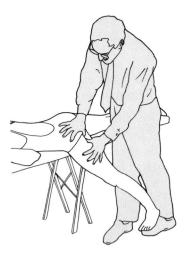

Fig. 9.5 Palpation of the sciatic nerve through the buttocks

and vein. Posterolaterally at the knee, the common peroneal nerve can be palpated medial to the tendon of biceps femoris. From here, it can be followed down to where it wraps around the head of the fibula.

The tibial nerve is again palpable at the level of, and posterior to, the medial malleolus (Fig. 9.6). Here it is still rather thick, up to 5mm or more and in some people stands out like a tendon, especially if the foot is dorsiflexed and everted. It can be traced towards the foot as the medial and lateral plantar nerves. On the dorsum of the foot, the superficial peroneal nerve is easily palpable. This nerve stands out readily, especially if the foot is plantarflexed and inverted. It can be followed up into the lower leg before it is lost

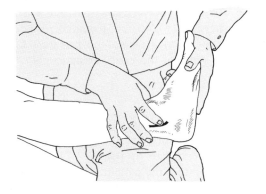

Fig. 9.6 Palpation of the posterior tibial nerve, posterior to the medial malleollus

in fascia. The deep peroneal nerve can be felt between the first and second metatarsal, some 4 cm proximal to the first web space. The difference in the hard round feel of the nerve compared to the softer tendon of extensor hallucis longus is evident. The sural nerve is palpable on the lateral aspect of the foot. Here, a thumb-nail can be carefully dragged across the nerve. This nerve can be followed upward, posterior to the lateral malleolus and up into the calf alongside the achilles tendon. In some individuals, the nerve can be clearly seen posterior to the lateral malleolus when the foot is dorsiflexed and inverted.

The femoral nerve enters the thigh approximately halfway along the inguinal ligament and lateral to the femoral artery. It can be palpated, although through considerable skin and fascia. At the level of the knee joint, its major branch, the saphenous nerve, is palpated between the tendons of sartorius and gracilis. The infrapatellar branch of the nerve is sometimes palpable using the twanging method on the upper tibia. The lateral femoral cutaneous nerve can be palpated deeply in the inguinal ligament about 1 cm medial to the anterior superior iliac spine.

Upper limb

The posterior cords of the plexus and the suprascapular nerve are palpable at the lateral base of the neck. If there is difficulty in identifying the plexus, it can be tightened by shoulder girdle depression and rendered more obvious. The suprascapular nerve can also be palpated deeply in the scapular notch. With anterior palpation of the cervical spine, tips of the fingers and thumbs cannot be far away from emerging spinal nerve. The response to this palpation will be different if the arm is in some abduction. By running a finger nail along the clavicle the subcutaneous supraclavicular nerves can be felt, especially if the cervical spine is laterally flexed away from the side tested.

In the lower axilla, the median and ulnar nerves are easily palpated. The radial nerve is a little more deeply placed. They can be identified by the distribution of the symptom response following palpation. Also, the ulnar nerve can be followed from the axilla to the medial epicondyle of the elbow, and the median nerve from the axilla, more anteriorly than the ulnar, to the elbow. They are both easy to identify if tightened up. If a thumb is placed in the axilla and the shoulder girdle depressed, movement of the hand will cause considerable movement and tension, particularly in the median nerve. The radial nerve can also be palpated here, a little posteriorly to the others, although a neural response is difficult to elicit. The radial nerve is also palpable a few centimetres below the insertion of the deltoid muscle where it emerges from the radial groove. This was a favourite target of the barefisted boxers before the wearing of gloves was enforced.

At the elbow, the radial nerve can be palpated where it is adhered at the radiohumeral joint. The median nerve can be palpated just lateral to the biceps tendon, and the ulnar nerve is very obvious in the ulnar groove. The ulnar nerve in the ulnar groove is a good area to practise and perhaps assess the use of palpation skills. Figure 9.7 shows a useful position to examine the ulnar nerve. Note that the nerve is hard and round, and with the elbow in extension, the nerve has some transverse movements available. This movement disappears as the nerve tightens up with elbow flexion.

In the forearm, the superficial radial nerve can be felt and twanged on the lateral and volar aspect of the radius. Compare the hard feel of nerve here to the softer tendon of brachioradialis next to it. This nerve can be followed into the anatomical snuff box and these branches of the superficial radial nerve palpated easily using a

fingernail to twang across them. Also, palpable in the hand is the ulnar nerve, just medial to the hook of hamate bone.

The greater occipital nerve can be palpated as it exits the fascia at the base of the skull.

Many other nerves are palpable, such as digital nerves in the fingers, especially if swollen or scarred. Obviously the techniques are easier in slimmer individuals. Interested readers should arm themselves with a good anatomy textbook and just see what nerves are actually available to skilled palpation. Better still, when a sensitive spot is elicited, think of the possible structures that underlie it and try to prove by symptom analysis and structural differentiation just what the sensitive structure is.

CLASSIFICATIONS OF NERVE INJURY

For many years, workable and useful classifications of nerve injury have existed in medicine and surgery. Some categories relevant to the kind of patients that manual therapists encounter are discussed below. Important existing classifications are:

1. Upper motor neurone and lower motor neurone injury.
2. Categories of peripheral nerve injury; the Sunderland (1951) numerical categories 1–5 and the Seddon (1943) categories of neuropraxia, axonotmesis and neurotmesis. This section also includes a suggested categorisation for physiotherapists.

Upper motor neurone/lower motor neurone

The signs and symptoms of both have been outlined in Chapter 6. The upper motor neurone deserves a closer look. It is not unreasonable to assume that minor, usually temporary cord injuries are part of the patient population who present for treatment. Also, a neuropraxic cord injury, as described by Torg et al (1986), or even less subtle injuries may commonly exist. The physiotherapist has no way of knowing whether there is a minor cord injury. If this encourages a higher index of suspicion in examination, it can only be

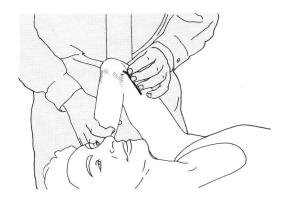

Fig. 9.7 A convenient position to examine the ulnar nerve

beneficial. Where there are definite signs of cord trauma, mobilisation is initially contraindicated. Such a patient requires assessment and treatment by a medical practitioner or specialist. However, in severe injury such as paraplegia where hamstring stretches are the norm, consideration of what such a stretch actually does to the nervous system has not really been considered. Where there are suspicious indicators, such as bilateral leg symptoms, but not absolute indicators, such as an upgoing Babinski response, the advice is to proceed with caution.

Classifications of peripheral nerve injury

Classifications of nerve injury have existed for many years. Seddon (1943) introduced the neuropraxia, neurotmesis and axonotmesis categories. Sunderland (1951) introduced a numerical classification that allowed three categories of the more severe nerve (axonotmesis) injury (Fig. 9.8). These classifications are based on failing nerve conduction and hence functional loss such as motor paralysis and sensory loss.

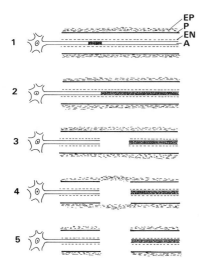

Fig. 9.8 Sunderland's five stage categorisation of nerve injury. EP epineurium, P perineurium, EN endoneurium, A axon. 1. conduction block, 2. transection of the axon with an intact endoneurium, 3. transection of axon and endoneurium inside an intact perineurium, 4. transection of all except the epineurial tissue, 5. transection of the entire trunk. From: Sunderland S 1978 Nerves and nerve injuries, 2nd edn. Churchill Livingstone, Edinburgh, with kind permission from the publishers and the author

These classifications are more relevant to severe nerve injuries and to treatment via surgery. However, they have a limited application to the majority of patients encountered by physiotherapists and to the sort of treatment physiotherapists administer. Indeed, they were never meant to apply to these patients. There are a number of reasons for this limitation:

• The majority of patients seen by physiotherapists do not have, or have only a minimal, loss of function related to failing nerve conduction. The main problem bringing them to a physiotherapist is usually one of symptoms.
• As discussed in earlier chapters, symptoms are not likely to be solely from alterations in the nerve fibre; there are the connective tissues to consider.
• While conduction may well be altered, manual neurological examination is usually all that is available to most patients. Not many physiotherapists or patients have the luxury or need of electrodiagnosis. The pitfalls of such diagnosis are well known (see Ch. 6), especially when the injury is not severe (Peterson & Will 1988). The classifications do not address these issues.

If consideration is given to the medical models and to the physiotherapy outpatient population with a component of adverse tension in their presenting disorder, then most of them belong in the area of Sunderland category 1, and in previously unnamed categories 'above' category 1. With these disorders assumed to be neuropathies, there is no real proof that the symptoms are neurogenic; there is only the support of clinical inference. The best title for many of these is 'occult neuropathies'. The exact pathoanatomical basis remains hidden.

In the next few sections, I have attempted to place nerve injuries in a classification suitable for physiotherapists. This classification must be used, where possible, with the medical model.

Attempts to classify the minor nerve injuries

Sunderland (1978) refers to a group of disorders which do not fit into his classifications. In these patients, conduction is normal but 'perversions of function' occur and he refers to these as 'irritative lesions'. Sunderland considers that these irritative lesions may arise from local pathology. More recently, Sunderland (in Jewett 1980) suggested the first degree lesion needs subgrades to accommodate differences between an ischaemic block and a demyelinating block. Jewett (1980) refers to the need for a 'zero degree' classification for similar reasons.

These issues have been taken up by Lundborg (1988). He defines two categories that are 'pre category 1' classifications. In the first category, the conduction block is due to an intraneural circulatory arrest leading to a metabolic block and being immediately reversible. The second category was a block occurring with intraneural oedema and reversible within days or weeks. Both these categories have ischaemia as the underlying cause and no nerve fibre injury. No attempt has been made to categorise minor injury to peripheral nerve connective tissue sheaths.

With these existing classifications as a background, more emphasis on symptoms and signs, and a link betwen that and the literature findings that have been discussed in Part I, a relevant classification for this patient group emerges. There are, however, some pitfalls which require acknowledgement before attempting the classifications:

1. Some overlap is inevitable.
2. There is always great difficulty relating clinical expression to pathoanatomy. This is especially difficult with the nervous system. There exists massive variations in the symptomatology related to peripheral nerve injury. An example of this is the variation from painless acute nerve compression, such as 'Saturday night palsy', to the horribly painful causalgic state. Simply, some nerve injuries are painful and some are not and the reasons are not fully understood. It must be continually realised that pain and dysaesthesias are peripheral and central phenomenons and that the clinical expression is particularly human. However, most of the relevant research is on animal models.

Classification is made easier by the fact that some physiotherapists have noted repeated patterns of tension test responses in disorders such as tennis elbow and hamstring pain. It does seem clear that once there is an injury in a nerve trunk, responses are often consistent with mechanical displacement during body movements.

Classifications for physiotherapists

I propose that physiotherapists should be able to identify and interpret the following categories of peripheral nerve injury:

1. The potential lesion
2. Physiological pain
3. The inflamed and irritated nerve —
   a. Irritation within the epineurium
   b. breach of the perineurium
4. Fibrosis of varying degrees —
   a. intraneural
   b. extraneural

Identification of a category will rely on symptomatology, physical signs, and the relationship between the two. It must also rely on what is known about nerve pathology.

The potential lesion

It is impossible to appreciate neurobiomechanics, pathology and consequent symptoms without consideration of the interfacing tissue to nerve. Peripheral nerve and the interfacing tissue form a complex motion segment. Normal nerve mechanics during movement depend on the mechanical integrity of the nerve and the surrounding tissue. These features are made more complex by the possible effects from nerve and interfacing tissue elsewhere along the trunk. Injury to the interfacing tissues or injury to the nervous system may create a potential injury situation for the nervous system at other sites.

Some examples of clinical situations which may predispose a nerve trunk to injury are oedema in the carpal tunnel (Faithfull et al 1985), blood around the tibial nerve after a hamstring tear, Colles' fracture (see Ch. 12), irritated sympathetic trunk (Lundborg 1988), and compartment syndromes (Mubarak et al 1989). In this category of potential injury, splint and plaster immobilisation must be included. There are many reasons for immobilisation, but trauma requiring immobilisation is likely to be severe enough to affect nerve. The immobile joint may predispose to a sub-clinical neuropathy that may in turn be precipitated by trauma to present clinically. Mobilisation may be such a trauma.

Other proven, but perhaps unrecognised injury situations include spasticity (Stone & Keenan 1988) and the hemiplegic shoulder (Chino 1981).

The clinical consequences are, firstly, a high index of suspicion in certain clinical situations. Secondly, in many disorders, the injury cannot be declared 'fixed' unless the mechanical integrity of the nerve has been tested. For example, in the patient with a hamstring tear, even if apparently muscular in origin, the full movement and tension capabilities of the sciatic nerve need checking before the patient is discharged. In the patient with cervical zygapophyseal strain, a check that ULTTs are clear is warranted. Postural advice should also include a consideration of its effects on the nervous system. If there is restriction in nerve mechanics, early intervention before irritation of the nervous system or, even worse, fibroblastic proliferation in and around the system, is desirable.

Physiological pain

The normal responses to tension tests involves particular kinds of symptoms; usually pain, and often discomfort. By structural differentiation, these symptoms can be inferred to be neurogenic or otherwise in origin. In the absence of injury, these symptoms are physiological symptoms and, if they can be proven to originate from the nervous system, can be considered neurogenic.

It seems likely that these responses are vascular in origin; thus, the response is metabolic. The likely scenario is hypoxic axons firing off ectopically, perhaps due to fibre dissociation resulting from the metabolic affects on the large fibres first (Noordenbos 1959) However, there are many other possible sources of pain (see Ch. 4). Blood flow to a nerve ceases at approximately 15% elongation, although it will begin to diminish at about 8% (Lundborg & Rydevik 1973, Ogata & Naito 1985). Neurones are particularly sensitive to blood flow and, from nerve elongation of approx-

imately 6% upwards, may fire off ectopically. It is not difficult to reconcile this with the likely elongation that a tension test allows. This is especially evident given Millesi's (1986) work in the upper limb where he showed that, from wrist and elbow flexion to extension, the median nerve has to comply with a nerve bed made 20% longer. Some of the 20% percent will be made up by sliding of the nervous system in relation to the interface. The rest will be made up by tension. Most of the movements we do in normal activities must involve less than 6% elongation. This category is the instantly reversible ischaemic block that Lundborg (1988) refers to.

There are other possible sources of these normal symptom responses than tension tests. The connective tissues of the nervous system are innervated and a possible source of symptoms. Some thought must be given to connecting and adjacent fascia and possible influences from neuronal pools in the ganglia, and neuraxis. It is quite possible that in a complex test such as the ULTT1, some of the symptoms may originate from the nerve fibre, some from the connective tissues, and even some from stretch on non-neural structures. Given the protection that the connective tissue offers the nerve fibre, it seems unlikely that the 'normal' symptoms come from mechanical effects on the nerve fibre.

These physiological symptoms may also be evident with a nervous system injury. Take note though that they may be some distance from the actual site of the disorder. Clinicians have gathered much useful data about the normal responses to tension tests (Chs 7 & 8). Great care is needed with its interpretation. An abnormal response to a tension test can be indicative of a site of adverse tension almost anywhere along the nervous system. For example, fibrotic tethering around a cord of the brachial plexus may lead to an ULTT symptom response that is brought on earlier in range and/or different to what is known to be normal. Because of pre-tensioning, the 6–15% or thereabouts critical value is reached with less movement. A tension test can only indicate that something is wrong, most likely affecting nerve. It is up to the skill of the experienced clinician to find out the site of the adverse tension. Usually all the clues are there if you ask enough questions of the patient and correlate them with what you find on physical examination. Those skilled in the examination of nerve interfacing tissue, such as joint or muscle, will be a step ahead.

The inflamed and irritated nervous system

There are two categories to consider, (a) where the process is confined to the epineurium and (b) breach of the perineurium.

Irritation within the epineurium. Epineurium is well vascularised and innervated. It is a particularly reactive tissue (Millesi 1986) and is not difficult to injure. Slight trauma, such as mild compression or friction, may result in an epineurial oedema (Triano & Luttges 1982, Rydevik et al 1984). Epineurial tears are common in injuries such as ankle sprains (Nitz et al 1985), and since it is the outer connective tissue sheath, it will always have the potential to rub against interfacing tissue.

Compared to nerve compression lesions, the consequences of irritation of the nervous system are poorly represented in the literature. Epineurial inflammation, unless severe and persistent, should not effect fascicular contents due to the perineurial barrier. The features of this barrier have been discussed in Chapter 1.

Clinically, it seems that if the inflamed epineurium is palpated or stretched, then pain could be evoked. There could be catches of pain as the irritated segment glides against an unyielding interface tissue. There may be little or no loss of range in the tension test although it may be pain provocative.

The main clinical consequence is to realise the state of the nerve and treat it to prevent the pathology becoming intraneural. As well as utilising postural, ergonomic, and perhaps electrotherapeutic techniques, this stage is also treatable by passive movement, as discussed in detail in the next chapter. Attention to an aggravating interface tissue, gentle through-range nerve/interface movements and perhaps some tension generation within the epineurium, are suggested.

Breach of the perineurium. If inflammation persists around the nerve, then an inflammatory reaction may begin from within. Sunderland (1976) has detailed a stage of events (see Ch. 3) that occurs with persistent irritation and pressure around a nerve. Essentially, with deprived blood supply and, as a later consequence, capillary damage and oedema, an intrafascicular inflammatory response occurs that is potentially damaging to the nerve fibre and to endoneurial tubules. Due to the perineurial diffusion barrier, the inflammatory response that finally gains access to the fascicle is also difficult to remove. There is potential for intrafascicular fibroblast activity. With a rise in the endoneurial fluid pressure, conduction is likely to be affected.

These patients may complain of persistent pains, usually in areas where the nervous system is vulnerable (such as where nerve branches or is in tunnels). On palpation, nerves may be tender and swollen. A tentative hypothesis is that patient complaints relating to peripheral nerve connective tissue are similar to other connective tissues in the body. However, the more bizarre descriptions (i.e., 'strangling', 'burning', 'crawling') may relate to the nerve fibre. Refer to Table 9.1.

The main clinical consequence is to recognise that, if the aggravating activity or material creating the pressure on the nerve is not removed, then damage, (perhaps irreversible) to neural and/or connective tissue elements is possible. Nerve pressure from a plaster of Paris cast is easily understood. Another example in the same category would be the secretary who continues to use a keyboard in the presence of swelling in the carpal tunnel. Awareness of the progression of pathology possible with peripheral nerve injury should be basic physiotherapy knowledge. Passive movement techniques can surely cause fluctuations in the intraneural pressures. 'Milking' of the nerve, especially where it can be mobilised through a tunnel, may help remove the excessive intraneural fluid (Elvey 1986). Patients with known carpal tunnel syndrome obtain relief from self mobilisation of the wrist; this may be a similar mechanism.

Fibrosis

Fibrotic reactions to the inflammatory phase may be intraneural, extraneural, or both.

As an inevitable consequence of persistent inflammation, fibroblasts may lay down scar tissue, either extraneural or intraneural. There may not be a measurable alteration in conduction, though this is far more likely than in the previous category, especially if there is intraneural fibrosis causing endoneurial tube destruction. Mackinnon & Dellon (1986) suggest that the worst fascicle may contribute to symptoms and an undamaged one may account for a normal electrodiagnostic test.

Fibrosis in and around a nerve can vary greatly, and will depend not only on the amount and type of trauma, but also on temporal and constitutional factors. A few patients encountered in this stage with severe nerve fibre disorganisation and destruction of endoneurial tubules could be classified as Sunderland grade 3. Others may just have a few immature axons caught in some endoneurial or perineurial scar and be difficult to classify.

Fibrosis may well be a part of any stage and not necessarily a progression. It is also possible to have different stages occurring along the same nerve. For example, the loss of extensibility in the median nerve within the carpal tunnel may precipitate an irritated nerve elsewhere.

The main clinical considerations are to prevent scar formation and to understand the potential for symptom development if an area of nerve is scarred. This has been discussed earlier. In scar development, there must be a stage where the effects of fibroblastic activity can be minimised, but also a later stage where some of the activity is irreversible.

Fibrosis may be extraneural, thus altering the ability of the nerve to glide in its bed, or intraneural, altering its ability to stretch. Massage of neuromas is a well accepted technique, but physiotherapists can greatly refine their techniques. Physiotherapists should be aware that they are capable of altering techniques to get at either form of fibrosis. These features are discussed in the next chapter.

In this stage, it is likely that nervi nervorum are caught in scarred epineurium or immature axons or neuromas could be caught in endoneurial or perineurial scarring thus leading to an abnormal impulse generating mechanism.

It has been stressed that, although physiotherapists have a familiar and recognised role in the management of severe nervous system injuries, it is the management of the more minor injuries to which this book is directed.

With the injuries that have been classified, it is important to note that clear scientific evidence allowing the linking of these categories to how patients present clinically is lacking, especially in the 'pre category 1' classifications. There are many pitfalls to declaring that a symptom is neuropathic in origin. There is clearly no histological proof because nerve biopsy is out of the question in minor injuries. Electrodiagnosis has great shortcomings with minor nerve injury and there is no proof available from biochemistry tests. Clinical inference, including structural differentiation and close attention to the area, behaviour and history of injury, extrapolation of data from animal studies, and extrapolation from anatomical studies have been used. Still, clinically it appears that tension testing is the most sensitive way to pick up a subtle nerve injury. Symptoms related to subclinical entrapment (Ch. 3) may also be reproduced by tension testing.

REFERENCES

Asbury A H, Fields H L 1984 Pain due to peripheral nerve damage: an hypothesis. Neurology (Cleveland) 34: 1587–1590
Buehler M J, Thayer D T 1988 The elbow flexion test: a clinical test for the cubital tunnel syndrome. Clinical Orthopaedics and Related Research 233: 213–216
Butler D S 1989 Adverse mechanical tension in the nervous system: a model for assessment and treatment. Australian Journal of Physiotherapy 35: 227–238
Chino N 1981 Electrophysiological investigation on shoulder subluxation in hemiplegics. Scandinavian Journal of Rehabilitation Medicine 13: 17–21

Clare H A 1989 The clinical testing of upper limb neural tissue in repetitive strain injury. In: Jones H M, Jones M A, Milde M R (eds) Manipulative Therapists Association of Australia, Sixth biennial conference proceedings, Adelaide
Cyriax J, Russell G 1977 Textbook of orthopaedic medicine, 9th edn. Bailliere Tindall, London, vol 2
Elvey R L 1986 Treatment of arm pain associated with abnormal brachial plexus tension. Australian Journal of Physiotherapy 32: 225–230
Faithfull D K, Moir D H, Ireland J 1985 The micropathology of the typical carpal tunnel syndrome. Journal of Hand Surgery 11B: 131–132

Jewett D L 1980 Functional blockade of impulse trains caused by acute nerve compression. In: Jewett D L, McCarroll H R (eds) Nerve repair and regeneration. Mosby, St. Louis

Kenneally M, Rubenach H, Elvey R 1988 The upper limb tension test: the SLR test of the arm. In: Grant R (ed) Clinics in Physical Therapy 17, The cervical and thoracic spines. Churchill Livingstone, New York

Lundborg G 1988 Nerve injury and repair. Churchill Livingstone, Edinburgh

Lundborg G, Rydevik B 1973 Effects of stretching the tibial nerve of the rabbit: a preliminary study on the intraneural microcirculation and the barrier function of the perineurium. Journal of Bone and Joint Surgery 55B: 390–401

Mackinnon S E, Dellon A L 1986 Experimental study of chronic nerve compression. Hand Clinics 2: 639–650

Mackinnon S E, Dellon A L 1988 Surgery of the peripheral nerve. Thieme, New York

Maitland G D 1986 Vertebral manipulation, 5th edn. Butterworths, London

Millesi H 1986 The nerve gap: theory and clinical practice. Hand Clinics 2: 651–663

Mubarak S J, Pedowitz R A, Hargens A R 1989 Compartment syndromes. Current Orthopaedics 3: 36–40

Nitz A J, Dobner J J and Kersey D 1985 Nerve injury and grade II and III ankle sprains. The American Journal of Sports Medicine 13: 177–182

Noordenbos W 1959 Pain. Elsevier, Amsterdam

Ogata K, Naito M 1985 Blood flow of peripheral nerve, effects of dissection, stretching and compression. Journal of Hand Surgery 11B: 11–14

Peterson G W, Will A D 1988 Newer electrodiagnostic techniques in peripheral nerve injuries. Orthopaedic Clinics of North America 19: 13–25

Philip K, Lew P, Matyas T A 1989 The inter-therapist reliability of the slump test. Australian Journal of Physiotherapy 35: 89–94

Rydevik B, Brown M D, Lundborg G 1984 Pathoanatomy and pathophysiology of nerve root compression. Spine 9: 7–15

Saal J A, Dillingham M F, Gamburd R S, Fanton G S 1988 The pseudoradicular syndrome. Spine 13: 926–930

Seddon H 1943 Three types of nerve injury. Brain 66: 237–288

Stone L, Keenan M E 1988 Peripheral nerve injuries in the adult with traumatic brain injury. Clinical Orthopaedics and Related Research 233: 136–144

Sunderland S 1951 A classification of peripheral nerve injuries producing loss of function. Brain 74: 491–516

Sunderland S 1978 Nerves and nerve injuries, 2nd edn. Churchill Livingstone, Edinburgh.

Sunderland S 1976 The nerve lesion in carpal tunnel syndrome. Journal of Neurology, Neurosurgery and Psychiatry 39: 615–616

Thomas P K 1984 Clinical Features and differential diagnosis. In: Dyck P J, Thomas P K, Lambert E H, Bunge R (eds) Peripheral neuropathy, 2nd edn. Saunders, Philadelphia, vol 2

Torg J S, Pavlov H, Genuario S E et al 1986 Neuropraxia of the cervical spinal cord with transient quadriplegia. Journal of Bone and Joint Surgery 68A: 1354–1370

Triano J J, Luttges M W 1982 Nerve irritation: a possible model of sciatic neuritis. Spine 7: 129–136

Treatment and treatment potential

PART III

Treatment and treatment potential

10. Treatment

HISTORY

The concept and techniques of mobilisation of the nervous system are not new. A form of surgical treatment known as 'nerve stretching' was in vogue late last century in France and England. This technique was usually applied to the sciatic nerve or the brachial plexus and was used for a variety of complaints ranging from sciatica to locomotor ataxy. In the case of sciatic stretching, the surgeons would make an incision at the gluteal fold or lower, attach a hook or place their fingers under the sciatic nerve, and then firmly pull on the nerve. Just how hard to pull was a matter of great debate, as was the direction to pull. There are reports in the British Medical Journal of 'the exposed nerve twice raised nearly 6 inches above the level of the skin and then violently stretched in its long axis' or 'the whole weight of the limb was supported by the nerve'. Others pulled on the nerve until a distinct effect occurred on the pulse (Cavafy 1881). An improvement at the time was thought to be 'M. Gillette's nerve stretcher'. This was a blunt flattened hook which was inserted under the nerve at right angles to its course. The limb was held down by an assistant and a dynamometer was connected to the instrument so that the force employed could be measured (Cavafy 1881).

The popularity of nerve stretching encouraged research on the breaking strains of cadaveric nerves. An example from cadaver studies of the time is the body of a cirrhotic 37-year-old man which sustained 100 lbs on its sciatic nerve without it snapping. However, its left sciatic nerve broke at 90 pounds. Another example is that of a tiny 17-year-old girl who died of 'waxy disease';

her body could only stand 84 lbs before the sciatic nerves snapped. The record in the literature was 240 lbs with the average weight before breaking being 140 lbs. From these studies, and no doubt, clinical findings, it was deduced that the therapeutic dosage should be between 30 lbs and half the person's body weight. With forms of ataxy, a pull downwards was considered best. However, for problems with low back pain, a pull in a rostral direction was thought to be most effective. Results ranged from apparently remarkable cures to the occasional death (Symington 1882, Marshall 1883).

Other than giving some indication of the tensile strength of peripheral nerve, such reports are of historical interest only. They have no place in the considerable skill required for safe and effective passive and active mobilisation of the nervous system. They should, however, serve as a reminder of the speed of change in medicine. It is interesting to think that nerve stretching was accepted 100 years ago, yet carpal tunnel syndrome has only been understood for a little more than 30 years, and the awareness of specific pathways for pain arose little more than 20 years ago. The present stage of the progression towards a total understanding of neuro-orthopaedic disorders remains unknown.

GENERAL TREATMENT POINTS

1. The nervous system cannot avoid being mobilised with any movement related treatment. In present day manual therapy, most physiotherapists mobilise the nervous system inadvertently. For example, in a

hamstring stretch, the sciatic nerve, its branches and part of the neuraxis and meninges will be moved and tensioned. In mobilisation of the end ranges of shoulder movements via a technique such as the quadrant (Maitland 1977), the brachial plexus, associated nerve roots and trunks will be mobilised. Even the gentlest breathing exercises mobilise the neural structures of the thoracic spine and the brachial plexus (McLellan & Swash 1976). Trapezius stretches and iliopsoas stretches will also involve stretch of associated nervous system. Patients' signs and symptoms have been improved by passive and active mobilisation techniques long before the ideas of nervous system mobilisation in this book were introduced. However, if the physiotherapist is in search of better results and of understanding of the limitations of treatment, consideration of what is now known about the nervous system is imperative. If it can be ascertained that the faulty structure requiring mobilisation is the nervous system, techniques can be more specific and more refined. For example, a SLR could be performed with ankle dorsiflexion and hip adduction in order to refine and hence bias the technique toward a particular nervous system structure. There are also precautions and contraindications that are specific to the nervous system. Prognosis making is part of the clinical reasoning process, and it will also differ depending on structures involved in a disorder.

2. Maitland (1986) emphasised that analytical assessment is the cornerstone of his concept. The techniques following the analysis are more than the implementation of a learnt technique. The actual delivery of a technique involves many factors such as handling skills, patient communication, knowledge of biomechanics and reassessment abilities. Prognostic knowledge can only come from skilled reassessments and an awareness of the pathology being dealt with. There are no set techniques, or recipe treatments for a particular diagnosis. The basis is clinical reasoning (Ch. 5).

3. The treatment techniques suggested are anecdotal and rely on clinical reasoning processes. At this stage, I am aware of only one study that has experimentally examined and compared nervous system mobilisation with other treatments. In a double-blind survey, Kornberg & Lew (1989) examined 28 professional Australian Rules football players with a grade 1 hamstring tear and compared the effects of traditional treatment of 16 players with 12 who received traditional treatment and nervous system mobilisation. Of the 12 players whose management included attention to the nervous system, only one player missed more than one match. All 16 players who were treated traditionally missed one or more matches.

4. Treatment via nervous system mobilisation is not a quickly acquired skill, nor is it an easy skill to learn. It could be argued that it is more difficult than a joint approach. There are no bony levers to push on, it is more difficult to visualise and it requires thinking that encompasses the whole body. The potential for a physiological response may be over a greater area and amplitude than for a joint. Probably what may make it more difficult is that, for most physiotherapists, it is a relatively new tissue to contemplate, at least in biomechanical terms, and basic knowledge of the structure is generally less than of joints and muscles.

5. After examination of the patient, if the physiotherapist decides there is a relevant tension component related to the patients disorder which needs changing, then there are three related ways of approaching it via movement:

• Direct mobilisation of the nervous system, usually via tension tests and their derivatives, but also via palpation techniques
• Treatment via interfacing and related tissues, such as joints, muscles, fascia and skin
• Incorporation into indirect treatment such as postural advice and ergonomic design.

In this and the next chapter, these three approaches are discussed. In this chapter emphasis is placed mostly on direct mobilisation of the nervous system.

BASIC PRINCIPLES OF MOBILISATION

Once the decision to mobilise the nervous system has been made, the actual treatment delivered can be chosen by relying on two main considerations:

1. The Maitland concept. That is, the treatment of the signs and symptoms based on the severity, irritability and nature of the disorder. Consideration of these factors is a basic tenet of the Maitland concept. In this regard, treatment via nervous system mobilisation is no different from the method espoused by Maitland for a joint. The clinical reasoning processes inherent in the concept will easily embrace treatments other than joint mobilisation.

2. Expansion of thoughts on, and the use of 'nature'. 'Nature' is a term used by Maitland (1986) but is more widely understood as pathology. With clinical reasoning processes, up to date pathological knowledge would be included and assessed by the process itself. Thoughts regarding pathology should include the site(s) of altered nervous system mechanics, the tissues of the nervous system involved and possible structures around and along the nervous system which could interfere with its normal mechanics. Other thoughts could include the proportion of altered mechanics with altered physiology. Already, so much is known about the nervous system, and it must be included in treatment decisions.

One important key to successful treatment is for the physiotherapist to think of mobilisation rather than stretch. If one thinks of all that mobilisation entails — an appreciation of resistance encountered, symptoms felt and their relationship during movement, the place of gentle and strong treatment, and the reassessment essentials — it can be seen that all of these aspects are just as applicable to nervous system mobilisation as they are, say, to joint mobilisation. We can do much better than just crudely stretching the nervous system.

Grading the technique

Many issues will determine which technique to use; these are discussed below. One way to ascertain the desirable vigour of technique is to determine the relationship between resistance to the movement and the symptoms perceived. This has already been well covered in terms of treating a joint (Magarey 1985, Maitland 1986). Readers unfamiliar with the idea should consult the relevant chapter in Maitland's text (1986). The movement diagram is as applicable to the nervous system as it is to the joint. It also serves the purpose of encouraging the physiotherapist to think more about resistance encountered during a movement rather than merely relying on symptoms. They encourage the development of 'feel' and an understanding of the importance of the association between symptoms provoked and resistance encountered. This applies to both nervous system and joint mobilisation alike.

The nervous system is capable of producing a far greater range of symptoms than are joints. This means that more information (for example paraesthesia, feeling of warmth, even nausea) is likely to be placed on the diagram. For example, in a patient with a non-irritable disorder where the movement could be taken to the end of range (IV ++), the Straight Leg Raise (SLR) is recorded on a movement diagram (Fig 10.1). The SLR at 40° reproduces a pain in the hamstring area, and at 75°, a feeling of headache. These

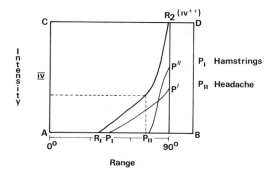

Fig.10.1 An example of a movement diagram for a SLR

symptoms can be recorded on the diagram. If the physiotherapist, considering all factors such as irritability and precautions, decided to perform a SLR as a treatment, with the technique stopping just short of reproducing the headache, this can also be placed on the movement diagram (dotted line). Note that the technique is therfore performed at about 70° and the technique will be about a grade IV–.

These movement diagrams are useful. Recorded on paper should be a clear representation of the physiotherapist's thought processes related to assessment and treatment. They are of particular value to students since they enable discussion over a visual representation of a technique.

Uses — pathomechanics and pathophysiology

Nervous system mobilisation is applicable for signs and symptoms whose origins may be biomechanical compromise (pathomechanics) or an inflammatory reaction (pathophysiology). These two situations will inevitably co-exist, although one will predominate and prioritise the treatment regime. A pathophysiological situation could lead to pathomechanics. A broad relationship occurs between pathology and irritability (Table 10.1). Irritability has been briefly discussed in Chapter 5. The concept of irritability is discussed in greater detail in Maitland (1986)

THE IRRITABLE DISORDER (PATHOPHYSIOLOGICAL DOMINANCE)

Treatment of the irritable disorder presents a challenge for physiotherapists. The dominant

Table 10.1 Relationship between irritability and pathology. The dominance of pathophysiological and pathomechanical responses in assessment and treatment. Adapted from Butler & Gifford (1989)

(Acute)	(Subacute)	(Chronic)
Irritable	Moderately	Non-irritable
Disorder	Irritable	

→ Decreasing dominance of pathophysiological response →

→ Increasing dominance of pathomechanical response →

symptom of such a disorder is constant pain which is easily provoked and can take a long time to settle. Some examples of irritable disorders which may be encountered by physiotherapists are certain stages of the whiplash syndrome, severe trauma, and acute inflammatory neuropathies such as Guillain-Barré. Rest plays an important part in the treatment. However, appropriate movement can be beneficial for symptoms, and perhaps more importantly, will lessen the chances of post inflammatory scarring. Some of the possible effects of treatment are summarised later in this chapter.

When an irritable disorder is traumatic in origin, there will usually be multi-tissue structural involvement. For example, in a whiplash incident, zygapophyseal joints may be strained, there could be fractured trabeculae in bone, and muscles and nerves are also likely to be damaged. Sorting out the contributions of each structure to symptoms and the relative importance of treatment to each structure can be difficult. Already the diagnostic value of being able to move the nervous system in isolation has been discussed (Chs 5 & 9). In an irritable disorder, clinically, there are advantages in being able to move one structure without interfering too much with others.

An example is used to illustrate guidelines to treatment. The patient sustained a whiplash injury three weeks previously. The amount of damage to cars and property suggested that substantial forces were involved. The patient presented with intermittent though easily aggravated headaches, constant central and right sided neck and shoulder pain. None of the symptoms were improving; if anything, the shoulder was getting a little worse. The patient was in a collar and had been resting. Cervical rotation to the left was limited to 30°. The patient was not palpated.

The beauty of examining this patient by techniques utilising components of the SLR or left ULTT should be clear since the disorder appeared highly irritable.

Guidelines to the starting technique

1. Use a technique well removed from the symptom area. For example, in the patient

example just given, a SLR or left ULTT technique could be used. Perhaps techniques such as left elbow extension in some shoulder abduction, or right wrist extension could be beneficial. Rather than the tradition SLR, knee extension in hip flexion or hip adduction in some degree of SLR could be useful techniques. In some irritable whiplash syndromes, just dorsiflexion and plantar flexion in some knee flexion may be a starting treatment. There is an array of available starting techniques.

2. The technique should be non-provoking initially, thus remaining short of any symptoms or increase in symptoms. It is best to undertreat initially until the irritability of the disorder related to treatment becomes apparent. There may be some latent responses.

3. The suggested grades of technique are large amplitude Grade IIs performed slowly and rhythmically through range with maximal respect to symptoms. Grade IV– techniques, just nudging at resistance with similar respect for symptoms are also a possibility (for those unfamiliar with grades, consult Maitland 1986). The largest amplitude of movement possible should be done. For example, if it is possible to do 20° of knee extension in hip flexion, why not do more if it can be done without aggravating the disorder?

4. The symptoms of the disorder must be continually monitored. This requires constant verbal and non-verbal communication with the patient. A dull constant ache should be avoided, and if the physiotherapist judges it is acceptable for some symptoms to be reproduced with the technique, these should be in rhythm with the technique.

5. It follows that, for the optimum movement of the nervous system in relation to interfacing tissues, the patient must be relaxed and comfortable. This may mean spending some time positioning the patient in a pain-relieving position. The most prevalent interfacing tissue to the nervous system is muscle. If muscles are contracted, it is possible that the sliding aspect of nervous system mechanics will be impaired. It is possible to change symptoms at the time of treatment, or they may change some hours later.

6. If the disorder is deemed less irritable, passive movement in a very gentle manner may be applied to the symptom area. In the example of a whiplash patient already discussed in these guidelines, depression and elevation of the right shoulder girdle would be an appropriate technique at a grade II. The rest of the body should be taken out of tension; the elbow is flexed, pillows are placed under the knees and the neck is laterally flexed towards the right. Again, the same guidelines as listed above are followed. With selection of the technique, thoughts should turn to the position of the interfacing tissues. Better movement of the nervous system can be achieved with the interfacing structures positioned in their inner- and mid-ranges. Thus, in the patient example, depression of the shoulder girdle may be a better technique than abduction of the shoulder.

Progression

1. There will be an infinite number of ways and directions in which techniques can be applied to influence the nervous system. Physiotherapists must carefully explore the therapeutic possibilities. No two patient's signs and symptoms will be the same and all patients will require different treatments. If an improvement is achieved with a particular technique, the physiotherapist should try to resist the temptation just to repeat that technique. While it may be beneficial, the physiotherapist does not know it is the best treatment available. The technique can be used in combination with another technique or it can be performed slightly differently and the responses reassessed.

2. The number of repetitions can be increased. In the irritable disorder, I prefer to perform a sequence of gentle oscillations, say for 20 seconds and then reassess the effect. The number of these sequences could be increased so the techniques last several minutes.

3. The amplitude of the technique can be increased. The technique could be progressed to a point where some symptoms are reproduced, or it could be taken to a point where some resistance to the movement is encountered.

4. The technique could be repeated with the nervous system in more tension. In the above example, knee extension in hip flexion could be performed with the cervical spine in some flexion. Similarly, the shoulder girdle depression technique could be performed with the neck laterally flexed away or with the elbow extended. Here, thoughts should be focussing on the source of the symptoms. If an intraneural component to the disorder is suspected, then it will be desirable to add more tension to the nervous system while performing the technique.

5. If using a distal technique, such as the knee extension in hip flexion, the technique could be moved closer to the source of symptom area. For example, the traditional SLR of hip flexion with the knee extended could be employed.

6. The effect of treatment on other structures involved in the disorder needs to be reassessed. Later in this chapter, the treatment of interfacing structures is discussed. It is very unlikely that the nervous system could be injured without injury to other structures. So, in our patient, after a technique is performed, an assessment of related joint (active movements, palpation signs), muscle (length, palpation, spasm) and other structures involved needs to be reassessed. This is a basic manual therapy tenet and one that is crucial to continued learning.

In this regard, the patient needs to be asked how his/her symptoms are changing. Remember that the nervous system can be responsible for a variety of symptoms, and you need to enquire about all symptoms. The patient in severe pain can easily forget alterations in more minor symptoms, and this information may be valuable to assist in progression of a technique. There could also be symptoms that at the initial assessment were not originally related to the adverse tension, such as stomach pain. These may alter with treatment, and the only way to find out is to enquire.

7. The nervous system also allows easy regression of a technique. If the symptoms are being provoked by the technique, then as well as the obvious considerations of performing the technique more gently or abandoning the technique for another, there exists the possibility of performing it in less tension. So, in the example of the patient in severe pain discussed earlier, shoulder depression could be performed with the neck in some lateral flexion towards the side treated, more knee flexion could be added and perhaps some spinal extension would also assist in a beneficial response from the technique.

THE NON-IRRITABLE DISORDER (PATHOMECHANICAL DOMINANCE)

The longer a disorder persists, the greater the likelihood of problems caused by disuse of structures and the products of an inflammatory response causing features of a pathomechanical nature. It follows that the only way to tackle a pathomechanical problem is to utilise techniques that address mechanics. Treatment such as drugs, bed rest and electrotherapy are unlikely to solve the problem. Surgery may be an option.

As with the irritable disorder, there are no set techniques but a multitude of therapeutic possibilities. Each technique is a hypothesis whose value has to be proven. Most patients seen in physiotherapy outpatient clinics will present with disorders at the more non-irritable end of the scale.

Guidelines to the starting technique

1. The initial technique performed will need to be into some resistance, i.e., through range grade IIIs and/or grade IVs. Techniques short of resistance are unlikely to alter mechanics. The technique initially performed should, however, be short of provoking pain.

Remember that a grade III mobilisation provides plenty of movement with a short, low dose of tension at the end of range for a given period. Conversely, a grade IV technique maintains tension at the end of range with very little movement. From the assessment, some pathologies and findings may make one technique more desirable than another. In pathological terms, a through range, large amplitude (grade III) movement should be employed where abnormalities of mechanics of the nervous system in relation to the interface exist (that is, extraneural disorders). The small amplitude, end range movements (grade IV) can be used where an intraneural disorder is thought to predominate. In general, grade IIIs will be less symptom provoking then grade IVs. Any symptoms provoked during treatment should subside immediately the treatment technique is released. For some reason in non-irritable disorders, paraesthesia may occasionally persist for a few minutes post treatment (see page 251).

2. The position and component selected for treatment may not be in a familiar base tension position. With the non-irritable disorder, the physiotherapist should have had more opportunity to explore the movements affected by the disorder. The idea of hunting out the best positions to treat, using clues from the subjective examination and knowledge of neurobiomechanics follows on from the physical examination as discussed in the previous chapter. If a technique is used which is not part of a base test, the base test can be used to reassess the effectiveness of the test. However, if symptoms are easily reproduced during a base test, this can be used as the technique, and perhaps use another base test for assessment of whether the tension component in the disorder has altered.

3. The irritability will again play a part in the treatment decision. The degree of irritability will differ in the group loosely termed 'non-irritable'. It may be desirable initially to stay a component away from the source of symptoms. For example if the hypothesis was that there was some limitation of movement of the brachial plexus, an initial treatment, keeping a component away might be, IN: pain productive ULTT position DID: elbow extension, or a cervical movement. With decreasing irritability and confidence in the treatment, the physiotherapist can move the component treated closer to the hypothesised source of tension.

4. After the initial mobilisation, all components of the disorder must be reassessed. This may mean examining the effect on all structural components and other nervous system components. The initial treatment selected can only be a hypothesis that has to be proven by reassessment.

Progression

1. If required, the starting technique can be performed for longer or it can be performed harder, i.e., further into resistance and thus with less respect for the symptoms provoked.

2. The same starting technique can be performed with other components in different positions, usually with an increase in tension.

3. The component utilised can be closer to the source of symptoms. If the source of the adverse tension is at the shoulder, while in a symptom provoking tension position, a technique involving shoulder movement rather than elbow movement could be used. IN: pain provoking tension position DID: shoulder external rotation.

From clinical studies (Ch. 2) and clinical experience, the technique that best accesses the nervous system will involve taking up the injured component that contains the hypothesised source of tension and then adding neural tension to it progressively. Then the injured component is treated. For example, if the deep peroneal nerve was involved in an adverse tension situation in the anterior aspect of the ankle, and plantar flexion and inversion of the ankle was the positive component, this movement could be taken up first, then the SLR added and the plantar flexion and inversion used as a treatment technique. If physiotherapists, familiar with aspects of mobilisation of the nervous system, consider how the Slump Test is commonly used in treatment of an adverse tension disorder originating in the lumbar spine, most will utilise the knee extension component. However, this is a component away from the spine, and ultimately a technique of moving the spine in the Slump position may be required.

4. As a progression, the other structural components of the disorder can be treated in a tension position. In the example above this may mean IN: Slump longsitting/plantar flexion inversion DID: antero-posterior pressure on the talus.

Some other aspects of progression are discussed below.

Aspects of treatment of the non-irritable disorder

1. The ultimate strength of treatment is discussed in the section 'Commonly asked questions' (see page 194). It is worth reiterating one point: if the base tests are exclusively used as the treatment, more vigour will usually be required to access the nervous system correctly than if the technique involved movements which reproduced signs and symptoms better. For example, while a SLR may be getting at a disorder in the lumbar spine, to access that disorder with less force, the spine could be placed in a position of lateral flexion and some of the sensitising movements of the SLR, such as hip adduction and medial rotation, could be used.

A corollary for joint dominant physiotherapists can be given. While strong postero-anterior pressures on the spinous process of a relevant cervical vertebrae may assist restoration of rotation, the same benefit may be achieved with much gentler unilateral pressures or combined physiological movements.

2. Clinical reasoning skills are required to answer the questions of how many, how much and how long? Treatment can be thought of as a session of slow oscillations, say 20–30 seconds in duration, or a number of repetitions. As a broad guide, the greater the concern about the irritability or severity of the disorder, the more likely that a session of oscillatory techniques will be used. It provides

the physiotherapist with a greater opportunity to question the patient about symptoms during the technique. In the more non-irritable disorder, where pathomechanics is the greater concern, the physiotherapist may prefer to perform just one or two firm repetitions of a technique. Here, a further progression is possible by sustaining the technique for a longer time. Anecdotally, the slow and sustained movements appear better. Perhaps this fits, in some small way, with the temporal properties of the nervous system with regard to stretch (Ch. 3). Some patients report a decrease in symptoms while the position is held. Oscillating may activate the muscles around the system, in which case it seems better to sustain the movement or very slowly oscillate. My suggestion is that a technique should not have to be sustained for longer than 20 seconds.

There are some patients where the technique needs to be performed at speed. The clues will come from the subjective examination. For example, there could be a pain on kicking or a catch of pain that only comes on during a tennis serve. I interpret this as being an inability of the nervous system to adapt at speed to the surrounding structures. The technique can be performed at speed to reproduce and alter the symptoms. Attention to the surrounding structures is also warranted in this kind of presentation.

3. It is sometimes easy to forget that the nervous system is a continuum. In most adverse tension disorders there will be axial and transverse tension considerations. It should be clear that if a person is to have optimum upper limb tension tests then they will require an optimum Slump (i.e, axial nervous system movement) and vice versa. They will also require an optimum ULTT of the other arm. Similarly to have the best possible Prone Knee Bend, the SLR will need to be optimal.

4. Treatment of the non-irritable disorder inevitably involves some discomfort. These symptoms provoked are one of the main guides to treatment. With nervous system mobilisation in the non-irritable disorder, no

matter how strong the treatment, the symptoms reproduced should disappear within seconds of stopping. This is most likely due to the instant replenishment of blood to nerve fibres rendered hypoxic by the stretch or compression. If residual symptoms persist, then other tissues may have been affected, or the nervous system treatment is too strong for that particular patient or stage of the disorder. That is, the irritability has been misread.

It is not uncommon for patients to say on reassessment 'My back is much improved from the treatment but my neck is very sore,' when the physiotherapist has not even touched the patient's neck. Unless handled correctly, this situation can result in an instant loss of communication. Consideration of biomechanics makes such a presentation feasible. If tension is altered in one area, an altered tension and nervous system relationship with interfacing structures is set up elsewhere. This may be symptom provocative and take some time for the patient to adjust to. It can also be a clue that these interfaces may need attending to.

It is probably therapeutic to give gentle, through range mobilisation of the same or similar movements to help limit the possibility of treatment pain. Knee extension in hip flexion is a nice technique to perform after vigorous SLRs or Slump treatments. Shoulder depressions and elevations appear useful after vigorous ULTTs.

5. A nerve, where accessible, or the fascia around a nerve can be treated by frictions or mobilised via oscillatory pressures. This is often better performed with the nervous system in tension. For example, the deep friction techniques used by many physiotherapists for tennis elbow are often more effective if performed in the ULTT2 radial nerve bias position. Palpation techniques have been discussed in Chapter 9.

6. It is of no use continuing a technique if it does not work. A technique performed should be reassessed immediately after its cessation. This should incorporate a subjective and a physical reassessment. As in the irritable disorder, it is worthwhile asking about all symptoms, even if they were symptoms you or the patient did not associate with the disorder. The nervous system is a continuum and the effects of treating part of it could be manifest anywhere in the body. Examples of symptoms often changed early in the treatment are feelings of swelling, night pain, and morning stiffness. Often the patient will not volunteer these important symptom alterations unless asked. Another interesting change may be 'nerve crepitus'. Noted more often in the upper limb, this appears to herald an improvement; the patient will report a creaking along the nerve during mobilisation, especially with large, through range movements.

A crucial point in reassessment, already stressed with regard to the irritable disorder, is the effect of mobilisation of the nervous system on other signs. It is a basic manual therapy tenet that, if you are mobilising a specific tissue, you need to know the effect on other tissues. This is the basis of a multifactorial approach.

TREATMENT OF THE INTERFACING STRUCTURES

A positive tension test does not constitute a definite indication that mobilisation of the nervous system will be required. If the pathological situation causing the positive tension sign is extraneural, alteration of that situation may lead to amelioration of the tension signs and related symptoms. In such a situation, the physiotherapist will need to closely monitor the tension signs to ensure they have cleared. The nervous system will rarely, if ever, be the only structure requiring mobilisation. The more skilled the physiotherapist is at examining and treating the interfacing structures, the better he/she will be at examining and treating the nervous system.

There are certain areas and interfaces that require more attention than elsewhere in the body. If symptoms or a source of symptoms are in these areas, the treatment of the interfacing tissues should be given high priority. These are the vulnerable points, listed in Chapter 3.

The physiotherapist who is unfamiliar with the concept of mobilising the nervous system, may initially prefer to treat the inevitable non-neural structures involved in the disorder and see what the effect the treatment has on the tension signs.

The relationship of the interfacing tissues with the tension test needs continual reassessment to evaluate which structures warrant priority in treatment. For example, in a disorder such as 'frozen shoulder', where the main physical signs could be a limitation in the range of the shoulder joint movements and a positive Upper Limb Tension Test; although joint treatment may be indicated first, the joint movement might improve to a point where it is the nervous system that is the main limiting structure. Both structures may need treating, for example in prone and ULTT1, a postero-anterior pressure can be placed on the humeral head.

If treatment of the interfacing tissues is required, it does not necessarily have to be in the neutral position for that structure. Better results could be gained if the interfacing structures can be treated in a position of tension. For example, if needed, wrist intercarpal movements could be performed with the arm in an ULTT position, the ribs could be mobilised in Slump or the knee could be mobilised in a SLR position.

It might be helpful to consider some of the limitless treatment possibilities available, if the nervous system is implicated:

• Nervous system mobilisation (NSM) in neutral (e.g., medial rotation of the hip)
• NSM with joint positioned (e.g., inversion of the foot in SLR)
• NSM with muscle positioned (e.g., ULTT1 with scalenei on stretch)
• NSM with fascia positioned (e.g., SLR/DF with plantar fascia stretched
• Joint technique with nervous system positioned (e.g., postero-anterior pressures on the head of the humerus in ULTT, unilateral pressure on a rib in Slump Longsitting)
• Muscle technique with nervous system positioned (e.g., contract relax of the hamstrings in SLR)
• NSM with nervous system positioned (Bilateral Straight Leg Raising in Bilateral Upper Limb Tension Test 1).

Other structures may also need attention if their function has been impaired by altered conduction or axoplasmic flow. Remember the aim of treatment is to clear all component signs. The optimum health of target tissues is beneficial to the function of the cell body and thus the entire nervous system (Farragher & Kidd 1987, Dahlin & Lundborg 1990)

In the next chapter (Ch. 11) the self-mobilisation aspect of mobilising the nervous system is discussed.

COMMONLY ASKED QUESTIONS ABOUT TREATMENT

Is it best to treat the joint or the nerve first?

The question could also be asked 'Is it best to treat the muscle or the fascia first'? This question has been answered in the text, particularly in Chapter 9. To summarise, if the limitation to the tension test appears due to extraneural sources, that extraneural structure (joint, muscle fascia, other) could be treated first. A trial and error approach could be used where one structure is treated first and the result assessed, then subsequent treatment of other structures involved and the result assessed.

Some examples where the nervous system could be treated first are:

• When it is the most comparable structure in the disorder i.e., when the neural signs are more relevant to the patient's symptoms than physical signs from other structures such as joint and muscle
• When the patient has had adequate treatment of other structures involved in the disorder
• When a familiar pattern of signs and symptoms or pathology known to the physiotherapist implicates the nervous system.

In some situations, the history may give overwhelming evidence as to the involvement of the nervous system and the need for it to be mobilised (see page 251).

How hard can you stretch the nervous system?

I usually admonish the person who asks this question and in return ask them to think of mobilisation of the nervous system and the structures around it rather than a crude stretch. This would be like asking a joint based physiotherapist how hard the neck can be tractioned. There is no easy answer. The ultimate aim in treatment is to perform a technique using the minimal force required to achieve a beneficial response.

Clearly, the cadaver experiments mentioned earlier in this chapter are of little use to this concept. The forces used in those experiments would be far greater than the forces a physiotherapist could place on the nervous system of a patient.

The answer to this question lies in clinical reasoning skills. The basis is the methodical approach of continual reassessment that should be inherent in any clinician using the Maitland approach. It will take a number of treatments to work up to any vigour and decisions will be based on results gained from earlier treatments. The clinician with more clinical reasoning experiences and with a greater knowledge base will quickly reach the optimum treatment. Nevertheless, the nervous system is strong, adapted to handle forces, and may require vigorous treatment, especially in the non-irritable disorder. Physiotherapists are encouraged to continually think when performing a strong technique if there is an easier, gentler way to perform the technique. For example, rather than performing a strong SLR, better and safer results could be achieved with the spine in some lateral flexion, and treating hip adduction with the SLR held on the point of symptom reproduction. Perhaps a more skilled treatment of the interfacing structures may be warranted before vigorous mobilisation of the nervous system is employed.

What about causing pins and needles or distal pain during treatment?

Pins and needles are a neural response, just as pain can be. In the tension tests, especially the median biased tests, pins and needles responses are quite common (Kenneally et al 1988). In most situations, a treatment technique should stop short of reproducing pins and needles. In some other situations, it is necessary to cause pins and needles. To get at a connective tissue disorder of the nervous system such a neural response may need to be provoked. However, the physio-

therapist will know before the application of that technique that the pins and needles are a non-irritable symptom and part of a non-progressive disorder. I would be less inclined to provoke pins and needles in a patient who had not complained of them previously than in one who had pins and needles as part of the disorder. Techniques must not cause a worsening or spread of any numbness. Just as in the second question, the process of deciding the vigour and kind of symptoms that may be reproduced is a result of methodical assessment and reassessment.

What about plateaux in treatment?

Analysing the prognosis is probably the first step in the commonly encountered clinical situation where the physiotherapist has improved the patient to a point but then his/her treatment progress has plateaued. There may well be a reason why the patient will not get any better, and the physiotherapist and the patient are wasting their time. There are a number of answers to this question:

• Have you been fair to yourself and interpreted the prognosis correctly? This important issue is discussed later in this chapter.
• Has the disorder been treated hard enough? (See page 194)
• Are the treatment techniques getting at the disorder adequately or do they need refinement?
• Have you considered other tension contributing sites along the system and remembered that the nervous system is a continuum? If a movement can alter symptoms, possible sources and contributions to that symptom can be anywhere between the part moved and the symptom. So, if a Passive Neck Flexion alters lumbar symptoms, although the lumbar spine area is the most likely source, contributions to the symptoms can be anywhere between the head and the lumbar spine. In general, physiotherapists need more confidence to examine further than the area of symptoms and known referral sites. Adverse tension in the nervous system gives a valid anatomical reason to examine further.

What is the difference between active and passive mobilisation of the nervous system?

Both modes of mobilisation have a role, but I lean towards passive movement as best to influence the nervous system. Most of the interfacing tissues to nerve are muscles. To get the best nerve/interface movement, it seems logical to move the nerve with the surrounding structures being as lax as possible. On the other hand, an abnormal nerve/muscle movement relationship may only be evident if the muscle is contracted. With a home exercise prescription, part of the exercises will need to be done actively. My observations of skilled exponents of the proprioceptive neuromuscular facilitation approach performing muscle techniques in positions of nervous system tension have made me realise the value of both treatment of a non-neural structure in a position of tension and the use of active movement in tension positions.

What about hypermobility and the nervous system?

The nervous system should be thought of like any other system involved in movement. Logically, the hypermobile person requires a more mobile and elastic nervous system than the hypomobile person. Not only the nervous system, the mobility must extend to skin, fascia, the circulatory system, joints and muscles. If one of these structures loses its mobility then the others may suffer.

How long will I continue to treat for?

This question can be answered by considering two distinct groups of patients. The first is the group where it can be decided, after a few treatments, that physiotherapy is not the optimum treatment for that stage in their disorder. The two main issues in that decision are related to the underlying pathology and the response to treatment. These patients may require surgery, drugs, counselling or nothing. The second group have perhaps had a chronic disorder for many years and begin to improve slowly with mobilisation of the nervous system. In their overall assessment, there should be the realisation that

there is no reason why this person should not improve. That is, there is no history of severe trauma or disease. In these patients, I believe that treatment over many months can be justified and makes economic sense. With long term treatment, much will be self mobilisation. The major indications however, come from continual reassessments of treatments. It is no use treating if the patient does not improve.

What do you think you are actually doing when you are mobilising the nervous system and how do you explain your results?

I do not know the answer to this question and can only offer a list of hypotheses. The exact mechanisms whereby surgical decompression of an entrapped nerve can ease symptoms at the entrapment site and elsewhere are not known either.

It should be clear that, to mobilise the nervous system, effectively, a complete understanding of the pathophysiological and pathomechanical processes behind disorders is not essential, nor is such information available. The clinical reasoning processes behind the Maitland concept allow for the delivery of an effective and low risk treatment (see Ch. 5). Nevertheless, as well as encouraging physiotherapists to at least 'have a go' at the site(s) of adverse tension and trying to prove that hypothesis, they should also attempt to consider or investigate the physiological and/or mechanical alterations their treatment may cause.

Mobilisation of the nervous system has a mechanical effect that must affect the vascular dynamics, axonal transport systems and mechanical features of the nerve fibres and connective tissues.

- It is easy to envisage that the 'stuck' peripheral nerve or dura mater surrounded by fresh blood and oedema would benefit from movement.
- Dispersion of an intraneural oedema could be enhanced by alteration of the pressures in the nervous system during movement (Ch. 2). This may explain the relief experienced by some sufferers of carpal tunnel syndrome when they self mobilise their wrists.
- It is not inconceivable that dysmyelination

could be beneficially altered by mobilising the nerve fibre.

• Restoration of normal mechanics of the connective tissues after injury lessens the possibility of the nerves being entrapped in their surrounding connective tissues. The sinuvertebral nerve could be caught in dural scar. Similar examples are the nervi nervorum caught in the connective tissue sheath or injured or regenerating nerve fibres caught in endoneurial scar.

• It is possible that the nervous system can be trained to lengthen. While some pure stretch is possible, more complex mechanisms probably occur. Bora et al (1980) showed that sutured rat nerve could become more compliant and suggested that this feature allowed repaired nerves to adjust to mobilisation. Perhaps the cell body can be signalled from an injury site (presumably by the retrograde axoplasmic flow) and 'requested' to alter the compliance of the nerve. Similar signalling could occur from target tissues. For example, stretch of the hamstring muscle may result in neuronotrophic messages requesting the compliance of the sciatic nerve to be altered. There is an interesting clinical study that would provide support for this hypothesis. Ramamurthi (1980) noted that tension signs in patients with surgically proven disc lesions were significantly more marked in westernised Indian men and women compared to those who followed a more traditional way of life where squatting and bending were more commonly adopted postures. He hypothesised that in the latter the nervous system had stretched over time.

• Where a rapid improvement occurs, at least some of this improvement could be due to improved blood supply to hypoxic nerve fibres. The pressure gradients around the nervous system are in a delicate balance. Treatment of interfacing tissues and mobilisation of the nervous system may normalise the gradients and thus normalise the blood supply. In this regard, the effect of mobilisation of the sympathetic trunk, either directly or via the ribs, cannot be underestimated. Distortion and angulation of the sympathetic trunk has not been associated with sympathetic maintained syndromes, although clear pathological evidence of alterations in the sympathetic trunk and ganglia has been provided by Nathan (1986). Marked neuroischaemia in rabbit sciatic nerve following stimulation of the lumbar sympathetic chain has been shown (Selander et al 1985).

• The circulation and percolation of cerebrospinal fluid would be assisted by normal movement. At least half of a nerve root's metabolic requirements come from the CSF (Ch. 1).

• Normal movement will optimise the axonal transport systems. This may be achieved by altering mechanical restraints on the axoplasm or improving the blood flow and thus increasing the energy available for axonal transport.

• Normalisation of the interface will affect the axoplasmic flow. Korr (1985) suggests that the afferent bombardment from a facilitated segment deprives the nerve fibres related to that segment of some of the energy required for axonal transport. Manipulation of the segment and improvement of the joint movement eases the energy demand from the facilitated segment.

There is also the question of whether mobilisation of the nervous system assists axons to regenerate:

• Longitudinally polarised scar may allow better contact guidance for regenerating axons (Lundborg 1988).

• More vigorous treatment may cause minor injury to nerve and stimulate neurite promoting factors such as nerve growth factor (NGF). The presence of these neuronotrophic proteins are necessary for active regeneration and neurite elongation. Heumann et al (1987) demonstrated that the level of NGF at a site of nerve transection was 15 times more than in the normal nerve. Lundborg (1988) has provided an excellent summary of neuronotrophic factors and their effects on neurones.

• After nerve suture, the most minimal tension on the suture site is considered best for the optimal proportion of regenerating axons to penetrate the scar. What has not been taken into account is that it is impossible to immobilise the nervous system. In the case of suture of the median nerve at the wrist and immobilisation of the fingers, wrist and elbow, the median nerve at the wrist will still be moved and tensioned by the movements of the shoulder and neck (Ch. 2).

These hypotheses and thoughts must be taken into account, with the fact that the nervous system, especially the peripheral nervous system, has considerable regenerating powers.

PROGNOSIS MAKING

I feel that physiotherapists can improve their skills in prognosis making and also the skills involved in making an adjustment to a prognosis during treatment. In many cases, the prognostic decision regarding physiotherapy treatment is made by, rather than in association with, other professionals. Without diminishing the value of interpretation of signs and symptoms and their responses to treatment, in many situations, decisions involving a prognosis for physiotherapy treatment will have to rely on what is known about the underlying pathology.

A useful exercise is to have a calculated guess, following the initial assessment, as to what percentage improvement in a certain period of time can be achieved. It is in retrospect, after the period of treatment, that some self-evaluation and learning will occur when the physiotherapist tries to work out 'Why did I think I could get that patient 80% better?'

The ideal result is 100%. In terms of a patient who has been painfree and unhindered in any way prior to injury, this means complete freedom from any manifestations of the injury. In another patient with a reinjury of a chronic complaint, 100% may mean returning him or her back to the previous level (though hopefully better) prior to reinjury. Patients can put a percentage improvement on their own treatment, so too can the physiotherapist, by analysis of changes in signs.

Factors that may lessen the ideal result

1. Severity of the injury. Severe trauma to the nervous system may lead to irreversible fibrosis and alterations in conduction. Severe trauma, such as a fall from a height or a velocity accident such as a motor vehicle accident, inevitably injures many structures. As well as an injury to the nervous system, products of injury, such as blood and oedema from other structures, could combine to worsen the original nervous system injury. Mobilising the nervous system can be more difficult because surrounding structures might be too painful or stiff to move.

2. Site of the injury. If a pathological process has gained access to the nervous system, either intrafascicular or intradural, especially if there is scarring, then part of this process may be irreversible. If injury occurs at vulnerable sites, such as the T6 vertebral level where the spinal canal is smallest, the clinical implications may be worse than if the injury were elsewhere. The vulnerable sites are listed and discussed in Chapter 3.

3. An unremitting interface. Alterations in the structure next to the nervous system may not allow the greatest improvement that the nervous system is normally capable of. Common examples are spinal stenosis, fixed unphysiological postures such as the 'dowager's hump', angulations post fracture, myofascial bands across nerves, and congenital abnormalities.

4. The patient. For a multitude of reasons, the patient may not be allowing you to access the problem. Reasons could range from low pain thresholds, the physiotherapist's poor communication skills, malingering, possible financial gain, and the psychological content of the symptoms. There also appears to be a 'nervey' person just as there are 'jointy people' (Maitland 1986). The mechanisms are probably similar. Perhaps lower thresholds for stimuli interpreted centrally as pain occurs in the 'nervey person'. In a disorder with a large psychological component, the potential for alteration of the physiological component on the psychological component is not usually considered.

5. Spread of symptoms. It can be more difficult to achieve a 100% result in patients who complain of widespread symptoms than in those who complain of localised symptoms. However, the physiotherapist should be optimistic at first. In some situations (such as a double crush (Ch. 3)) relief of tension at one site along the nervous system can lead to symptomatic relief at the other site. Clinically, it appears that restoration of normal movement of thoracic spine structures can relieve a widespread variety of symptoms such as abdominal pain, headache and vague limb symptoms, all part of the so called 'T4 syndrome' (McGuckin 1986).

6. Spread of signs. A patient who presents with a bilateral limitation of SLR to 30° and limited ULTTs will clearly be more difficult to help than a patient with the only tension sign being a unilateral SLR limitation to 60°.

7. Chronicity. The longer a disorder has been present, the greater are the chances of further anatomical, physiological and psychological involvements. It takes time to breach the defences of the nervous system such as the perineurial diffusion barrier.

8. Occupation. The demands of certain occupations could predispose the worker to further injury, or could have created changes in the nervous system that may contribute to a component of irreversibility. Examples are sustained postures, repeated movements, repeated movements of part of the body with the rest of the body static (keyboard operator) or association with forces such as vibration (jack-hammer operator).

9. Post surgery. Occasionally, symptoms persist or may even worsen following surgery. One of the the main reasons for this is the connective tissue proliferation that occurs with the trauma of surgery. Failed surgery would further worsen the prognosis.

10. Congenital abnormalities. Known or unknown congenital abnormalities in the nervous system or the surrounding structures could predispose a person to the development of an adverse tension syndrome and also lessen the treatment potential. Some of these anomalies are discussed in Chapter 3.

11. Disease. Co-existing disease processes may lessen the chances of an optimum result. Common examples are diabetes and herpes zoster. While treatment via mobilisation may offer some assistance by easing symptoms, it clearly does not offer any cure.

12. Response to treatment. A poor response to early attempts at mobilisation could lessen the prognosis.

A prognosis should change as treatment progresses, depending on the response to treatment (subjectively and objectively) and also as various features of the disorder are clarified over time. Note that the matters listed above are all features which may influence the 100% outcome. They do not have to.

After a period of treatment, if prognostic goals are not being realised, some consideration should be given to the possibility of underlying sinister pathologies.

Thoughts on prognosis should not be limited to what the physiotherapist can achieve. Mobilisation may be in association with treatment from related fields such as surgery, medicine, podiatry and psychotherapy.

COMMUNICATION

Communication skills and their importance are well discussed in Maitland's text (1986). I have no doubt that the ultimate skill in manual therapy is the communication involved in applying the treatment to the patient. Moreover the best physiotherapists have the ability to adapt their communication skills to the many different kinds of patient who present for treatment. The idea of mobilising the nervous system raises a few more aspects of the physiotherapist's communication skills.

It is often difficult for patients to comprehend that their nerves are being mobilised. To some extent, and as a gross generalisation, patients understand joints and muscles, but the nervous system is quite a mystery. In my experience, most patients when asked how big the major nerve to the hand is, will say that it is about the size of a piece of cotton. If a patient is told, without any explanation, that the treatment will be 'mobilising the nerves' or worse, that their nerves are going to be 'stretched', rather odd images will flood into the patient's mind, many of which may distort the communication processes. Some education will be necessary. For example, patients can be told that the nerve in their buttocks, where they sit on it, is as thick as their little finger. Also, the demonstration and explanation of

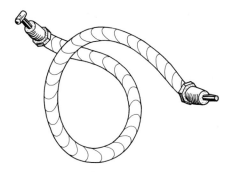

Fig.10.2   The brake cable analogy

why cervical extension can ease pain in the hamstring area during a Slump manoeuvre takes little time and could be a crucial step towards the patient's acceptance of the treatment.

I sometimes find an analogy to a brake cable useful in treatment (Fig. 10.2). The nervous system is the cable and the interfacing structures are the sheath. Treatment can be by moving the cable through the sheath and/or by treating the sheath. The cable has to have a range of movement in relation to the sheath and the sheath itself has to have a certain mobility.

Patients' lack of knowledge about the nervous system also extends to cognitive symptoms as well as those arising from physical injury to the nervous system. A recent study by Aubrey et al (1989) found that laypersons were well aware of the possibility of physical injury after a whiplash incident, but hardly aware of the common cognitive symptoms such as loss of emotional control and depression.

Communication skills are closely allied to the physiotherapist's understanding of the underlying responses to treatment. Patients' acceptance of the symptom alterations, good and bad, during a treatment, rely on good communication skills that must be based on knowledge. For example, it is hoped that a physiotherapist who has read this text and who is mobilising the nervous system could give a reasonable answer to these questions posed by a patient:

Why do I sometimes get a headache after you do those Straight Leg Raise techniques? *or* You say that I am getting better, but why do I have this new pain in my good arm now?

Some chronic disorders with a large pathomechanical contribution may initially be aggravated by treatment. There is a particular communication skill in relating this to the patient. As in the questions asked above, it will often be the need arises for an explanation for symptoms worsening elsewhere. With mobilising the nervous system, this is more likely to occur than mobilising other structures, the reasons being related to the fact that the nervous system is a mechanical and physiological continuum. Always be aware that, although subjectively patients may report they are worse, the statement will need clarification. Make sure they are referring to all symptoms and also be aware that, initially, patients could have improved physical signs yet complain of increased symptoms. I sometimes think it can be painful to acquire a movement that may not have been available for a long time. The feeling can sometimes be likened to the discomfort experienced after having a long run for the first time in years.

A big part of communication is tolerance. Symptoms are not always pain; nervous system thinking underlines this. For example, patients will describe an ache, and insist that it is not a pain. Injury to the nervous system could be responsible for a plethora of symptoms, especially if the neural elements and connective tissue elements are considered. Some patients experience great difficulties adequately expressing their symptoms. Sometimes, use of the word 'discomfort' when discussing symptoms will help. It is far more open than 'pain' and will help the patient to describe their symptoms in their own language.

Communication with other professionals

It is a difficult thing to explain what mobilisation of the nervous system entails. The concept is very new and perhaps alien to many medically oriented professionals, including physiotherapists. As far as possible, the disorders need to be expressed in pathoanatomical terms. For example, if a doctor received a letter that included a sentence such as 'This patient was treated for some adverse mechanical tension in the nervous system by using a derivative of Upper Limb Tension Test 3', most recipients of the letter would shake their head in bewilderment and probably discard the letter. Terms such as scar, neuroma, tethered dura, neuritis, arachnoiditis, entrapment, neuropathy, neuropathic, neurogenic, double crush, etc., are far better. It also encourages physiotherapists to have a calculated guess at the pathological pro-cesses involved. If an injury to the nervous system is evident as a part of the patient's presenting disorder, all changes found at neurological exam-ination such as weakness and changes in vibration sensation should be reported. This assists with the inference that a neurogenic process is in-volved.

The ultimate communication with other pro-fessionals is to write, research and publish.

REFERENCES

Aubrey J B, Dobbs A R, Rule B G 1989 Laypersons' knowledge about the sequelae of minor head injury and whiplash. Journal of Neurology, Neurosurgery and Psychiatry 52: 842–846

Bora F W, Richardson S, Black J 1980 The biomechanical responses to tension in a peripheral nerve. Journal of Hand Surgery 5: 21–25

Cavafy J 1881 A case of sciatic nerve-stretching in locomotor ataxy: with remarks on the operation. British Medical Journal Dec 17: 973–974

Dahlin L B, Lundborg G 1990 The neurone and its response to peripheral nerve compression. Journal of Hand Surgery 15B: 5–10

Farragher D, Kidd G L 1987 Eutrophic electrical stimulation for Bell's palsy. Clinical Rehabilitation 1: 265–271

Heumann R, Korsching S, Bandtlour C et al 1987 Changes of nerve growth factor synthesis in non-neuronal cells in response to sciatic nerve transection. Journal of Cell Biology 104: 1623–1631

Kenneally M, Rubenach H, Elvey R 1988 The upper limb tension test: the SLR of the arm. In; Grant R (ed) Physical therapy of the cervical and thoracic spine, Clinics in Physical Therapy 17. Churchill Livingstone, New York

Kornberg C, Lew P 1989 The effect of stretching neural structures on grade 1 hamstring injuries. The Journal of Orthopaedic and Sports Physical Therapy June: 481–487

Korr I M 1985 Neurochemical and neurotrophic consequences of nerve deformation. In: Glasgow E F et al (eds.) Aspects of Manipulative Therapy, 2nd edn. Churchill Livingstone, Melbourne

Lundborg G 1988 Nerve injury and repair. Churchill Livingstone, Edinburgh

Magarey M E 1985 Selection of passive treatment techniques. In: Proceedings fourth biennial conference, Manipulative Therapists Association of Australia, Brisbane

Maitland G D 1977 Peripheral manipulation, 2nd edn. Butterworths, London

Maitland G D 1986 Vertebral manipulation 5th edn. Butterworths, London

Marshall J 1883 On nerve stretching for the relief or cure of pain. British Medical Journal 2: 1173–1179

McGuckin N 1986 The T4 syndrome. In: Grieve G P (ed) Modern manual therapy of the vertebral column. Churchill Livingstone, Edinburgh

McLellan D L, Swash M 1976 Longitudinal sliding of the median nerve during movements of the upper limb. Journal of Neurology, Neurosurgery and Psychiatry 39: 556–570

Nathan H 1986 Osteophytes of the spine compressing the sympathetic trunk and splanchnic nerves in the thorax. Spine 12: 527–532

Ramamurthi B 1980 Absence of limitation of straight leg raising in proved lumbar disc lesion. Journal of Neurosurgery 52: 852–853

Selander D, Mansson L G, Karlsson L et al 1985 Adrenergetic vasoconstriction in peripheral nerves in the rabbit. Anesthesiology 62: 6–10

Symington J 1882 The physics of nerve stretching. British Medical Journal 1: 770

11. Self treatment

INTRODUCTION

Treatment contact time with a physiotherapist will rarely provide maximum benefit unless the patient can apply therapeutic movement and principles at home and elsewhere.

There are two main aspects to self treatment. The first is self mobilising techniques, either as a treatment alone or more likely as a progression and continuation of hands on treatment. The second aspect is postural adaptation and awareness with an orientation toward the nervous system. In both areas, just as with the delivery of a technique, the type, timing and amount of self treatment will differ with each patient. A basic tenet of the Maitland (1986) concept worth reinforcing at this stage is that 'technique is the brainchild of ingenuity'.

Self mobilisation of the nervous system should not differ greatly from mobilisation of other structures. Indeed, it is difficult to self mobilise one structure without affecting others. With a knowledge of precautions and contraindications, neurobiomechanics, and pathologies, the application of exercises should not be difficult. There is no strengthening of course (unless of a target tissue); the skill is in mobilisation.

SELF MOBILISATION

There are a number of suggested principles and guidelines.

1. Before self mobilisation is prescribed, the physiotherapist and patient must be aware of the likely affect of mobilisation. This can be ascertained in the clinic. If treatment techniques are having the desired response, then similarly performed home mobilisation should also produce desired responses. It may be that four or five treatment sessions pass before the clinician knows enough about the disorder and hence the best treatment direction.

2. The technique must fit the patient. There can be no uniform prescription, or exercise handout (mass produced handouts surely cannot enhance compliance). If active treatment is designed to fit the patient then so should the self treatment. All necessary guidelines are included in the previous chapters on assessment and treatment.

3. Only a small proportion of patients who are prescribed exercises will actually do them as prescribed. If extrapolations were made from the drug and exercise compliance literature it would seem that at least 50% of patients prescribed simple exercises will fail to do them (Stone 1979, Peck & King 1982). Within the 50% who do the exercises, a considerable percentage will underdo them, overdo them, or manage somehow to do a completely different exercise. It is important to identify and control all categories. However, I believe that compliance to a nerve mobilising programme is better than to a muscle strengthening programme. Nervous system self mobilising usually involves only one or two manoevres, it does not take long (perhaps a few minutes a day) and the patient does not usually perspire, and often will feel better after.

Some factors that increase compliance are simplicity of the prescription (Stone 1979), non-patronising manner of the physiotherapist (Bradshaw et al 1975), patient awareness of the effects of non-compliance (Peck & King 1982), specific information about the exercises such as how many to do, how often to do them, and when to stop (Glossop et al 1982, Peck & King 1982). Experts probably underestimate their intelligence and as a consequence, patients' knowledge may be overestimated.

4. Self mobilisation can be adapted for the irritable as well as the non-irritable disorder. Great care will be needed with an exercise prescription for a patient with an irritable disorder. There is, however, a kind of patient and a kind of disorder where it is best to let the patient do the technique for him or herself. Some whiplash presentations come immediately to mind. With some acute traumatic disorders the physiotherapist may be unable to ascertain the contribution of the various structural components present. With analysis of the symptomatology and history, involvement of the nervous system may be presumed. Similar principles for the prescription of exercise for the irritable disorder exists as for the hands-on treatment delivered by the physiotherapist (see previous chapters on examination and treatment).

5. In the more non-irritable and chronic disorders, a caring spouse, family member or friend can be of assistance. In nearly all cases, the Upper Limb Tension Test manoevres are too complex for the untrained. However, there will always be special cases for the adaptable physiotherapist. For example, if a man lived on a sheep station at Oodnadatta in South Australia, some 1500 kilometres from the nearest physiotherapist, a lot of effort would be justified in teaching his wife how to do an ULTT technique whilst in the city for their annual visit. Slump Longsitting techniques are good examples where an assistant is useful. If a partner assisted technique is prescribed then the idea of an 'escape valve' is worth using. For example, in the Slump Longsitting technique, the patient should have control over the neck flexion. If the assistant is too enthusiastic, the patient has control of neck extension to get away from the tension caused in the nervous system. This technique is illustrated later in the text (refer to Fig. 11.7).

6. I feel that the mechanical pain principle, as espoused by McKenzie (1981), is best for self mobilisation. This means that during an exercise the patient can cause symptoms (the amount and kind of symptoms will have been clearly defined in the clinic) as long as those symptoms stop on releasing the mobilisation. Patients should follow the principle of 'do the exercise until you feel the desired pain, release the stretch, and as long as the symptoms ease then it is safe to continue'. If this simple principle is followed together with the physiotherapist's advice, the technique can be gradually performed harder and for longer.

7. The decision of how much, how many and when to perform the exercises must be based on clinical reasoning. There is no exact answer. There will be different goals other than achieving mere muscle power such as range of movement, functional abilities and painfree movement. Broadly, as for passive mobilisation by the physiotherapist, the optimum treatment application should be the use of the least force for a safe and definite improvement in physical signs. In some pathophysiological states, repeated gentle mobilisation may be beneficial whereas, in a chronic pathomechanical states, one or two strong mobilisation may be optimal, but may need to be carried out over a long period of time. It may be thought that a severe fibrosing reaction which has gained access to the nervous system will be irreversible. While there may be a component of irreversibility, my experience is that, with continual mobilising both at home and in the clinic, some benefit may be gained. One only has to think of the effects of pressure garments on deformed skin post burn trauma even after many years to get the stimulus to continue such a low risk and potentially beneficial therapy. It seems that the nervous system, particularly peripheral nerve, has the ability to adapt over a long period of time as witnessed by the usually easy adaptation to leg lengthening procedures. It may be assumed that, given the difficulty the nervous system has clearing an intraneural reaction, a potentially harmful intraneural oedema may persist long after the apparent resolution of the injury. Persistence with a

simple manoevre taking perhaps a couple of minutes a day could be useful prophylaxis. Where there is an irreversible component, self mobilisation is likely to be useful as a maintenance therapy.

8. Similar progression principles as suggested in the previous chapter are applicable. However, compromise will always be necessary and appropriate application relies on the physiotherapist's flexibility. There are tension tests or components of them that are hard to self mobilise. For example, ULTT2 can be difficult to self mobilise, but in self treatment, ULTT1, even if not as positive, could be used. In many situations it is likely that active movements rather than passive, or assisted active, movements are all that are available. It should not be difficult for a thinking physiotherapist to apply techniques to sporting or aerobic activities. For example, the freestyle swimming stroke could be analysed as alternate left and right Upper Limb Tension Tests. The bouyancy of water assists active exercises and is likely to be beneficial for more irritable disorders such as whiplash. Other thoughts about adapting exercises may include self hold/relax techniques in tension and the use of restraints such as belts.

SOME USEFUL TECHNIQUES

The techniques illustrated and described are variants and additions to the base tests. They are a selection of techniques only and it would be disappointing if physiotherapists were to think that this were a final list. The possibilities and variations are endless.

Straight Leg Raise techniques

Physiotherapists have prescribed SLR stretches for many years, in some situations to stretch the sciatic nerve and its roots, but more often ostensibly to stretch the hamstring muscles. To turn a hamstring stretch into a nervous system stretch may require no more than a little lateral thinking. More likely, fine adjustments can be made to existing techniques to get at the nervous system more effectively. For example, if a SLR stretch were performed with the hip in medial rotation,

a known sensitising manoeuvre for the nervous system, this would allow better access to the neural tissues and take some of the emphasis off muscle

Some spinal and leg disorders may benefit from a derivative of the SLR such as knee extension in hip flexion (Fig. 11.1). This could be useful for lumbar symptoms with an element of irritability because the component used (knee extension) is some way from the source of symptoms. It is thus a convenient starting point for a SLR self mobilising technique. Take care with those patients who have arm symptoms. This is especially so if the symptoms are linked to the lumbar symptoms as holding the thigh in flexion may aggravate the arm. There will be situations where a marked, painful restriction of the SLR exists. This will require components of the SLR to be employed, such as dorsiflexion or hip medial rotation, before the hip is flexed. Remember that when a patient is supine and at rest, there is already a good deal of tension in the sciatic tract because the knee is extended. I have encountered a number of patients, usually post trauma such as whiplash or a fall from a height, where dorsiflexion of the ankle has to be the starting position for cervical pain.

For stronger techniques, try using the open doorway (Fig. 11.2). This is useful as long as the patients' SLR is not over 90°. This technique can be directed more toward the nervous system by adding in sensitising tests such as ankle dorsiflexion, hip medial rotation and cervical flexion. A towel could be used to hold the ankle dorsiflexion. A towel gives better control of the whole foot, including the toes, than a belt or a rope does. In this position, plantar flexion and inver-

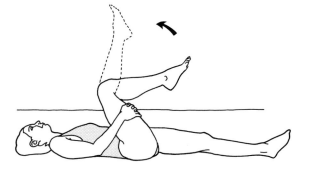

Fig. 11.1 In hip flexion, active extension of the knee for a moderately irritable lumbar spine

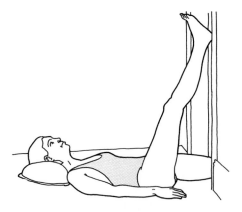

Fig. 11.2 The SLR in an open doorway

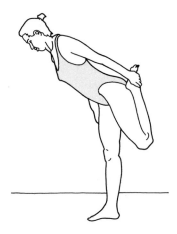

Fig. 11.4 'Quadriceps' in standing

sion of the ankle can be added by the patient performing the movement actively. Other techniques are described below.

Bilateral SLR techniques (BSLR) can be mobilised by using a wall. If one SLR is limited more than the other, this leg can be mobilised in BSLR. With two legs on the wall the knee of the more limited will flex. This leg can then be mobilised by pushing the knee into extension. Perhaps a little powder on the heel will facilitate the sliding (Fig. 11.3).

Contract/relax techniques to the hamstring muscles can be readily integrated and seem clinically worthwhile. Presumably, as well as lengthening the hamstrings, this allows better access to the nervous system by eliminating the muscle tightness component to the limited SLR. There will be some situations where there appears to be a nerve/muscle relationship disorder

and the best way to approach it is to do a muscle technique such as contract/relax with the nervous system in the desired amount of tension.

Prone Knee Bend

When the quadriceps muscle group is stretched, so will the upper part of the femoral nerve. Like the SLR, no more than a little lateral thinking may be needed to turn a quadriceps stretch into a femoral nerve stretch. An easy quadriceps/femoral nerve stretch is the standing stretch shown in Figure 11.4. Another stretch can be performed by sitting on the haunches and then leaning backwards.

Combination Slumps

Adding spinal movements onto the SLR and the PKB

Slump Longsitting is a useful base technique which can be easily refined and sensitised further for use at home. I often select it for home use for disorders with a Slump component. Patient can easily see how far their foreheads are from their knees and this can give them a goal. Ankle dorsiflexion can be added by putting feet against a wall (Fig. 11.5) or plantar flexion/inversion by sitting with the foot forced into inversion in the corner of a room. Medial rotation of the hip and spinal lateral flexion can be easily added to this position.

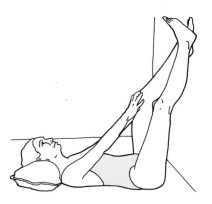

Fig. 11.3 Bilateral Straight Leg Raise on a wall

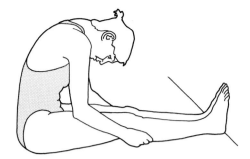

Fig. 11.5 Slump Longsitting with ankle dorsiflexion

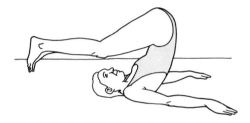

Fig. 11.6 Slump roll over

A more vigorous Slump technique without having to call on an assistant is shown in Figure 11.6. I find it useful for tension disorders that originate from or have components in the upper thoracic and cervico-thoracic junction. More mobile patients may need to have their head on a pillow. Take care with this technique — it is aimed at a younger patient with a non-irritable disorder. With techniques requiring this vigour, an assistant is often required. The Slump Longsitting can be done with the assistant bowing the spine and further flexing the hips. The concept of the 'escape valve' was discussed earlier in the principles of exercise prescription (Fig. 11.7). If required, knee extension can be maintained with straps.

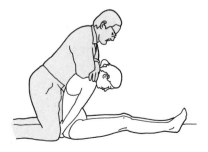

Fig. 11.7 Slump Longsitting with an assistant

Slump Longsitting requires the SLR part of the slump to be taken up first. Some disorders require the Slump sitting technique. A helper may be needed to mobilise the leg, although I have had one ingenious patient who found she could effectively mobilise the leg with a foot on a skateboard as illustrated in Figure 11.8. Such ingenuity does not only have to come from the physiotherapist. If the required mobilisation is demonstrated to a patient and the patient asked to find a way to mobilise it, the response can be very helpful and the physiotherapist will inevitably learn new techniques.

Often a patient, especially if at work, cannot lie down during the day. Similarly, the patient may want to mobilise while waiting on the side-

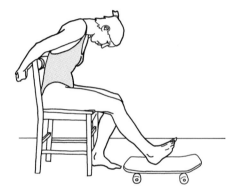

Fig. 11.8 Slump sitting with a skateboard to assist the knee extension component

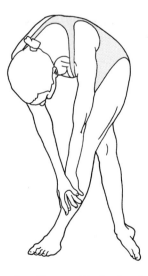

Fig. 11.9 Standing Slump with the foot in plantar flexion and inversion and the knee held extended

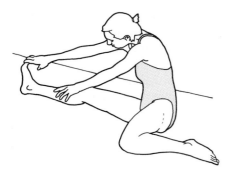

Fig. 11.10 The hurdler's stretch — combining Prone Knee Bend and the Straight Leg Raise

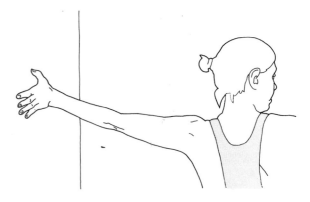

Fig. 11.11 Standard ULTT1 on a wall

line at a sporting event. This useful standing technique (Fig. 11.9) utilises hip adduction and medial rotation and various foot and spinal positions.

If needed, a PKB can be added to the Slump positions. The hurdler's stretch (Fig. 11.10) is one method.

The Upper Limb Tension Tests

Unfortunately, the upper limb provides more difficulties for a self mobilisation programme. Due to the greater complexity of upper limb neuroanatomy, techniques to get at the disorder need far more refinement than they would in the lower limb. Greater caution needs to be taken as it is much easier to aggravate the upper limb than the lower.

For a more acute and irritable disorder, a single component of the tension test could be utilised as a technique. For example, if neurogenic neck/shoulder symptoms worsen in shoulder abduction of 40°, gentle elbow extension in a lesser range of shoulder abduction could then be a technique possibility. More likely in an irritable disorder, techniques away from the site of symptoms such as using the other arm or a leg will be used. Shoulder girdle movements, often forgotten in the joint and muscle based exercise programmes, are useful techniques for this kind of irritable disorder. Shoulder girdle depression with combinations of protraction and retraction could be done in lying or even in a bath where the bouyancy and warmth of water will assist the technique.

Wall based techniques can come reasonably close to replicating ULTT1 positions. The position shown in Figure 11.11 could be thought of as a starting point with many possible variations in position and in the component used to mobilise. These can be listed:

- Both lateral and medial rotations of the shoulder can be easily added.
- Shoulder range of abduction and horizontal flexion and extension can be altered.
- The forearm can be supinated or pronated.
- The mobilisation can then come from the neck, body or the elbow.

A problem with self mobilisation using the Upper Limb Tension Tests is that shoulder depression is difficult to maintain. The patient may have to hold the depression component by using the other arm (Fig. 11.12).

The ULTT2 is a more difficult test to self mobilise. The best way I have found is the behind back combinations seen in Figure 11.13. If shoul-

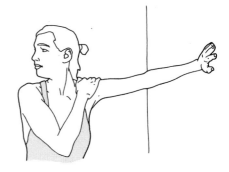

Fig. 11.12 ULTT1 maintaining the shoulder girdle depresion component

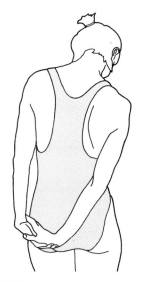

Fig. 11.13 ULTT2

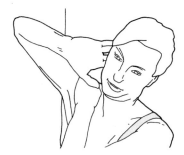

Fig. 11.14 ULTT3

der depression is the main component requiring mobilisation, standing and holding onto the side of a table and extending the knees can be done. ULTT3 is not difficult to replicate. The patient can simply place his/her hand on or about the ear and then use abduction of the shoulder, wrist flexion and elbow flexion to refine the technique (Fig. 11.14). The technique can be made more vigorous by the patient attempting to flatten the axilla towards the wall.

The Klapps crawling position is a useful way to treat a disorder requiring bilateral ULTT's (see Ch. 13). In this position, neck flexion and lateral flexion can be incorporated.

POSTURE

With an appreciation of the biomechanics and the continuum of the nervous system, some pos-tural considerations that may not have been previously contemplated, become rather clear. There are three areas to consider:

1. Static postures with the nervous system on full stretch
2. Repetition as part of dynamic posture
3. Combinations of static and dynamic posture.

There are many clear examples of postures which place the nervous system on full stretch. For example, the patient who complains of symptoms whilst reading in bed is open to immediate postural analysis and likely correction because the longsitting position adopted replicates a Slump position (Fig. 11.15). The sidelying position adopted by many people to read in bed is similar to an ULTT3 position (Fig. 11.16). Some sustained postures, such as spinal flexion from driving or thoracic flexion from using a keyboard, while not being at the very end of nervous system elasticity, still place the system on some stretch.

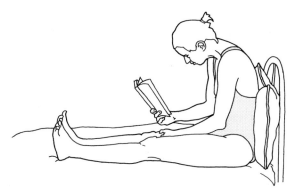

Fig. 11.15 Reading longsitting in bed replicated the Slump Longsitting position

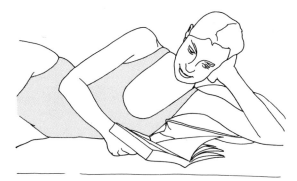

Fig. 11.16 Reading in bed sidelying replicates the ULTT3

Over a period of time, the amount of stretch could ultimately cause or contribute to symptoms.

Repetition as part of a dynamic posture needs analysis. The effect of repetition on the nervous system has been discussed in Chapter 12 with the suggestion that it may be an underestimated aetiology in nerve injury. In this regard, postural adaptations such as pause gymnastics during work involving sustained postures could be thought of as taking the nervous system through a range of movement, not just exercise for muscles and joints.

Combinations of static posture and repetition are probably the worst. An example is the secretary who types with the spine in some degree of thoracic flexion and perhaps a poked chin posture and who persists with this posture after work — perhaps driving home, and sitting in a low chair while watching television. Typing may be potentially injurious to the median nerve in the carpal tunnel. This may be further compounded by the sympathetic trunk being on some stretch in the typing posture (Ch. 2) perhaps even inhibiting blood flow into the median nerve at the wrist. If this person does not take part in out of tension activities but prefers to go home and knit or watch television after work then there is a potential for further injury in this rather insidious way.

PROPHYLAXIS

Joint and muscle stretches are almost universally regarded as an injury preventive. The question must be asked, 'What about mobilising exercises for the health of the nervous system?'. There are a number of answers to this. First of all, the nervous system is unavoidably mobilised in routine stretches. Some of the benefits from those exercises could well be attributed to the mobilisation of neural structures with consequent benefits for target structures. This would be as relevant in the warm-up as well as the warm-down. There are physiological reasons for neural mobilisation as a prophylactic measure. A healthy, mobile nervous system is necessary to allow the non-neural structures to be used to their full extensibility. As a speculation, the flushing of the intraneural vascular system due to stretch may enhance the supply of oxygen for the action potential and also for the axoplasmic transport systems.

REFERENCES

Bradshaw P W, Kensey J, Ley P et al 1975 Recall of medical advice, comprehensibility and specificity. British Journal of Social and Cllinical Psychology 14: 55–66
Glossop E S, Goldenberg E, Smith D et al 1982 Patient compliance in back and neck pain. Physiotherapy 68: 225–226
Maitland G D 1986 Vertebral manipulation, 5th ed. Butterworths, London
McKenzie R A 1981 The lumbar spine: mechanical diagnosis and therapy. Spinal Publications, Waikanae
Lewit K 1985 Manipulative therapy in rehabilitation of the locomotor system. Butterworths, London
Peck C L, King N J 1982 Increasing patient compliance with prescriptions. Journal of the American Medical Association 248: 2874–2877
Stone G C 1979 Patient compliance and the role of the expert. Journal of Social Sciences 35: 34–59

PART IV

Selected disorders and case studies

12. Adverse neural tension disorders centred in the limbs

INTRODUCTION

In this chapter, differing aspects of the role of adverse neural tension in selected disorders centred in the limbs is discussed. In Parts II and III, I have suggested the bases for examination and treatment of the nervous system. This chapter includes:

1. Disorders involving the extremities. A detailed analysis is presented outlining the necessary depth of anatomical knowledge and specific assessment and treatment techniques. Much of the information is relevant to all sites of adverse tension.

2. The sources and contributing factors which need to be examined in the thoracic outlet syndrome are listed. The importance of examining the mechanics of the nervous system is discussed.

3. Meralgia paraesthetica is presented as an isolated case of nerve entrapment.

4. Peripheral nerve surgery is discussed. A surgical case study is presented and the symptoms analysed in terms of the examination procedures in this book.

5. Muscle tears, concentrating on the hamstring tear, are discussed. The role of the nervous system in management and assessment is outlined.

6. The analysis of adverse neural tension in repetition strain injury (RSI) is discussed. Aspects of the presentation of the disorder are discussed.

THE EXTREMITIES

Certain features of the hand and foot make them susceptible to the development of adverse neural tension syndromes. These features are:

- The hands and feet have great mobility.
- Many nerves in the hands and feet are cutaneous.
- The structures have a richer innervation than elsewhere.
- Proximal sites of injury can have a marked effect.
- There is a greater awareness of nervous system injuries in the extremities since they are easier to diagnose.

The examination principles of nervous system mechanics in the hand and the foot are similar. Although the base tension tests are used, often the tests will have to be performed in reverse. For example, taking up a hand or foot component first, then progressively adding on nervous system tensioning movements.

As in other body areas, the importance of the nervous system is believed to be underestimated. In 1960 Kopell and Thompson wrote:

A concurrent neuropathy is often overlooked and all the complaints and dysfunctions are attributed to ligamentous or joint residuals.

More recently, a reawakening of interest in the peripheral nervous system has been evident. To some extent, an exposé of some disorders is occurring. De Quervain's disease is a good example where recent research (Saplys et al 1987) has supported the clinical suspicions of others (Rask 1978) that involvement of the superficial radial nerve is often mis-diagnosed as de Quervain's disease. Injury to the superficial radial nerve is discussed later in this chapter. It is important to realise that, by the time a nerve injury earns the label of entrapment, the injury will be reasonably severe and probably in a well known site. Although there are known vulnerable sites, we must consider the more minor injury and the fact that injury can occur anywhere along the nervous system.

THE FOOT AND ANKLE

Disorders involving the peroneal nerves

The deep peroneal nerve descends infero-medially on the fibula. A couple of centimetres above the ankle joint, it exits from beneath the muscle belly of the extensor hallucis longus. The nerve then passes beneath the superior and then the inferior extensor retinaculum. This area, referred to as the anterior tarsal tunnel (Marinacci 1968), also contains the anterior tibial blood vessels. Beyond the tunnel, the nerve branches, with the lateral branch giving motor supply to the extensor digitorum brevis and nearby joints. The medial branch accompanies the dorsalis pedis artery, supplying the cutaneous sensation in the space between the first and second toes (Fig 12.1). Kopell & Thompson (1963) identified an entrapment neuropathy of the deep peroneal nerve

under the inferior extensor retinaculum. Mackinnon & Dellon (1988) reported an additional site of entrapment as being distal to the anterior tarsal tunnel, overlying the junction of the first and second cuneiforms with the metatarsals. Here, the medial (sensory) branch is crossed by the extensor hallucis brevis. Mackinnon & Dellon (1988) identified an aetiological factor as being the straps from a particular design of womens' shoes (Fig. 12.2). This could be regarded as a form of external double crush. Note, too, the plantarflexion induced by high heeled shoes places the peroneal nerves on some tension. Tight shoes, as an aetiological factor, have also been identified by Borges et al (1981) and Gessini et al (1984).

From under the peroneus brevis muscle, the superficial peroneal nerve pierces the deep fascia of the lower leg some 10–12 cm above the lateral malleolus. It then divides into intermediate and medial dorsal cutaneous nerves that cross the dorsum of the foot (Kosinski 1926). The nerve supplies the dorsum of the foot with the exception of the web space between the first and second toes. It does have a motor supply to the peroneus brevis and longus, but this branch exits much higher than the exit through the fascia. The most common sites of injury are where the nerve passes through the fascia and as part of ankle sprains and other ankle trauma. Tight fitting shoes could compress the nerve on the dorsum of the foot. Increases in the pressure within the compartments of the lower leg have been shown to interfere with nerve function (Hargens 1989).

A report on incisional neuromas by Kenzora

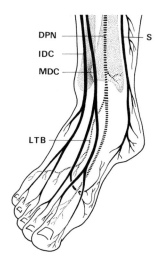

Fig. 12.1 The saphenous and peroneal nerves in the foot. DPN deep peroneal nerve, IDC intermediate dorsal cutaneous, LTB lateral terminal branch (motor), MDC medial dorsal cutaneous (IDC and MDC are branches of the superficial peroneal nerve) S saphenous nerve

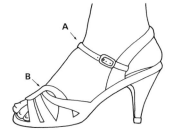

Fig. 12.2 A common design of womens' shoes places the straps over two anatomically vulnerable sites for the deep peroneal nerve. In A the nerve is in the anterior tarsal tunnel and in B the nerve is under the tendon of extensor hallucis brevis (adapted from Mackinnon & Dellon 1988)

(1984) highlighted the vulnerability to injury of the cutaneous nerves on the dorsum of the foot. He reviewed 17 patients with 25 highly symptomatic neuromas on the dorsum of the foot following routine orthopaedic surgery in that region. He noted that 76% occurred in a zone on the upper dorsum of the foot which he called the 'neuromatous zone'. This zone corresponds to an area of greater ankle movements and also an area prone to compression from tight or ill-fitting footwear. The peroneal nerves are also at risk from ankle sprains (Nitz et al 1985).

Examination directed at the nervous system

Symptoms of adverse tension, as discussed in Chapter 4, may exist. A clear outline of any sensory changes and recognition of any paralysis is required to help differentiate between nerves involved and also any injury to the L5 nerve root (see Table 12.1). A neurological examination is performed routinely. Look for any signs of trophic changes (redness, shininess, puffiness, sweating). I find it useful to palpate over the anterior tarsal tunnel, the emergence from the fascia of the superficial peroneal nerve, the branches of the superficial peroneal nerve on the dorsum of the foot and the common peroneal nerve at the knee (see Chapter 9). Swelling or fullness may

Table 12.1 Some features that allow differentiation between sites of injury along the common peroneal nerve. More than one disorder may exist. CPN common peroneal nerve at the fibula head, DPN deep peroneal at the anterior tarsal tunnel, SPN superficial peroneal nerve at the distal anterolateral leg

Site of Injury	Weakness	Symptoms
L5	All L5 innervated muscles including tibialis posterior and gluteus medius	Lateral lower limb, dorsum of foot, back
CPN	Ankle dorsiflexors, evertors, toe extensors	Lateral leg, dorsum of foot, more clearly defined than L5
DPN	Extensor digitorum brevis	First web space
SPN	None	Dorsum of foot excluding web space

be evident in the antero-lateral compartment if the contained muscles have been overused.

The tension tests, as well as the base tests, can be done in reverse as this appears to allow better access to the nervous system in the foot. For the superficial and common peroneal nerves, plantar flexion and inversion of the ankle and foot will be involved with the SLR further superimposed. This has been described and illustrated in Chapter 7. Further sensitisation can be added by hip adduction and medial rotation. If these hip movements alter the foot pain, then some involvement of the nervous system can be inferred. If a spinal component to the symptoms is suspected, the Slump Test, either in sitting or in longsitting, utilising plantarflexion and inversion may be more sensitive.

With a foot injury, the mechanics of the peroneal nerves in the foot are often interfered with. I find that most inversion ankle sprains have a component of altered nervous system mechanics as part of their symptoms. In a pilot study, Mauhart (1989) examined 20 patients with chronic ankle sprain and found that, compared with a control group, the experimental group showed a decrease in the painfree range of PFI/SLR. It seems inevitable that with inversion fractures, the peroneal nerves will be affected either directly or indirectly by pressure from blood, oedema and plaster casts.

Remember in examination that clinical physiological pains (Ch. 9) could be indicative of nervous system involvement. For example, on PFI/SLR on the left leg, the symptom response could be in the hamstring but to the PFI/SLR on the right leg it is in the calf. This response, even if not reproducing the patient's pain, still indicates that something may be wrong with the nervous system. In some patients, the disorder may need sensitising. For example, it would be preferable to examine a patient who complains of symptoms after considerable activity, directly after such activity. As in all disorders, the nervous system cannot be examined alone. The relevant joints and muscles also need examination.

Treatment directed at the nervous system

In the early stages of injury, where the disorder

may be severe or irritable, treatment via gentle through range movement out of tension, such as plantarflexion in knee and hip flexion, would be called for. As a progression, stronger treatment in tension and in various positions related to the interface would be called for. To place maximal tension on the nerve, the foot is plantarflexed and inverted, then the SLR and further sensitising movements such as hip adduction and medial rotation are added. Then, PF/I is added again as a treatment technique (Fig. 12.3). The toes can also be plantar flexed. If there is a component of the disorder in the spinal canal or the enclosed neuraxis and meninges, then slump techniques can be introduced. If there are difficulties in examination and treatment in SLR, the slump longsitting position can be utilised. This is also a good position for self mobilisation. Likely extraneural sources of tension, other than at the ankle, are at the head of the fibula, the low lumbar spine and the mid thoracic spine.

Advice regarding footwear can have a quick effect. Here an interfacing force can be instantly removed. Be aware of the potential for injury to the peroneal nerves in the unconscious patient or patient with a denervated foot who is put to bed with tight sheets holding the foot in plantar flexion and inversion.

For peroneal nerve injuries out of the reach of physiotherapy techniques, an excellent response to surgery is nearly always possible. Mackinnon & Dellon (1988) have summarised the literature

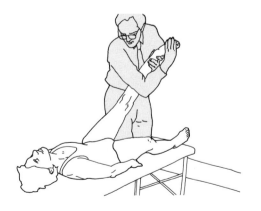

Fig. 12.3 Increasing the tension on the peroneal tract by plantarflexion/inversion, knee extension, hip medial rotation and adduction

and report nearly 100% successful results without complications.

Disorders involving the tibial nerve

The major reported site of entrapment is the posterior tarsal tunnel. This tunnel involves the flexor retinaculum bridging the space between the medial malleolus and the calcaneus. It can be considered analogous to the carpal tunnel because the tunnel contains tendons and blood vessels together with the tibial nerve. There is further analogy because, like the carpal tunnel, there is an increasing awareness of the potential for this area to cause symptoms such as those of plantar fasciitis or metatarsalgia (Mackinnon & Dellon 1988). Within the tarsal tunnel, the posterior tibial nerve bifurcates into the medial and lateral plantar nerves and usually a calcaneal branch (Dellon & Mackinnon 1984). Hence, divisions occur in areas of great mobility which can only make the nervous system more vulnerable at that point (Ch. 3).

Other reported areas of injury to the medial and lateral plantar nerves are where the nerves travel under the abductor hallucis muscle, commonly known as 'jogger's foot' (Oh & Lee 1987), and injury to the interdigital nerve to the toes, usually between the third and the fourth metatarsal. This interdigital nerve is often involved in a well known entrapment, Morton's neuroma. This is characterised by pain on weight-bearing, especially in high heel shoes and on toe extension. The disorder is unique amongst neuropathies because the usually successful surgical treatment is to excise the affected segment of nerve. This has allowed pathological analysis. Lassman et al (1976) found that the interfascicular epineurium and perineurium were thickened with some large fibre destruction and Wallerian degeneration depending on the amount of compression. These findings are not typical of a neuroma.

Of course, injury is possible anywhere. By structural differentiation and palpation examination, I have noted medial heel pain of neurogenic origin in an athlete who ran with pronated heels. I feel many cases of plantar fasciitis are neurogenic. They are often related to the posterior tarsal tunnel, but also small cutaneous branches of the plantar nerves may be caught in the fascia.

Examination directed at the nervous system

Distribution of symptoms may suggest compromise of individual branches. For example, calcaneal pain could implicate the calcaneal nerve. There could be shooting pain along any individual nerve. Weightbearing, particularly in high heel shoes, may aggravate a Morton's toe neuroma.

Palpation of the tarsal tunnel may reveal swelling. Pressure or tapping the tibial nerve may cause a neural response elsewhere along the tibial track. If the medial plantar nerve is involved, the neural response could be felt in the big toe, the lateral plantar in the little toe or any other areas of entrapment. Knowledge of the cutaneous innervation fields is helpful (Ch. 6). Palpation can be performed in and out of tension. Try to follow the nerve down into the foot.

The adverse tension component can be examined by putting the foot into a pain reproductive position and then altering a distal component, usually the hip component of the SLR. The alternative would be to put the patient in SLR or Slump and then add the symptom provoking manoeuvre. Being the tibial nerve, dorsiflexion and eversion of the ankle will be required. Superimposed on this, pronation of the foot would be expected to stress the lateral plantar nerve (Fig. 12.4) and abduction and pronation would stress the medial plantar nerve. Dorsiflexion of the toes will add further tension. The heel can be further abducted to place more tension on the calcaneal branch.

Another method, useful for examining a disorder such as heel spurs, is to find the painful spot by palpation (even use the blunt end of a pen). Then, with the pressure from palpation held on, change the tension in the nerve by adding a SLR or a Slump. If there is a nerve component, the pain will alter; if there is a symptomatic heel spur, the pain should stay the same. Remember too that palpation can be used to differentiate the source of symptoms. The painful position is held and then the tibial nerve is palpated or twanged

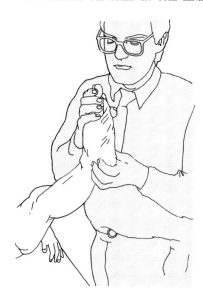

Fig. 12.4 Tension on the lateral plantar nerve. In SLR/ankle dorsiflexion/eversion/forefoot pronation

posterior to the ankle. This may reproduce the symptoms in the foot. Palpation techniques have been discussed in Chapter 9.

Any findings related to muscle or joint examination can be differentiated. For example, if the metatarsal row is compressed, symptoms of metatarsalgia may be reproduced. The source could be joints or nerves. If increasing nerve tension alters the symptoms, then a neurogenic component must be evident.

Treatment directed at the nervous system

Before pathological changes put treatment beyond the range of physiotherapy, anecdotally, excellent results can be obtained with mobilising the nervous system and the structures around the nervous system.

Figure 12.5 is an example of a combined joint/nerve technique for Morton's neuroma. In Slump Longsitting and ankle dorsiflexion, an intermetatarsal glide of the third and fourth metatarsals is performed. This technique could also be performed in the SLR position. Some flexible patients may be able to perform this technique on themselves.

Other sites along the tibial tract which come to mind when considering tension potentiating

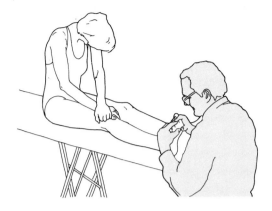

Fig. 12.5 An example of a joint treatment with the underlying nervous system in tension, for metatarsalgia. IN: Slump LS/DF DID: Intermetatarsal glides of the third and fourth metatarsals

sites are the knee, possibly the piriformis, the lower lumbar spine, the mid thoracic spine, and any areas of previous injury.

Always be aware that treatment of interfacing structures, such as the ankle joint, or pathological interfaces, such as oedema, can dramatically alter the tension test. A simple measure such as a heel raise will take some tension off the tibial nerve.

Involvement of the sural nerve

This nerve arises from both the peroneal and tibial nerves in the popliteal fossa. It is often neglected, yet by its innervation, is a potential source of lateral heel, foot or calf pain. The first cases of entrapment were reported by Pringle et al as recently as 1974. They reported four cases; one post ankle injury, two associated with ganglions and one from an unidentified source. A test has been described where the foot is inverted and dorsiflexed, then the SLR added to it (Ch. 7). The nerve can be palpated laterally in the foot and laterally along the achilles tendon. Potential sites of entrapment include its emergence from the fascia some 16 cm proximal to the lateral malleolus, and anywhere around the foot where the nerve lies on bone. I feel it is forgotten in the rehabilitation of injuries such as Achilles ruptures, fractures and ankle sprains. Biopsies may leave permanent numbness and paraesthesia (Dawson et al 1983). Smith & Litchy (1989) reported on 46 cases where the sural nerve was implicated by electrodiagnosis and the area of symptoms. The cases were mainly traumatic but the vein stripping operation and wearing tightly laced high topped footwear were also causative factors. While the nerve is only sensory, it is a source of symptoms, and if damaged, means a loss of sensory information. Similar assessment and treatment procedures apply as for the tibial and peroneal branches, although the sural nerve tension test will need to be utilised to adequately get at the nerve. Because the nerve arises from both branches of the sciatic nerve, injury in these branches could predispose or contribute to the maintenance of sural nerve injury.

The other nerve which could possibly contribute to disorders at the foot is the saphenous nerve. The examination of this nerve has been discussed in Chapter 7.

THE HAND AND WRIST

Of the injuries to the nervous system at the hand and wrist, I have selected the effects of fractures, the carpal tunnel syndrome, and entrapment of the superficial radial nerve. All three show different aspects of syndromes associated with tension testing.

Colles' fracture

The mechanism of injury usually involves a fall with the hand outstretched, the elbow in extension and the shoulder externally rotated and abducted to some degree. Some hyperextension of the wrist could occur as the body weight falls over the hand. Treatment usually involves rest in a plaster of Paris cast for approximately six weeks, perhaps manipulation of the angulated bones and internal fixation. The incidences of nerve compression or neural related complications such as 'shoulder hand syndrome' from the injury or the treatment is reported at between 10–17% (Cooney et al 1980, Stewart et al 1985, Aro et al 1988). Carpal tunnel syndrome is by far the most common neurologically based complication post Colles' fracture.

If the joint positions during the fall are analysed, most are nervous system tension increasing positions. The median nerve seems most at risk. Other complicating features are that the injury happens at some speed and that the age group of sufferers is likely to have some degenerative changes in the neck with perhaps some nerve root adhesions (Edwards & La Rocca 1983) which could pre-tension the nervous system. Most patients who sustain a Colles' fracture are female and approximately in their fifties (Frykman 1967). The patient could also end up in a Slump position or at least a forced bilateral SLR after their fall. The high incidence of neurological complications reported is not surprising considering the possibility of injury in other areas of the nervous system and injury sequelae at the wrist such as callus formation, bleeding, and oedema in and around the carpal tunnel. Primary nerve trauma from stretch or involvement with a sharp piece of bone is possible. However, the incidence of neurogenic symptoms complained of after the injury and during the rehabilitation phase must be higher than the percentages recorded. This is based on my assertions, that minor injuries are not counted or realised, and that the connective tissues of the nervous system, as possible sources, are neglected. A small pilot study (Young 1989) has shown that the ULTT1 may reproduce symptoms post Colles' fracture and that the nervous system may be responsible for some range of movement limitations in up to 35% of Colles' fracture sufferers.

The issue of an adverse tension disorder ensuing post fracture raises some new thoughts regarding management. These same thoughts can apply to post fracture management elsewhere.

• With trauma, all tissues in the injured area will be affected in some way. Some of the presenting symptoms may be neurogenic or part neurogenic in origin.
• Loss of the muscle pump and the immobilisation may allow further fibrosis in and around the nerve. A plaster cast, although usually necessary, could possibly form a pathological interface.
• The injury is such that other areas of nervous system, such as nerve roots, could contribute to the wrist symptoms.
• The injury may leave a residual abnormality in nerve or interfacing structures.

Although the patient may be symptom-free and considered cured, I speculate that this injury could predispose the nervous system to injury in the future by pretensioning it more than normal.

Physiotherapy management

In the rehabilitation phase, the source of symptoms and signs requires analysis. Some patterns suggesting an adverse neural tension component (Ch. 4) may be evident. The obligatory neurological examination may reveal patterns of sensory and motor deficits. As well as the usual joint and muscle examination, the ULTT needs examination, with special consideration to the median nerve (ULTT1 and ULTT2 median bias). If the patient can describe the mechanism of the fall, these components can be used in the tension test. As in the foot, tension testing from the other end can be utilised in all these patients. Here, the limited or symptomatic wrist and hand movement is taken up with supination, elbow extension, shoulder lateral rotation and abduction further added. If there is suspicion, either due to the symptomatic area or a motor deficit, of radial or ulnar nerve involvement, then the tension test can be biased towards these nerves: ULTT3 for the ulnar nerve and ULTT2 with a radial bias for the radial nerve.

There should also be a heightened awareness of the possibility of injury elsewhere along the nervous system, including the spine. It is recommended that the thoracic spine is examined in all symptomatic post Colles' fractures. This is especially so if there are hints of altered autonomic nervous system activity as part of the disorder. Irritation of the sympathetic trunk could contribute to the maintenance of symptoms in the hand.

In treatment, more than the wrist may require attention. Be aware that, although a limitation to wrist extension may be from the radiocarpal or intercarpal joints, once these are freed, increased tension could be placed on the nervous system and on muscles. Conversely, if the nerves and muscles are freed a little, the next limiting structure could be joint. The multifactorial approach is as essential with apparently simple disorders as it is with the more complex.

It seems logical that the maintenance of shoulder and elbow range of movement during the plaster stage is also beneficial to the nervous system at the wrist by applying some movement and tension. If beneficial to the nervous system, then the target tissues will also benefit. Hence, with careful monitoring of symptoms, in shoulder abduction or shoulder girdle depression, patients can self-mobilise their nervous systems at the wrist by extending their elbows.

Maitland (1977, 1991) described techniques to mobilise the many joints that make up the wrist joint and hand. If required, these techniques can be performed in tension. For example, techniques such as intercarpal mobilisation and radiocarpal mobilisation could be performed with the arm in an ULTT position. Note that different responses can be produced if the joint is moved in a position of tension compared with the nerve moved in a joint position (e.g., IN: ULTT position with wrist held at a position of symptom reproduction DID: elbow extension).

Carpal tunnel syndrome (CTS)

This is the most common and most studied entrapment neuropathy. It presents as a model for other neuropathies.

Mackinnon & Dellon (1988) neatly visualise the carpal tunnel when they suggest it as an upside-down table with the carpal bones as the table top and the legs as the hook of hamate, pisiform, tubercle of trapezium and the distal pole of the scaphoid. The transverse carpal ligament runs across the upturned feet of the table. The median nerve runs lateral to the flexor digitorum superficialis of the long and index fingers and medial to the flexor carpi radialis. This has been illustrated in Chapter 3. The transverse carpal ligament, the only 'soft' boundary, presents a sharp edge at the entrance and exit to the tunnel.

The syndrome begins when the space in the tunnel decreases or the contents enlarge. The median nerve when pretensioned by injury elsewhere along the nerve such as in the pronator muscles, may be predisposed to the development of the syndrome. Using the wick catheter techniques described in Chapter 3, Gelberman et al (1981) measured the mean pressure in the carpal tunnel of normal volunteers as 2.5 mmHg compared to 32 mmHg in patients with carpal tunnel syndrome. Werner et al (1983) found similar figures. These pressures in the CTS group are well above those shown to alter axonal transport and intraneural circulation (see Ch. 3). Of relevance to the repetition disorders, discussed later in this chapter, Werner et al (1983) found that maximal contractions of the wrist and fingers elicited by tetanic stimulation could at least triple the pressure in the carpal tunnel.

There are comprehensive chapters on CTS in Sunderland (1978), Dawson et al (1983), Mackinnon & Dellon (1988), Lundborg (1988) and Szabo (1989) among others.

Diseases and situations contributing to CTS are listed below. There is no reason why similar situations could not occur in other entrapment sites.

• Non-specific tenosynovitis (Phalen 1966, Faithfull et al 1986). The swollen tendons and synovium take up a greater amount of space within the tunnel and consequently increase the tunnel pressure.
• Rheumatoid Arthritis (Herbison et al 1973).
• Congenital anomalies, such as aberrant muscles in the tunnel (Lakey & Aulisino 1986)
• Tumours within the carpal tunnel, including ganglia.
• Hormonal factors. The condition is more prevalent in middle aged women and is also associated with pregnancy. In these situations either fluid retention or a swollen synovium may be causative (Massey 1978).
• Occupations associated with repetitious activities. The use of vibratory tools has been associated with the onset of CTS (Cannon et al 1981). Lundborg (1988) suggests that when a male presents with CTS, the occupational factors should be strongly suspected.
• Post wrist fractures. Kongsholm & Olerud (1986) measured carpal tunnel pressures of 36 mmHg in association with Colles' fracture. Colles' fracture has already been discussed in this chapter.
• Increased susceptibility of the nerve to compression. This may involve disorders

elsewhere along the median nerve trunk and roots. Perhaps the first crush of a double crush syndrome where the carpal tunnel becomes the second crush or systemic peripheral neuropathies such as diabetes mellitus.

Physiotherapy management

Physiotherapy is often overlooked as a treatment for carpal tunnel syndrome. This is not surprising because electrotherapy and splints, while offering perhaps some symptomatic assistance, are inadequately addressing the pathophysiology and pathomechanics involved in the nervous system and the surrounding structures. For example, if the problem is intrafascicular oedema inside a nerve, associated with a constricted tunnel from hypomobility of the carpal bones, in my opinion this requires movement not rest.

Treatment techniques have been discussed in the previous section on Colles' fracture. The keys to successful treatment of CTS via physiotherapy, as I see it, are:

- Intervene early, before pathological changes put the disorder out of the reach of physiotherapy
- Address all structural components including muscles, joints, nerve and skin
- Examine and treat, if needed, sites along the nervous system
- Be aware of the potential of sympathetic epiphenomena with the thoracic spine postulated as a common source
- If surgery is required, mobilise the neurolysed nerve as soon as possible after surgery (Mackinnon & Dellon 1988).

De Quervain's tenosynovitis and the superficial radial nerve

The superficial radial nerve (SRN) branches from the radial nerve at the level of the lateral epicondyle. Unlike the posterior interosseus nerve, it does not have to contend with the radial tunnel. However, distally in the arm, it emerges to become subcutaneous between the tendons of extensor carpi radialis longus and the brachioradialis

tendon about a third of the way between the wrist and the elbow. When the forearm is pronated, these tendons squeeze the nerve in a scissor-like action (Dellon & Mackinnon 1984). Due to its unprotected position on the radius, the SRN is also subject to external compression from objects such as wrist-watches (Linscied 1965) and handcuffs (Massey & Pleet 1978). The nerve is sensory only and supplies the dorsoradial aspect of the thumb and thenar eminence, the dorsum of the index, long and ring fingers as far as the proximal interphalangeal joints.

De Quervain's disease provides an example of the possible relationship between tendon, tendon sheath inflammation and adjacent nerve. Mackinnon & Dellon 1988) believe that entrapment of the superficial radial nerve is underdiagnosed. A retrospective review of their patients was carried out by Saplys et al (1987). Seventy-one patients had been treated for entrapment of the superficial radial nerve and 82 for neuromas of the superficial radial nerve and the lateral antebrachial cutaneous nerve. Seventeen patients in the first group had been diagnosed as de Quervain's disease, as had 24 in the second group. None of these patients improved following surgical release of the first extensor compartment.

Physiotherapy management

Here, the ULTT2 radial nerve bias test (Ch. 8) is appropriate. Because the site of the disorder is most likely distal, the distal components (thumb flexion, wrist ulnar deviation and forearm pronation) can be taken up first. The superficial radial nerve can be palpated and twanged across where it lies on the radius (Ch. 9). This may also assist in diagnosis. Finkelstein's test (1930), whereby the thumb is grasped in the fingers and the wrist ulnar deviated, must be considered a test of both the superficial radial nerve and for first dorsal extensor tenosynovitis. If this manoeuvre reproduces the patient's symptoms, differentiation of the source is possible if the elbow were extended and then the shoulder depressed or abducted. If shoulder abduction or shoulder girdle depression alters the symptoms, then the source of the symptoms is unlikely to be tendon or tendon sheath, but more likely neurogenic in origin.

Other areas to consider are previous injury sites proximally and distally in the hand, the elbow joint especially the radiohumeral joint, the shoulder, the first rib, and the C5,6 intervertebral level.

Principles of mobilisation have been discussed in Chapter 10.

THORACIC OUTLET SYNDROME

Cherington (1986), Cherington et al (1986), and Phillips & Grieve (1986) questioned whether the thoracic outlet syndrome is a true clinical entity. As Phillips & Grieve (1986) note when discussing the syndrome, 'comprehensively examining every structure from which symptoms could be arising is enlightening and rewarding'. This basic tenet of clinical reasoning is the key to the thoracic outlet syndrome. To me, it is the nervous system which has been inadequately examined in the past, allowing an explicable group of signs and symptoms to persist in being considered as a syndrome.

It is difficult to find agreement in the literature regarding what constitutes a case of thoracic outlet syndrome. Pratt (1986) describes it as 'a generic diagnosis that is assigned to those patients who exhibit symptom characteristics of entrapment of the brachial plexus and the subclavian axillary vessels'. By nature, the symptomatology must be complex. The plexus is close to the meninges and neuraxis and entrapment could affect any of the nerve trunks. There are many differing structures to consider and analyse. Sunderland's (1978) descriptions of the anatomical arrangements in the cervico-brachial region associated with thoracic outlet syndrome are recommended reading. Lundborg (1988) and Toby & Koman (1989) have provided a summary of current thought and surgical management.

Both blood vessels and nerves at the thoracic outlet can be compromised. According to Toby & Koman (1989), however, approximately 90% of cases of thoracic outlet syndrome are neurological in origin. There must also be some combined vascular/neurogenic disorders.

The structures a physiotherapist should examine when assessing a disorder with the symptoms of a neurogenic thoracic outlet syndrome are listed. A multifactorial approach to examination is required.

All tension tests should be performed. Because the lower trunks are more at risk and are more commonly part of the syndrome, the ULTT3 should not be forgotten. The effects of lateral flexion towards and away from the sided tested needs examination. Tension tests on the opposite arm and a Slump Test, both in longsitting and in sitting, is suggested to investigate for any spinal canal components of adverse tension. Examination of the first and second rib joints, the zygapophyseal joints, especially in the lower cervical and upper thoracic spine, are needed. The length of the scalenes in particular need assessment.

The examination cannot stop with these local sources. There are other remote sources and contributing factors. The acromioclavicular, glenohumeral and possibly elbow and wrist joints need examination. This would be particularly so if a double or multiple crush syndrome were evident. Muscles such as the trapezius, levator scapulae, pectoral, and short cervical flexors need an examination of their length and strength. I feel the contribution of sympathetic epiphenomena, either due to irritation of the lower trunk where the bulk of sympathetic fibres destined for the arm lie, or in the trunks and ganglia, can be tested, in part, via the tension tests described.

Physiotherapy treatment must be based on an adequate examination of these structures. It is not enough to merely identify possible structures and contributing factors. The physiotherapist must have the skills to analyse whether each structure exhibits physical signs comparable to the signs and symptoms. Although this text has concentrated on the nervous system factor, the need to treat muscles and joints cannot, of course, be overlooked.

MERALGIA PARAESTHETICA

Entrapment of the lateral femoral cutaneous nerve (LFCN) or meralgia paraesthetica has been described since 1895 (Sunderland 1978). This in itself is interesting when carpal tunnel syndrome has only been recognised for a little more than 30 years. Also of historical interest is that Sigmund

Freud had the disorder and it appears he first thought thought it had psychological cause, although in later years he changed his mind (Dawson et al 1983). Sunderland (1978) and Dawson et al (1983) have provided a detailed summary of the syndrome

The LFCN is entirely sensory and is a branch of the upper lumbar nerve roots. It emerges from the lateral margin of psoas major, courses through the pelvis and passes beneath the inguinal ligament near its attachment to the anterior superior iliac spine. It then enters the fascia lata tissue. Variations at the region of the anterior superior spine are common (Sunderland, 1978). The fascial arrangement means the nerve is relatively fixed in the fascia, especially where it divides into anterior and posterior divisions (Sunderland 1978).

Symptoms are usually quite mild and consist of unpleasant paraesthesias, aches and burning in the anterior and anterolateral thigh, usually well delineated. Often hip extension and walking aggravate symptoms and hip flexion, as in sitting, eases symptoms (Sunderland 1978, Dawson et al 1983). Although the area supplied by the LFCN is quite large, the area of symptoms may be only as large as the patient's hand.

The nerve may be implicated in abdominal surgery scar or irritated by tight fitting corsets or seatbelt trauma. Often patients cannot give a predisposing factor. The literature points to the inguinal ligament as the main source of the irritation/compression (Murphy 1974, Sarala et al 1979). A recent study (Guo-Xiang et al 1988) describes 13 patients with meralgia paraesthetica who had evidence of stenosis at the L3,4 spinal level on myelograms. Surgical decompression at the surgical level was therapeutically effective. Kopell and Thompson (1963) originally thought the disorder was initiated by a derangement in the lumbar spine leading to a tightness of the fascia lata, consequently trapping the LFCN.

The nerve is also one where evidence of subclinical neuropathy in humans has been found. Disturbances of the myelin sheath at the inguinal ligament in normal autopsy specimens has been found by Jefferson & Eames (1979). Edelson (1975) reported that 51% of adult cadavers had a pseudo-ganglion in the nerve where it passed under the inguinal ligament.

Physiotherapy management

Often patients with this disorder are not considered for physiotherapy. However, logically, and indeed anecdotally, therapeutic movement can eradicate the symptoms as long as pathological changes are not irreversible.

Be wary initially of the diagnosis. Sources of symptoms in the innervation field of the LFCN could include the hip, femoral nerve neuropathy, or referral from the upper lumbar intervertebral joints and nerve roots. Due to the nerve being entirely sensory, the clear delineation of sensory changes should assist.

Palpating or tapping the nerve in the inguinal ligament can reproduce complaints of tenderness compared with the other side, or reproduce symptoms in the distribution. To tension test the nerve, the Prone Knee Bend needs to be modified. It should be performed in hip extension with some hip adduction. As well as the entry into the thigh through the inguinal ligament, the L2 to L4 vertebral levels and the psoas major muscle should be investigated as possible sources of tension. Once the symptoms have been reproduced, that position can be used as treatment and either the knee flexion or the relevant hip movements used to mobilise.

THE NERVE LESION IN LOWER LIMB MUSCLE TEARS

There are three main considerations regarding the role of the nervous system in a muscle tear:

• There may be symptoms originating from nerve damaged directly or made hypoxic from the pressure of blood around it.

• It comprises a structure whose mechanics must not be implicated in any traumatic and inflammatory exudate from the muscle.

• It may have been a cause of the muscle tear. One postulated mechanism is that injury to neurones elsewhere in the leg may have altered axoplasmic flow, leading to changes in the target structures, thereby weakening them (Ch. 3).

Hamstring tears

There have been recent reports that the Slump Test is often positive for footballers with torn hamstrings (Bourke et al 1986, Kornberg 1987, Barrett 1987, Kornberg & Lew 1989). This suggests that the nervous system may have been directly or indirectly injured in the incident or possibly was injured before the muscle injury. These studies cited are Australian studies. Most literature supports factors such as lack of strength and flexibility in hamstring muscles (Sutton 1984).

Physiotherapy patients with hamstring tears can be divided into two groups. One is where the tear is obvious in terms of history, bruising and swelling, the other is where the mechanisms of the disorder are not clear. There may be no bruising, a painful spot difficult to palpate, the injuring mechanism unclear, and rather suspicious associated complaints of spinal pain. An adverse tension syndrome should be suspected. Similar reasoning is evident in the case of groin and calf tears. Patients, particularly sportsmen and women, often complain of a 'run of injuries'.

There is some evidence that nervous system mobilisation could be helpful in returning footballers to the field faster (Kornberg & Lew 1989). The mobilisation performed in this study was a Slump Longsitting stretch. Of course, footballers are not the only group prone to muscle injuries. The principles of treatment could be applied to any muscle injury. If the principles suggested in Chapter 10 are followed, a treatment regime in a moderately severe hamstring tear could be based on a very broad guide as suggested below. The major determinant to progression will be the healing rates of the interfacing structures.

Day 1. Attend to interfacing structures. Mobilise dorsiflexion/plantarflexion in some knee flexion if needed. Passive Neck Flexion or passive neck and upper thoracic flexion could be useful. Address any contributing spinal interfaces.

Day 2. Repeat and progress. Assess and treat if required, dorsiflexion and plantarflexion in knee extension, hip medial rotation and adduc-

tion. Techniques of knee flexion and extension can be done in prone. The quadriceps could be worked.

Day 3. Repeat and progress the dorsiflexion and plantar flexion components to be performed in Slump longsitting. Other possibilities are knee extension in some hip flexion and hip adduction in a few degrees of SLR.

Note, up to Day 3, the attention has been on selective mobilisation of the nervous system. The hamstrings have only been minimally stretched but the nerve has been mobilised independently of the hamstrings. The through range movements are indicated initially, then some tension is added towards the third day. These techniques can be performed with any other modality such as ice and electrotherapy. The patient should be able to perform self mobilisation using the foot or cervical spine movements. Progression must be tailor-made for the individual patient.

Treatment 4. Progress knee extension in a greater range of hip flexion. Perform dorsiflexion and plantar flexion in some SLR. Progress the Slump longsitting with the addition of hip adduction and medial rotation.

Treatment 5. Slump sitting and longsitting combinations. Hold relax contractions to assist regaining the SLR.

Any of the exercises could be adapted into self mobilisation for the patient. The rationale is clear. Pain may be eased by the treatment, post inflammatory and post injury exudate will not be allowed to scar (see the case study below), the physical movement of the nerve through the haematoma will help clear that bleeding. It is not inconceivable that early restoration of normal nerve function will assist the best healing of the muscle. It is important to appreciate that the nervous system is a continuum because it makes the physiotherapist look for contributing sources further afield. This may also allow the discovery and treatment of sites important to the prevention of reoccurrence of the hamstring injury.

PERIPHERAL NERVE SURGERY

It is logical that restoration of sound mechanics of a segment of peripheral nerve, post surgery, would be a factor in the successful surgical outcome. In simple straightforward surgery this would occur with normal movement and perhaps exercises given by the surgeon. In other cases, physiotherapy is recommended. Any such physiotherapy must be in conjunction with the surgeon who performed the operation and would require particular skills and knowledge. There are four main kinds of nerve surgery performed:

1. External neurolysis where fibrous bands across nerve or scarred epineurium are divided.

2. Internal neurolysis where the fascicles are divided. This involves an epineurectomy and, depending on the nerve and the kind of injury, division of the internal epineurium.

3. Transposition of nerves.

4. Suture of resected nerves and nerve grafts. Both epineurial repair and fascicular repairs are performed. There is no evidence suggesting one technique is superior to the other (Mackinnon & Dellon 1988). The aim is to match fascicles as well as possible to allow correlating axons to meet. If a segment of nerve is lost from the injury, a graft can be placed. The sural nerve and the lateral antebrachial cutaneous nerve are favoured donor sites. This is the area of the specialist hand physiotherapist working in close conjunction with the surgeon. Like the surgeon, the physiotherapist needs knowledge of nerve biomechanics and an appreciation of the sequelae that may follow altered mechanics.

Case study

In order to discuss peripheral nerve surgery and to consider some examination techniques in relation to surgical findings, the following successful surgical case study, reported in the Journal of Neurosurgery (Søgaard 1983), is utilised.

A 51 year old man was admitted with a three year history of 'toothache-like' pain and paraesthesia extending from the back of the calf to the heel. If the patient sat for 10 minutes or lay down, symptoms were aggravated. He knelt to eat and fortunately, had a job which involved standing. The patient reported no low back pain or symptoms in the other leg. He complained of falling down a stone staircase three months prior to the commencement of symptoms, landing on the left buttock. Excision of an exostosis near the lesser trochanter gave him some relief for a couple of months. EMGs of the left gastrocnemius were normal.

The surgeon found no abnormality in motor or sensory conduction and Leseague's sign was negative on both sides. Percussion over the middle third of the thigh produced paraesthesias which descended towards the heel. An external neurolysis was performed at this site and the operative findings are shown in Figure 12.6. The patient was relieved of symptoms. At a five month review, he was still symptom-free.

There are interesting aspects of the examination. The patient had negative Leseague signs, yet from the aggravating activities and the surgical findings, it would be expected that symptoms would be reproduced by tension tests. Perhaps

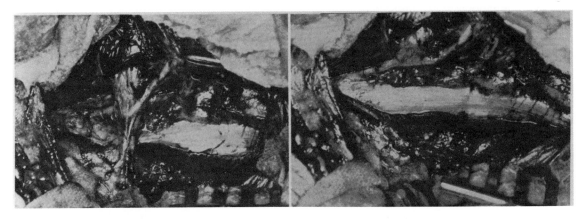

Fig. 12.6 Operation photographs. On the left, the sciatic nerve is compressed by a myofascial band including a branch to the biceps femoris muscle. On the left side is the nerve after decompression. It appears slightly swollen. The case study has been described in the text. From: Søgaard I 1983 Sciatic nerve entrapment. Journal of Neurosurgery 58: 275–276, with kind permission from the publishers and author

with the addition of the SLR sensitising movements, symptoms would be reproduced. With his complaint of pain on sitting, the Slump Test may have reproduced symptoms.

This case study shows the importance of palpation of the nervous system. In this case, operative management proceeded in the absence of measurable neurological loss.

The question arises as to whether mobilisation of the nervous system could have prevented the situation evident in the operative photograph on the left. At this stage it is doubtful whether more than a small measure of relief could be given with nervous system mobilisation. However, at an earlier stage, techniques addressing this probable traumatic haematoma, by treating the hamstring interface and the nerve movement in relation to the hamstring, could very likely have prevented this situation.

Suture of resected peripheral nerves raises an important point relevant to physiotherapists. The outcome of suturing depends on the scar formation at the suture site and the number and kind of axons that neurotocise the scar and meet up with like axons in the other segment of the nerve. There is an optimal amount of tension at the suture site that will allow this process to occur. Research conducted by Millesi & Meissl (1981) shows that a tension free zone is best. While minimal or no tension may be optimal, this does not take into account the fact that it is impossible to immobilise the nervous system. In the case of a median nerve sutured at the wrist, even with wrist and elbow immobilisation, movements of the shoulder and neck will still mobilise the nerve. Lundborg (1988) suggests that a little tension and movement at the site is helpful. One mechanism by which regenerating axons will grow is by guidance from the surrounding structures. Lundborg (1988) suggests that longitudinal polarisation of the fibrin clot from a small amount of tension is beneficial in this regard. Similar mechanisms may occur when nerve injuries are in continuity, even in chronic disorders, where some scar stretch may facilitate axonal regeneration. Nerve fibres trapped in a neuroma for years are capable of some regeneration once freed (Holmes & Young 1942). These thoughts may provide part of a rationale for some of the long term benefits of nerve mobilisation when the injury is 'in continuity'.

REPETITION STRAIN INJURY (RSI)

Repetition strain injury (RSI) is the common name given to the symptom complex of upper limb and trunk pain, also known as cumulative trauma disorder, where the aggravating factor appears to be repetitious activity. In Australia keyboard operators appear more vulnerable than anywhere else. The issue has become emotive with many practitioners doubting the existence of significant organic pathology in the disorder (Ireland 1988, Barton 1989).

Why has RSI collected such a bad image? One reason, I feel, is that a consistent pattern of signs and symptoms have not been recognised. Another is that while the joint and muscle components of the disorder were usually well examined, the nervous system component was neglected. I believe one underestimated factor in the disorder is abnormal physiology and mechanics of the nervous system during movement. There are a number of factors supporting this contention.

1. A clinical study by Elvey et al (1986), where 60 patients were examined, found a positive ULTT1 in 59 of the patients. It also noted that palpation of the neck over the neural tissue, at the exits from the cervical transverse gutters, revealed tenderness on the symptomatic, or more symptomatic side. This clinical study was later updated by Quintner et al (1987). One hundred and sixty five patients referred with a diagnosis of RSI or 'overuse injury of the upper limb' were seen consecutively. Patients were included if, on standard physical examination, there was no evidence of a local pathological condition which could give rise to the symptoms. Of the 165, there was an abnormality of the ULTT1 in 146. Forty-six percent also had a positive Slump Test. The authors also noted a high prevalence (50%) of the poked chin posture.

To these figures, I add my anecdotal clinical assessment and treatment findings in an estimated 130 patients diagnosed as RSI between 1986 and 1990. All had positive

Upper Limb Tension Tests, though not necessarily ULTT1, nor were the findings completely relevant to their disorder. That is, ULTT2 or ULTT3 were often more positive and some had more relevant muscle and joint signs than signs of adverse tension. Attempts to link the pattern of symptoms present in these patients to physical signs and to allocate anatomical and physiological bases for the symptoms, provided much of the clinical reasoning experiences discussed throughout this book.

2. An anatomical basis for the symptoms and signs is possible and has been presented in Part I. Such a basis includes recognition of the potential for both connective tissues and neural tissues to contribute to symptoms, of the potential for different parts of the system to contribute simultaneously and of the contribution of non-neural structures. Recent research, discussed in Chapter 3, where the ease of altering axoplasmic flow by mechanical means and/or by minimal deprivation of blood supply, provides a basis for at least some of the symptomatology. If axoplasmic flow is altered, there may be repercussions for the target structures (perhaps hypersensitivity). There may also be repercussions along the neurone, including an increased potential for the development of double crush or multiple crush type symptoms (see Ch. 3).

3. There is a recognisable pattern of symptoms (see Ch. 4). The pattern is unknown to those who suffer solely joint and muscle afflictions and is in the presence of signs of adverse neural tension. Anecdotally, the pattern will change, usually beneficially, when the physical signs of adverse tension are addressed.

4. The beginnings of a change in opinion, whereby the nervous system has been implicated in some disorders, can be noted. Saplys et al (1987) provided surgical and electrodiagnostic evidence to show that entrapment of the sensory radial nerve may be misdiagnosed as de Quervain's disease. Quintner (1989) pointed to the very high incidence of positive Upper Limb Tension tests, post whiplash injury. Mackinnon &

Dellon (1988) reported the common finding of entrapment of the posterior tibial nerve in the posterior tarsal tunnel being misdiagnosed as plantar fasciitis. More attention has been focussed on the more minor nerve injuries: the pre-neuropraxias (Ch. 9), (Loeser 1986, Lundborg 1988).

5. The literature burgeons with examples of neuropathy from repetition related activities. Some examples from occupations are rock drillers (Chatterjee et al 1982), interpreters for the deaf (Meals et al 1988) and professional musicians (Fry 1986).

In keeping with other structures, the nervous system must have a finite reserve to deal with physical stresses such as repetition. Repetition and the resultant friction injuries to the nervous system are probably the least understood and poorly researched. Compression of the nervous system has been studied, but not intermittent compression. Initially there must be a physiological deficit and perhaps a mechanical deficit that is subclinical.

Repetition injuries to nerve provides an example where the existing injury classifications of Sunderland, and Seddon are not very helpful to physiotherapists. Clinicians may find the classifications suggested in Chapter 9 more helpful. To this classification of peripheral nerve injury, other sources, such as the cervical spine and peripheral joints and remote contributing factors such as the sympathetic nervous system and the posture demanded by the occupation, will have to be added.

Wilson (1990), in a discussion on sympathetic maintained pain, refers to a group called 'pain dysfunction syndrome'. This involves sympathetic changes which are secondary to an initial and often insidious injury. Wilson notes that the clinical picture of RSI sufferers as described by McDermott (1986) and Fry (1986) fits a picture of sympathetic involvement. I feel this sympathetic involvement could be due to postural stresses placed on the sympathetic trunk, as described in Chapter 2. An initial minor injury, such as overuse of structures in and around the carpal tunnel, is maintained by irritation caused by postural stresses or an old injury of the sympathetic trunk. The hypothesis of the sympathetic trunk requiring a normal range of movement and elasticity to function correctly has been presented in Chapter 2. Clinically, involvement of the thoracic spine, as tested by the Slump Test and joint tests via combined movements and passive accessory movements as described by Maitland (1986), is very common. Remember that the cervical part of the sympathetic trunk originates from the thoracic spine.

Aspects of treatment

The irritable, and the irritable/chronic, nervous system, as seen in RSI, is difficult to treat. This is a multifactorial disorder with multi-tissue involvement. Together with this, external factors must be addressed: the work environment, the consequences of the label 'RSI' and the consequences of no one believing a person is capable of having such symptoms. The treatment suggested in Chapters 10 and 11 represents aspects of the physiotherapy treatment only. These patients respond at different rates. Some postural changes, altered work practices and mobilisation of any relevant structures may be all that is necessary in those diagnosed early enough. There is a large group who have symptoms for some time, yet are not reported or diagnosed early enough. Anecdotally, the majority of these will respond to prolonged management of which physiotherapy is only part. All involved structures must be attended to. It can be envisaged that symptoms may worsen if joints and muscles are treated and the nervous system neglected. At the other end of the spectrum, there is the patient who will not get better. Malingering clearly exists in some instances. However, the patient who does not improve is often the person whose language is not that of the country where he/she works, who has persisted with his/her job for fear of losing it and who often works in ergonomically unsound environments. Often, there are too many of the poor prognostic factors (Ch. 10) in evidence.

In Australia, the numbers of new patients reporting the signs and symptoms are declining (Ferguson 1987). The disorder is not new and has been occurring in some form for hundreds of years (Chatterjee 1987). It is still prevalent and probably always will be. While mental factors in the syndrome have been relatively easy to analyse, it has been difficult to research the physiological aspects of a particularly human and benign disorder. Repetition strain injury and its management are clearly complex issues that inevitably relate to work practices, treatment practices, social factors and compensation systems. I propose that better recognition of the nervous system as one of the structures involved will unravel some of the management problems associated with this disorder and many others.

REFERENCES

Aro H et al 1988 Late compression neuropathies after Colles' fracture. Clinical Orthopaedics and Related Research 233: 217–225

Barrett P G 1987 The hamstring injury in footballers. Unpublished thesis, South Australian Institute of Technology, Adelaide

Barton N 1989 Repetitive strain disorder. British Medical Journal 229: 405–406

Borges L F, Hallett M, Selkoe D J, Welch K 1981 The anterior tarsal tunnel syndrome. Journal of Neurosurgery 54: 89–92

Bourke A, Alchin C, Little K et al 1986 Hamstring symptoms and lumbar spine relationship in sports people: a pilot study. Proceedings of the Australian Physiotherapy Association National Conference, Hobart

Cannon L J, Bernacki E J, Walter S D 1981 Personal and occupational factors associated with carpal tunnel syndrome. Journal of Occupational Medicine 23: 255–258

Chatterjee D S 1987 Repetition strain injury: a recent review. Journal of the Society of Occupational Medicine 37: 100–105

Chatterjee D S, Barwick D D, Petrie A 1982 Exploratory electromyography in the study of vibration-induced white finger in rock drillers. British Journal of Industrial Medicine 39: 89–97

Cherington M 1986 Surgery for the thoracic outlet syndrome? New England Journal of Medicine 314: 322

Cherington M, Happer I, Machanic B et al 1986 Surgery for the thoracic outlet syndrome may be hazardous for your health. Muscle & Nerve 9: 632–634

Cooney W P, Dobyns J H, Linscheid R L 1980 Complications of Colles' fractures. The Journal of Bone and Joint Surgery 62A: 613–619

Dawson D M, Hallett M, Millender L H 1983 Entrapment neuropathies. Little, Brown, Boston

Dellon A L, Mackinnon S E 1984 Tibial nerve branching in the tarsal tunnel. Archives of Neurology 41: 645–646

Dellon S E, Mackinnon S E 1984 Susceptibility of the superficial sensory branch of the radial nerve to form painful neuromas. Journal of Hand Surgery 9B: 42–45

Edelson E G 1986 Meralgia paraesthetica: an anatomical interpretation. Journal of Bone and Joint Surgery 58A: 284

Edwards W C, La Rocca H 1983 The developmental segmental sagittal diameter of the cervical spinal canal in patients with cervical spondylosis. Spine 8: 20–27

Elvey R L, Quintner J L, Thomas A N 1986 A clinical study of RSI. Australian Family Physician 15: 1314–1319

Faithfull D K, Moir D H, Ireland J 1986 The micropathology of the typical carpal tunnel syndrome. Journal of Hand Surgery 11B: 131–132

Ferguson D A 1987 RSI:putting the epidemic to rest. Medical Journal of Australia 147: 213–214

Finkelstein H 1930 Stenosing tenovaginitis at the radial styloid process. Journal of Bone and Joint Surgery 12A: 509–539

Fry J H 1986 Overuse syndrome in the upper limb in musicians. Medical Journal of Australia 144: 182–185

Frykman G 1967 Fracture of the distal radius including sequelae: shoulder-hand-finger syndrome, disturbance in the distal radioulnar joint and impairment of nerve function: a clinical and experimental study. Acta Orthopaedica Scandinavica (Suppl) 108: 1–155

Gelberman R H, Hergenroeder P T, Hargens A R et al 1981 The carpal tunnel syndrome: a study of carpal tunnel pressures. Journal of Bone and Joint Surgery 63A: 380–383

Gessini L, Jandolo B, Pietrangeli A 1984 The anterior tarsal tunnel syndrome. Journal of Bone and Joint Surgery 66A: 786–787

Guo-Xiang J, Wei-Dong X, Ai Hao W 1988 Spinal stenosis with meralgia paraesthetica. Journal of Bone and Joint Surgery 70B: 272–273

Hargens A R 1989 Measurement of tissue fluid pressure as related to nerve compression syndromes. In: Szabo R M (ed) Nerve compression syndromes. Slack, Thorofare

Herbison G J, Teng C, Martin J H, Ditunno J F 1973 Carpal tunnel syndrome in rheumatoid arthritis: a preliminary study. Americal Journal of Physical Medicine 52: 68–74

Holmes W, Young J Z 1942 Nerve regeneration after immediate and delayed suture. Journal of Anatomy 77: 63–93

Ireland D C R 1988 Psychological and physical aspects of occupational arm pain. Journal of Hand Surgery 13B: 5–10

Jefferson D, Eames R A 1979 Subclinical entrapment of the lateral femoral cutaneous nerve: an autopsy study. Muscle & Nerve 2: 145–154

Kenzora J E 1984 Symptomatic incisional neuromas on the dorsum of the foot. Foot and Ankle 5: 2–15

Kongsholm J, Olerud C 1986 Carpal tunnel pressure in Colles' fracture. Acta Orthopaedica Scandinavica 57: 258–259

Kopell H P, Thompson W A L 1963 Peripheral entrapment neuropathies. Williams & Wilkins, Baltimore

Kopell H P, Thompson W A L 1960 Peripheral entrapment neuropathy of the lower extremity. New England Journal of Medicine 262: 56–60

Kornberg C M 1987 The incidence of positive slump in Australian rules football players with grade I hamstring strain. Proceedings of the 10th International Congress, WCPT, Book II, Sydney

Kornberg C, Lew P 1989 The effect of stretching neural structures on grade I hamstring injuries. The Journal of Orthopaedic and Sports Physical Therapy, June: 481–487

Kosinski C 1926 The course, mutual relations and distribution of the cutaneous nerves of the metagional region of the leg and foot. Journal of Anatomy 60: 274–279

Lakey M D, Aulicino P L 1986 Anomalous muscles associated with compression neuropathies. Orthopaedic Review 15(4): 19–28

Lassman G, Lassman H, Stockinger L 1976 Morton's metatarsalgia: light and electron microscopic observations and their relation to entrapment neuropathies. Virchow's Arch (A) 370: 307–321

Lincheid R L 1965 Injuries to the radial nerve at the wrist. Archives of Surgery 91: 942–946

Loeser J D 1985 Pain due to nerve injury. Spine 10: 232–235

Lundborg G 1988 Nerve injury and repair. Churchill Livingstone, Edinburgh

Mackinnon S E, Dellon A L 1988 Surgery of the peripheral nerve. Thieme, New York

Maitland G D 1977 Peripheral manipulation, 2nd edn. Butterworths, London

Maitland G D 1986 Vertebral manipulation, 5th edn. Butterworths, London

Maitland G D 1991 Peripheral Manipulation, 3rd edition. Butterworths, in press

Marinacci A A 1968 Neurological syndromes of the tarsal tunnels. Bulletin of the Los Angeles Neurological Society 33: 90–100

Massey E W 1978 Carpal tunnel syndrome in pregnancy. Obstetrical and Gynaecological Survey 33: 145–154

Massey E W, Pleet A B 1978 Handcuffs and cheiralgia paresthetica. Neurology 28: 1312–1313

Mauhart D 1989 The effect of chronic inversion ankle sprains on the plantarflexion/inversion straight leg raise test. Unpublished thesis, South Australian Institute of Technology, Adelaide

McDermott F T 1986 Repetition strain injury: a review of current understanding. Medical Journal of Australia 144: 196–200

Meals R A, Payne W, Gaines R 1988 Functional demands and consequences of manual communication. Journal of Hand Surgery 13(A): 686–691

Millesi H, Meissl G 1981 Consequences of tension at the suture line. In: Gorio A, Millesi H, Mingrino S (eds) Post traumatic peripheral nerve regeneration: experimental basis and clinical implications. Raven Press, New York

Murphy J P 1974 Meralgia paraesthetica: a nerve entrapment syndrome. Maryland State Medical Journal 23: 57–58.

Nitz A J, Dobner J J, Kersey D 1985 Nerve injury and grade II and III ankle sprains. The Americal Journal of Sports Medicine 13: 177–182

Oh S J, Lee K W 1987 Medial plantar neuropathy. Neurology 37: 1408–1410

Phalen G S 1966 The carpal tunnel syndrome: seventeen years experience in diagnosis and treatment of 654 hands. Journal of Bone and Joint Surgery 48A: 211–228

Phillips H, Grieve G P 1986 The thoracic outlet syndrome. In: Grieve G P (ed) Modern manual therapy of the vertebral column. Churchill Livingstone, Edinburgh

Pratt N E 1986 Neurovascular entrapments in the regions

of the shoulder and posterior triangle of the neck. Physical Therapy 66: 1894–1900

Pringle R M, Protheroe K, Mukherjee S K (1974) Entrapment neuropathy of sural nerve. The Journal of Bone and Joint Surgery 56B: 465–468

Quintner J, Elvey R L, Thomas A N 1987 Regional pain syndrome. Medical Journal of Australia 146: 230–231

Rask M R 1978 Superficial radial neuritis and de Quervain's disease. Clinical Orthopaedics and Related Research 131: 176–178

Saplys R, Mackinnon S E, Dellon A L 1987 The relationship between nerve entrapment versus neuroma complications and the misdiagnosis of de Quervain's disease. Contemporary Orthopaedics 15: 51–57

Sarala P K, Nishihara T, Oh S J 1979 Meralgia paresthetica: electrophysiological study, Archives of Physical Medicine and rehabilitation 60: 30–31.

Smith B E, Litchy W J 1989 Sural mononeuropathy: a clinical and electrophysiology study. Neurology 39 (Suppl 1): 296

Søgaard I 1983 Sciatic nerve entrapment. Journal of Neurosurgery 58: 275–276

Stewart H D, Innes A R, Burke F D 1985 The hand complictions of Colles' fractures. The Journal of Hand Surgery 10B: 103–106

Sunderland S 1978 Nerves and nerve injuries. Churchill Livingstone, Edinburgh

Sutton G 1984 Hamstrung by hamstring strains: a review of the literature. Journal of Orthopaedic and Sports Physical Therapy 5: 184–195

Szabo R M 1989 Superficial radial nerve compression syndrome. In: Szabo R M (ed) Nerve compression syndromes. Slack, Thorofare

Toby E B, Koman L A 1989 Thoracic outlet compression syndrome. In: Szabo R M (ed) Nerve compression syndromes. Slack, Thorofare

Werner C O, Elmqvist D, Ohlin T 1983 Pressure and nerve lesions in the carpal tunnel. Acta Orthopaedica Scandinavica 54: 312–316

Wilson P R 1990 Sympathetically maintained pain: diagnosis, measurement and effiacy of treatment. In: Stanton-Hicks M (ed) Pain and the sympathetic nervous system. Kluwer, Norwell

Young L 1989 The upper limb tension test response in a group of post Colles' fracture patients. Unpublished thesis, South Australian Institute of Technology, Adelaide

13. Adverse neural tension disorders centred in the spinal canal

In this chapter a variety of disorders with an adverse tension component centred in the spinal canal have been selected for discussion. The assessment and treatment principles, in general, have been discussed in Parts II and III. This chapter includes:

1. Acute and chronic cervical and thoracic nerve root disorders. Details of the features of these disorders are discussed and techniques particular to them are outlined.

2. Loss of lumbar extension. A possible role and treatment of adverse neural tension in this common examination finding is discussed.

3. Whiplash. I feel that injury to the nervous system is underestimated and this issue is discussed.

4. Epidural haematomas are discussed as a possible source of unexplained spinal pain, where positive tension tests are obvious yet changes in conduction and the symptom distribution are not specific.

5. Coccydynia and spondylolisthesis. The importance of recognition of the adverse tension component in these disorders is emphasised.

6. Post lumbar spine surgery. Both the acute and chronic post-operative situations are discussed. A suggested procedure for the acute post-operative patient is presented.

7. Headache. An attempt to delineate dural headache has been made and some precautions and advice in treatment are presented. Post lumbar puncture headache is discussed.

8. T4 syndrome. If a multifactorial approach was applied to this group of signs and symptoms, the 'T4' syndrome can be debunked.

9. Neurological disease and central nervous system injury. Some thoughts regarding the application of adverse neural tension concepts to the management of head injury and inflammatory disorders, such as Guillian Barré, are given.

NERVE ROOT INJURIES

In the absence of frank nerve trauma, injuries to nerve roots usually occur from some change or trauma to extraneural structures. Neighbouring zygapophyseal joints and disc are prime suspects. Once injured, processes within the nerve roots themselves can lead to ongoing irritation and symptomatology, both locally and in the innervation field (see Ch. 3). An important distinction here is that the nerve root irritation/compression can lead to more symptoms than the underlying cause. Extraneural structures, such as the disc, can refer symptoms, and there may be some potentially confusing overlap with referral from the nerve root.

There is a wide clinical spectrum of cervical nerve root injuries. Some injuries require completely different handling, treatment, and thoughts on prognosis from others. They are best discussed under the headings of the acute and chronic injuries to allow emphasis of the marked differences in presentation and handling.

Acute cervical nerve root injury

There is an easily recognisable pattern of signs and symptoms in patients with an acute nerve root injury. They may present with pain in the whole dermatome, often worse distally. This distal pain is usually dominant. Patients sometimes look ill, and the disorder can be disturbing enough for them not to sleep. Some of the terms used by patients to describe their pains are 'unpleasant', 'deep', 'burning' and 'surging'. Often the pain cannot be eased by any position and after a small movement there may be a latent period before pain begins again or worsens. Sometimes, they complain of paraesthesia.

These patients require, and indeed can only tolerate a small amount of gentle examination. Symptoms often behave in accordance with the extraneural structure. For example, on cervical rotation or extension, the intervertebral foramina are closed down and this may aggravate an enclosed swollen nerve root. Some of the anti-tension postures described in Chapter 4 may be evident. A common example is the patients with apparent C5,6 nerve root injuries who obtain relief by elevating their arms and placing their hands on their heads.

It is usually not necessary to palpate the spine. One or two active movements, a tension test modified for the irritable disorder (see Ch. 9) and a neurological examination comprise the necessary components of the physical examination. Clinically and logically, the Upper Limb Tension Tests will be positive. With tension testing, the contralateral arm could be tested or even the SLR examined. An essential part of examination is to ensure that the signs of altered nerve conduction do not worsen. A neurological examination must be performed daily to monitor these.

Treatment

For these patients, static traction in the position of comfort has been the long held treatment of choice (Maitland 1986). For some patients one or more treatment modalities including rest, electrotherapy, heat, anti-inflammatories, analgesics and a collar are prescribed or advised. Early responses to treatment can be unpredictable.

Mobilisation of the nervous system can add another dimension to treatment of the acute nerve root injury. There are two aspects to consider. Firstly, whether some of the tension on the compromised nerve root can be altered by treatment elsewhere along the nervous system. Secondly, whether direct mobilisation of the nervous system is applicable.

In the first situation, some easing of symptoms may be achieved by treatment above and below the injured level. Here, the thoracic spine could be mobilised or manipulated resulting in the easing of some tension in the cervical spine. Sympathetic epiphenomena related to thoracic spine could conceivably be eased. Perhaps possible peripheral sites of tension such as the carpal tunnel, the cubital tunnel or the first rib could be examined and treated if considered relevant. If nerve tension in the periphery could be lessened, the nerve root may become less mechanosensitive. It may also lessen the potential for the development of a double crush syndrome. Simple postural advice with an anti-tension basis is logical in these patients.

Consideration should be given to mobilising the injured nerve root. Perhaps this could be performed in conjunction with traction or the treatment of the interfacing structures. The earliest possible movement of the nerve to assist dispersal of an intraneural and/or extraneural oedema or blood seems imperative. This can be done very gently. Mobilisation via careful tensioning of the contralateral arm is a good technique to try. If the cervical spine is placed in a painfree or relatively painfree position (this could be traction or positioning with pillows), gentle mobilisation of the affected arm can be attempted. A suitable technique could be IN: pain relieving cervical spine position DID: gentle elbow extension in 20° or 30° of shoulder abduction. Even the more irritable disorders may lend themselves to mobilisation. Gentle mobilisation of the hand on the affected arm or the SLR may be tried. Elvey (1986) has also discussed and illustrated useful techniques for this kind of disorder. Great care is needed, and it is essential that techniques are non-provoking and stay short of increasing any symptoms. I think it is best for the patient to be undertreated at first to ascertain any latent responses to treatment. The list of precautions in Chapter 5 and precautionary questions in Chapter 6 should be reviewed.

The settling cervical nerve root disorder lends itself to stronger techniques and self mobilisation such as the technique illustrated in Figure 13.1

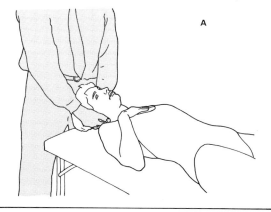

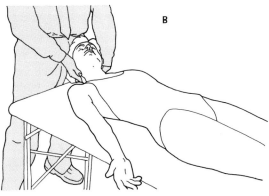

Fig. 13.1 Mobilisation for a non acute, nerve root disorder. Note that the technique takes the nervous system from a complete anti-tension posture through to a position involving considerable tension being placed through the system

A,B. Observe that the technique begins in an anti-tension position, then as the neck is laterally flexed or laterally shifted, the patient extends her elbow (flopping the elbow on the bed makes for more of a passive movement). This would be easy to progress by performing the technique with the arm in a greater range of abduction. Most patients should be able to do such an exercise themselves. There are useful techniques described by Elvey (1986) as progressions for the settling nerve root disorder.

Unfortunately, some patients with an acute nerve root injury will not respond to physiotherapy at the acute stage of their disorder. Overwhelming pathology of the interfacing structures is probably the main reason. These patients are candidates for surgery or some invasive treatment. There will always be the patient who cannot be helped or only partly helped. Such

people require referral on to other practitioners or back to their referring doctor.

Chronic cervical nerve root injury

Patients with a chronic cervical nerve root injury present with pain in similar areas to the acute nerve root injury. The pain is more patchy with less emphasis on the distal pain. Often the symptoms are of annoyance value only. However, on questioning, patients often say they are never 100% free of the pain and often remark that they 'have learnt to live with it'. While some patients can demonstrate a particular aggravating activity, others require an accumulation of activity, such as a long run or walk, to reproduce the symptoms.

The disorder may be a leftover from an acute injury that never completely recovered or could be part of an injury such as a whiplash. The important thing regarding assessment and treatment of the chronic nerve root injury is to ascertain whether or not the disorder is stable. These patients often require vigorous treatment and because of this, information about the behaviour of the disorder over the last few months and the sorts of daily activities that the patient can manage are vital. The physiotherapist needs to know whether the disorder is progressive or stable.

In many chronic nerve root injuries there will be a significant pathomechanical component of the disorder requiring alteration if there is to be any long lasting benefit for the patient.

Treatment of the joint, muscle, and nerve components of the disorder in their mid positions may not provide the optimum results. For the best techniques, the positions of the structural components will have to be combined. Some examples of treatment for these non-irritable disorders are discussed below.

Treatment

I find it beneficial to treat the cervical spine in tension positions. The ULTT1 is the most convenient and can be utilised in three ways. The patient can place his/her arm in a tension position or an assistant can hold the arm in a desired position, or the physiotherapist can hold the patient's arm between his knees. This can be done by standing astride the patient's arm with one thigh on either side of the elbow, maintaining the extension. Either lateral or medial rotation of the shoulder can be maintained in this manner. A good example of a technique from this position is to perform cervical lateral flexion in the ULTT1 position (Fig. 13.2), the technique being always easier with an assistant (Fig. 13.3). A shift manoeuvre can also be performed. Here the technique can be localised to a particular level by the ulnar border of the physiotherapist's hand. A unilateral antero-posterior pressure can be performed on the cervical spine in ULTT1 as well. The palpation findings in this technique will differ dramatically depending on the amount of neural tension under the palpating fingers. If the patient slides up to the end of the bed, a technique stretching the anterior muscles and fascia can be performed in ULTT1. Here, an assistant

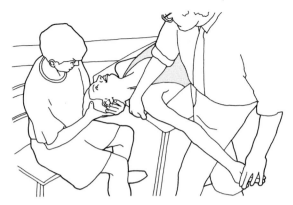

Fig. 13.4 In ULTT1, mobilisation of the anterior structures of the cervical spine

is recommended (Fig. 13.4). By use of the automatic muscle contractions of breathing, gentle hold-relax techniques can be used. All techniques can be performed in bilateral ULTT if required.

Maximal effect on the nervous system can be gained by following the suggested sequence of addition of components. This is where the component containing the source of tension is taken up first, then tension is added and the first component taken up is treated. Sometimes this sequencing is not possible. It usually suffices to place the patient in the tension position and treat via the neck movement.

For C7, C8 and T1 nerve root disorders, the ULTT3 can be used (Ch. 8). With an assistant, the ULTT3 can be taken up and held in position. With the ULTT3 maintained by an assistant, it is possible for the physiotherapist to place the neck in a certain position, say flexion and lateral flexion away from the side tensioned, and do an accessory movement on the relevant posterior zygapophyseal joints.

In this category, the role of adverse tension in the fixed head forward posture (dowager's hump) can be considered. This posture, illustrated in Chapter 4 could be considered an anti-tension posture because the upper cervical extension lessens tension on the neuraxis, meninges and nerve roots. When combined with the postural demands of so many sedentary occupations, this posture can become fixed. I have noted in the ULTT1 position, that attempts to correct the deformity increase symptoms reproduced by the ULTT1. Similarly, if the deformity is corrected,

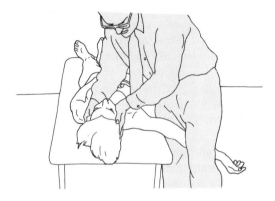

Fig. 13.2 In ULTT1/cervical lateral flexion away

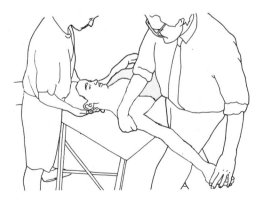

Fig. 13.3 In ULTT1/cervical lateral flexion away, with an assistant

the addition of ULTT1 will often increase any reproduced symptoms. As a technique, in ULTT1, or in bilateral arm tension, retractions of the cervical spine can be performed with the patient's cervical spine over the edge of the bed or with a wedge at the desired thoracic level. These techniques should not be seen as recipes and they require adaptation to individual patients.

These are strong techniques and must be applicable to the non-irritable disorder. Irritability is discussed in Chapter 5 and in more detail in Maitland (1986). Mobilisation of the nervous system is not a universal panacea. These techniques merely add and expand the treatment repertoire of physiotherapists and are part of a multifactorial approach. There are surely better techniques available for constructive physiotherapists. An accurate prescription of home exercises will be required. Some ideas and suggestions are given in Chapter 11.

Thoracic nerve root syndromes

Root syndromes in the thoracic spine are probably underestimated. There is little literature on the subject, and it is difficult to show a neurological deficit from one thoracic nerve root. Yet, given the forces placed through the thoracic spine during normal movements and the common occurrence of root syndromes in the cervical and lumbar spines, it seems likely that thoracic root syndromes exist and thus form a possible source of thoracic, chest and abdominal pain. The same pattern for lumbar and cervical nerve roots probably exists where the distal pain is worse. Such pains may obtain a diagnosis of 'torn rib cartilage' or 'snapping rib'.

According to Marinacci & Courville (1962) root irritation at the T6,7 level could produce epigastric pain, at the T7,8 level gall bladder pain could be caused, at the T9 level pain in the kidneys could result and at the T11,12 level, irritation could produce pain in the urethra and bladder. Clearly, not all chest wall pain will be nerve root in origin. Presuming that symptoms from structures in the abdomen and mediastinum have been excluded, the ribs, intercostal nerves and intercostal muscles are also possible sources.

Treatment

Sometimes treatment of the interfacing structure, such as mobilisation and/or manipulation of the relevant spinal segment will suffice. However, for a faster response and a better approach to some of the syndromes that are a little tardy, if involved, the nervous system can be mobilised, usually in combination with other structures. Here, combinations of the Slump Test are recommended together with some experimentation with spinal lateral flexion and rotation required to best access the nervous system. I find it worth testing both the Slump Test and the Slump Longsitting positions. In some of these positions, the effect of deep breathing on symptoms is worthwhile analysing. I have found the best way to mobilise a non-irritable disorder, involving a right thoracic nerve root, is to place the patient in the Longsitting Slump position. Then, overpressure the thoracic flexion component, perhaps laterally flex and rotate the spine away from the painful side and mobilise one of these positions, such as the rotation, as the treatment. A similar position has been illustrated in Figure 13.6 for the T4 syndrome (see page 243).

Although discussion has been limited to the cervical and thoracic nerve roots, similar principles apply to acute and chronic lumbar nerve root syndromes.

LOSS OF SPINAL EXTENSION

While most disorders involving adverse tension are characterised by symptoms aggravated when the nervous system is elongated, this is not always the case. Already in this text, I have discussed the possible relation between an interfacing structure and the nervous system, whereby symptoms are provoked on release of movement (Chs 4 & 9). When this situation occurs, the necessity of careful examination of the interface has been expressed. I feel good examples of apparent release of tension causing symptoms and ultimately limitations can be seen in some cases of loss of lumbar extension.

The nervous system is under some tension in all positions. The neuraxis and the meninges need to adapt to extension as well as flexion (Ch. 2). If these adaptive mechanisms are affected, then symptoms could be elicited as the movement is attempted. Perhaps the dorsomedian septum or the dural ligaments are, in some way, pathologically involved to limit the anterior and posterior dural theca movement in the spinal canal.

I first became clinically aware of this when I noted that SLR techniques often improved lumbar extension in both acute and chronic low back pain patients.

The chronic low back pain patient to which I am referring fits into the McKenzie 'dysfunction' pattern (1981). Attempts to regain extension via the manoeuvres advocated by McKenzie or postero-anterior pressures, even in lumbar extension as advocated by Maitland (1986), may not have satisfactory results. SLR, PNF and the Slump Test should be examined in these patients. SLR and PNF can be examined in lumbar extension if a manipulation couch is used to position the spine in extension.

If techniques are applicable, they need to be vigorous and some alteration in extension will be evident immediately. As well as the Slump Test and the SLR, SLR in lumbar extension can be a useful technique. By pulling the dura anteriorly in the spinal canal, the posterior aspect of the dura and its attachments onto the ligamentum flavum are probably mobilised.

Mobilising the nervous system has an application for the more acute lumbar spine presentations, such as possible acute disc injury. The beauty of nervous system mobilisation is that it can be performed with minimal effect on the interfacing structures. So, for example, if a disc injury is suspected, with a technique such as IN: Hip Flexion DID: knee extension, the disc and surrounding joints do not have to be moved. The technique is also useful where there is multi-tissue damage such as could occur post whiplash injury. Here, only one of the pain sensitive structures involved is moved.

In some of these patients, the Prone Knee Bend may be relevant and can be used as treatment and aid in the restoration of extension as well as improving the SLR.

WHIPLASH

With severe injury, damage to the nervous system is inevitable. The injury could be the result of direct trauma to the nervous system or its vasculature. It could also be a result from injury to non-neural structures, for example, pressures around the nervous system could be increased from blood and oedema from injury to these structures. In later stages, parts of the nervous system could be involved in scar development in the non-neural structures. Whiplash is such an injury.

Implicating the nervous system in whiplash

The pathology of injury to the nervous system has been summarised in a review paper by Bogduk (1986). Outside the brain, there are few references to nervous system injury. I feel that the injured nervous system in the whiplash accident is underestimated. Points which lend support to such an hypothesis are discussed below.

1. There are mechanics that implicate the nervous system. The initial movement is one of uncontrolled cervico-thoracic extension which may compromise the neuromeningeal tissue in the area of the intervertebral foramen. The second phase involves uncontrolled spinal flexion which causes movement and tension throughout the whole system. Many whiplash incidents are not pure flexion/extension movements. Lateral flexion and rotation of the cervical spine may be involved due to the position prior to impact or the direction of the impact. Lateral flexion has been shown to alter tension both within the spinal canal and in the brachial plexus (Breig 1978).

The whiplash injury occurs at some speed. Hence multi-tissue damage is more of a possibility and the nervous system has less time to call upon all its tension deployment mechanisms. For example, in the whiplash injury, rapid forces may be placed on the nervous system in the head, neck and thorax and the distribution of forces may be less in the arms and legs.

2. The brain can be injured by the whiplash accident (Ommaya et al 1968). Given the continuum of the nervous system, if forces are adequate to injure the well protected brain

and brainstem, then cord injuries are also possible. Haemorrhage around the cord in experimental injuries in monkeys has been noted (Ommaya et al 1968). It also seems reasonable to assume that the spinal cord could undergo a similar contra-coup injury as does the brain. There is no reason why the meninges and the neuraxis could not be injured in the flexion phase of whiplash as the spinal canal lengthens rapidly. The whole length of nervous system in the spinal canal is at risk.

3. The cervical sympathetic trunk and ganglia, lying forward of the axis of flexion and extension, could be torn in the extension phase of whiplash. This has been shown experimentally in monkeys (MacNab 1971). The sympathetic trunk in the thoracic spine must also be at risk, not only from the spinal flexion but by its connections to the nerve roots.

4. With severe injury to non-neural structures, secondary involvement of the nervous system seems inevitable. In cadaver studies, Clemens & Burrow (1972) found that intervertebral disc and anterior longitudinal ligament rupture were most common at the C4,5 to C6,7 levels; the area in the cervical spine where the spinal canal is narrowest. Wherever there is haemorrhage, nerve root compromise leading to fibrosis could theoretically occur (Bogduk 1986). Scalene muscles that are torn or in spasm would have repercussions for the cords of the brachial plexus passing through them.

5. The common presentation of symptoms seen in whiplash gives some support to the hypotheses presented in this book. The pattern of cervical pain associated with mid thoracic pain and then occasionally lumbar symptoms is quite common. Clemens & Burrow's (1972) study showed that most injury occurred at the C5,6 tension point level. A study by Maimaris et al 1988 showed that whiplash sufferers who reported interscapular pain in the first three weeks post whiplash had a worse prognosis than those who complained of only cervical pain.

6. In my clinical observations of an estimated 150 whiplash sufferers, I feel that altered mechanics of the nervous system play a large part in the symptomatology following the whiplash injury. Structural differentiation is the key to this inference. In apparently moderate to severe whiplash injuries, SLR will very often reproduce headache and neck pain. With the arm in a position of tension, wrist extension will often alter cervical symptoms. These pains must, in some way, be associated with the nervous system or structures to which the nervous system is attached.

Quintner (1989) reported that the brachial plexus tension test was positive in 55 out of 61 symptomatic arms in 37 patients complaining of arm pains post whiplash. This lends support to Bogduk's suggestion that nerve roots may be implicated in post haemorrhage scarring.

Aspects of treatment

In Chapter 10, the principles of treatment have been outlined. The acute whiplash injury provides an example where the nervous system can be treated by the use of remote components. In the acute and irritable disorder, it offers a pain relieving treatment and logically should prevent or limit scarring of the nervous system. Other structures inevitably involved must also be addressed.

Prognosis, whiplash and the nervous system

The pattern that follows many whiplash injuries is well known. Symptoms may persist for many years and the patient may have bouts of symptoms; some that settle with time and others that require treatment. Physiotherapists must consider some possible irreversibility of signs and symptoms, primarily due to the extent of trauma involved, but also to pre-existing conditions and the kind of patient. I believe that much of this irreversibility is due to the damaged nervous system. Once an inflammatory reaction is intraneural or intradural, then resolution may be very slow and may lead to irreversible changes in the form of scar (Murphy 1977, Ford & Ali 1985, Fernandez & Pallini 1985). Even very minor intraneural swelling inside nerve may take months to disperse (Triano & Luttges 1981). Early movement intervention may prevent some of the irreversibility. Presumably, healing rates of target tissues are in some way influenced by the composition and flow of axoplasm to and from that target tissue. The injured nervous system with the axonal transport systems affected may slow down healing rates.

EPIDURAL HAEMATOMAS

There are many kinds of injury that could possibly affect the neuraxis and meninges. Spinal epidural haematomas are reported occasionally in the literature. I have included it as an example of a possible explanation for marked signs and symptoms of adverse neural tension in patients following minimal trauma where there is little or no evidence of conduction changes. The advent of magnetic resonance imaging (MRI) has made the condition easier to diagnose (Pan et al 1988). These injuries are believed to originate from the venous plexus of the epidural space. The thin walled veins in the epidural space could be torn by traction forces or perhaps sudden increases in intravenous pressure (Scott et al 1976). The aetiology is uncertain however and many of the reported haematomas appear spontaneously without a clear cause (Wittebol & van Veelen 1984).

Many cases can recover spontaneously over days or weeks as the extraneous material is reabsorbed. Others may need surgical evacuation. Attention to restoration of normal movements of the neuraxis and meninges via therapeutic movement or surgery before any tethering occurs seems warranted. Any mobilisation should be done with full knowledge of referring doctors.

COCCYDYNIA AND SPONDYLOLISTHESIS

These two disorders are used as examples of spinal disorders where a large adverse tension component is often evident, yet I believe underexamined and undertreated.

Not all pains in the coccyx come from the local structures that comprise the coccyx. There are two distinct patterns of coccydynia presentation.

The first group has clear evidence of coccygeal involvement. For example, the patient may have fallen heavily with the coccyx landing on an object, the patient could have been kicked in the coccyx, or it could have been injured during childbirth. There may be radiological evidence of fracture. Still, while the source of local symptoms is obvious, there could still be secondary structures injured and contributing to the symptoms and/or maintaining some of the symptoms. The second group complain of coccygeal pain, yet on questioning, there seems to be no reason for the pain. Richards (1954) reviewed 102 cases of coccydynia of which less than half gave a history of injury. He believed the cause to be a central disc prolapse at a low lumbar level.

Sometimes patients may volunteer nervous system implicating information. They may get pain when they sit, but when they flex their head forward the pain increases. Indeed, this test could be performed in all coccydynia patients. The patient is asked to sit and find the pain, then see if cervical flexion (or extension) will change the pain. Also assess if the position of the legs can alter the pain.

In treatment, while Slump techniques are useful, attention to interfaces such as the spinal tension point areas and the sacro-iliac joints may also be needed. There could be referral into the coccyx from low lumbar joints. The coccyx can be mobilised by the patient or the physiotherapist. This can be done in Slump Longsitting if required.

I hypothesise that the relationship of adverse tension syndromes with coccydynia is due to the filum terminale attaching to the dorsal coccygeal surface. If the filum is the sensitive monitor of tension in the neuraxis and meninges (Ch. 1), then it and its attachments may be particularly reactive to tension elsewhere along the neuraxis and meninges.

Patients occasionally complain of pain in the coccyx after vigorous Straight Leg Raising or Slump mobilisation resistance. This usually only persists for a day or two and appears to be a good indication that something has moved and the coccyx is now taking some tension. In the absence of any local coccyx pathology, this pain usually disappears over a couple of days.

Spondylolisthesis

Many physiotherapists are aware of tight hamstrings associated with spondylolisthesis. Inevitably I have wondered if these are really tight hamstrings. Logically, a spondylolisthesis that alters the dimensions of the spinal canal could alter the nervous system mechanics, either directly or as a by-product of neuroischaemia. This may worsen with age as repeated inflammatory episodes begin to lead to pathomechanics. I have noted in patients with spondylolisthesis that a tightness exists spinally as well. Also, the spinal tension points of C5,6 and T6 are often involved.

Mobilisation of the nervous system may offer a way of treating pain and maintaining movement of the nervous system at the site of the spondylolisthesis. Techniques have an advantage in that they can move the nervous system without moving the joint structures. If altered mechanics of the nervous system are included in the hypotheses associated with spondylolisthesis, the examination of higher levels of the spine is essential. Some tension may be released from the symptomatic site by attention to the spinal interfacing structures affected.

POST LUMBAR SPINE SURGERY

Inevitably, the normal physiology and mechanics of the nervous system will be affected post spinal surgery. Even if the dural theca has not been surgically manipulated, blood, oedema and connective tissue proliferation from cut ligament, muscle and bone could involve the dura mater and dural sleeves. Following spinal surgery and in coordination with the surgeon, mobilisation of the nervous system is suggested. Post laminectomy and post fusion are the two most common situations. Following some spinal fractures, similar principles could be applied.

There are two distinct groups of patients to consider — the acute early post operative situation where the techniques could be employed from the first postoperative day, and the chronic disorder where the techniques many be applicable for many years after the original surgery. The main aims are to treat pain and minimise any post laminectomy scarring. It seems such a shame that the success of surgery could be marred by failure to follow a few simple post-operative procedures, which may even be pain relieving. There have been a number of investigations into substances, both biological, such as fat, and non-biological, such as silastic membranes, to minimise post laminectomy scarring (Mikawa et al 1986). Logically, early movement of the nervous system should also be seen as potentially minimising post laminectomy scarring. In this light, it should receive the same experimental exposure.

A general term used to describe the scarring which occurs post spinal canal invasion is 'spinal fibrosis' (de la Porte & Seigfreid 1983). This broad term is also used to describe intermeningeal fibrosis, for example between the arachnoid and dura or the nerve root and arachnoid. The term 'arachnoiditis' is similarly included as part of spinal fibrosis. Spinal fibrosis is also loosely used to describe dura fibrosed onto the spinal canal structures. The difference needs to be understood. If the cord is pathologically adhered in any way to the connective tissues with resultant cord signs, this invites a different treatment approach, prognosis and precautions. In such a case, the techniques I am advocating in this text may be inappropriate.

It does appear that once the continuity of the dural sac is opened or an inflammatory process is intradural then, for some reason, connective tissue proliferates (Fernandez & Pallini 1985, Hoyland et al 1988). Some common identified causes are:

- Post-myelogram. This was more common with the use of oil based contrast materials (Quiles et al 1978, Benoist et al 1980).
- Surgery into the spinal canal (Hoyland et al 1988).
- Trauma. A disc prolapse may tear the dura mater and cause an intradural rupture (Blikra 1969, Lee & Fairholm 1983). In a motor vehicle accident, torn dura is a possibility. Both of these situations probably relate to the fact that the dura is weak in the transverse direction (Ch. 1).
- Degenerative disc disease (Ransford & Harris 1980) and canal stenosis (Clark 1969).

The inflammatory by products of these processes, if not cleared, may lead to fibrosis.

Much has been written on the failed back syndrome. One of the main reasons for the syndrome is given as intra-spinal canal and meningeal fibrosis. This scar tissue is very obvious on viewing a re-laminectomy. Hoyland et al (1988) suggests that individuals who are prone to scar development, such as those who develop keloids after skin injury, are prone to spinal fibrosis. Impaired fibrinolytic activity, leading to poor clearance of fibrin deposition, has been shown to occur in chronic back pain patients compared with matched controls. This may be a feature of the failed back patient (Pountain et al 1987). These authors also suggest that reduced physical activity in back pain patients may produce a fibrinolytic defect.

In 1966, Farhni presented three of his post spinal surgery patients. He recommended gentle SLRs post surgery and thought that rather than prevent adhesions, it would keep adhesions in a lengthened state. Louis (1981) has probably undertaken the largest and most exhaustive examination of neuromeningeal biomechanics. He states that 'to avoid painful sequelae due to epiduritis following surgery of the lumbosacral canal, one must assure the mobility of the roots of the cauda equina'.

The acute post-surgical patient

By necessity, the acute post surgical patient is treated quite differently to the patient who may present many months or years after surgery. A basic programme is suggested. This would be in association with routine physiotherapy such as mobilisation and breathing exercises and with the cooperation of the surgeon who performed the operation. In many patients, there is no reason why mobilisation of the nervous system could not begin immediately post-operation.

Day 1. Large through range movements of ankle dorsiflexion and plantar flexion, hip abduction and adduction, hip rotations in neutral, passive neck flexion.

Day 2. Repeat the manoeuvres of day one plus progress to perform some through range knee extension in some hip flexion. Minimal movements of the spinal canal have occurred but the nervous system has been tensioned and moved. Some patients may tolerate a SLR.

Day 3. Repeat techniques. Progress by performing the knee extension in a greater range of hip flexion. Also techniques of hip adduction in some degree of SLR are suggested.

Day 4. Repeat techniques. Add techniques of hip adduction and medial rotation in a higher range of SLR.

The features are that, initially, the techniques do not move the spine, as a SLR would do, although the nervous system is mobilised. There is no use putting tension on the nervous system, it needs movement. Tension can be added as the disorder improves. Such a programme must be individually tailored to the patient.

Patients vary and the aims will be different for each patient and for each post-operative day. If surgery is around the L2,3 levels, some attention to the Prone Knee Bend will be required.

The aim should be first to treat pain and symptoms from the surgery, while at the same time, to limit post laminectomy scarring in any of the intraneural or extraneural tissues. It can be done in a gentle, non-provocative way.

As the patient begins to mobilise and sit out of bed, attention to the nervous system is still necessary. For example, in sitting, self mobilisation via cervical and thoracic flexion can be performed. The patient can also flex and extend the knee with the body in a part slumped position. While physiotherapists are aware of the value of mobilising the SLR in these patients, usually not enough attention is placed on the head end or the initial use of gentle movements.

The chronic post-surgical patient

Post-spinal surgery pain and limitations are common. It must be remembered that patients who are finally operated on will have multi-structural problems and the surgery often only addresses one or two of these structures.

In many of these patients, vigorous mobilisation and self mobilisation can be attempted. All involved structures, and levels well above the site of surgery, will need to be addressed. However, in nearly all cases, there will be some irreversibility in the disorder. To achieve the best results, the involved structures need to be placed in combined positions to access the movement limitations best. A good example is the technique suggested by Stoddard (1969) of lumbar rotation with the upper most leg in SLR. There may be some benefit in performing SLR manoeuvres in lumbar traction. Through range techniques and end range tension techniques are recommended. To achieve the best results, the patient will have to be conscientious with self-mobilising exercises. Often another person will have to assist in the exercises. Although firm treatment can be employed in these patients, beware of spinal canal instability and also tethered cord syndrome (Ch. 5).

HEADACHE

Dural headache

The cranial and cervical dura are innervated (Ch. 1), therefore, the dura can be considered a source of headache (Bogduk 1986, 1989). Irritation of the cervical dura mater could conceivably cause headache, as noted anecdotally by Cyriax (1978) and as inferred from extrasegmental referral patterns from the lumbar dura mater (Smyth & Wright 1958, El Mahdi et al 1981). The term 'dural headache' is commonly used by physiotherapists. However, it is very difficult to ascribe a clear pattern of signs and symptoms. Much care is required before suggesting that the symptoms emanate from the dura. It seems unlikely that the dura could be the sole source of symptoms. As Bogduk (1989) has clearly described, activity in the trigemino-cervical nucleus is necessary for the perception of pain in the head. The trigeminal nerve is not the only nerve that terminates in the nucleus. Nociceptive afferents from the dura mater and intracranial blood vessels are examples of others (Bogduk 1989). Activity in the trigemino-cervical nucleus could be triggered by movement of the nucleus (Breig 1978).

A tentative attempt to categorise the signs and symptoms of a dural headache can be made. Possible symptom of a dural headache may include the following:

- Symptoms may be non dermatomal. For example patients may complain of caps of pain, non-dermatomal strips, 'tightness' and 'fullness' of the head.
- Symptoms will often alternate sides, more than headaches referred from a zygapophyseal joint. Symptoms are more commonly bilateral and central.
- Symptoms may be brought on by tensioning movement of the nervous system. An example is sitting in a longsitting position in bed.
- There will be a pattern of symptom presentation elsewhere that may indicate the presence of adverse neural tension, for example, tension point area pain, or coccygeal pain (Ch. 4).
- A previous and perhaps disregarded history of nervous system injury is nearly always present. Whiplash is a common experience together with post epidural and post lumbar puncture headaches.

Possible signs of a dural headache may include the following:

- Tension tests may be positive or display clinical physiological symptoms. The SLR, Slump, Slump longsitting and ULTTs should be performed depending on the irritability. In some disorders, ankle dorsiflexion or Prone Knee Bend will reproduce headache.
- Often a resistance to tension tests can be perceived before any symptoms.
- Joint signs are present at tension points during some stage of the disorder.
- The signs elicited from other comparable structures, such as zygapophyseal joint and muscles, will not match the subjective complaints. Sometimes, a diagnosis can be made in retrospect after joint and muscle signs have been treated and altered, thus implicating the dura mater by default.

Treatment

The subjective examination must be detailed enough to clarify the pattern of headaches. There will often be associated symptoms. For example, the patient may describe a certain dull feeling in a limb, a feeling of tightness or a particular pain (perhaps in the trapezius) which precedes the headache. In disorders deemed more irritable, the treatment selected may have to be performed with great regard to this associated symptom.

The perception of resistance during the tension tests is also of great importance. Many physiotherapists have noted, with headaches suspected to be of dural origin, that aggravation of the headaches can occur if this resistance is neglected while tension testing.

A thorough investigation of the interfacing structures is required. This includes the tension points, areas between the tension points, muscles such as the scalenes and the erector spinae, and the coccyx. Do not be surprised if mobilisation of the lumbar spine alters a headache. For headaches suspected to be of nervous system origin, all tension tests must be performed, including the SLR and the PKB. If the patient does not present with a headache, some of the tests may reproduce one.

Take care when the hypothesis is one of a headache being dural in origin. Slump techniques can easily aggravate such headaches. It is suggested that the initial nervous system mobilising technique is non-provocative and be performed with great respect for resistance and for associated symptoms.

Post lumbar puncture headache

Physiotherapists may occasionally be called to treat headaches post lumbar puncture. These headaches also serve as an example of what can happen when the normal neurobiomechanics are affected. Post lumbar puncture headaches are quite common. Vandam & Dripps (1956) reported an incidence of 11% from 10 000 cases. Most of these headaches begin within 24 hours of the lumbar puncture. Patients complain of occipital, neck and retro-orbital pains. There may also be complaints of neck stiffness. A relationship exists to postural changes, with the symptoms usually eased by lying flat but made worse by standing or sitting. Most headaches resolve quickly, although Vandam & Dripps (1956) noted that some headaches persisted for between 7 to 12 months.

There is a considerable body of evidence to suggest the cause of the headaches is related to leakage of cerebrospinal fluid from the puncture. A caudal shift of the neuraxis occurs, placing traction forces on cranial nerves, blood vessels and dural attachments. The relief usually obtained from lying prone means that the neuraxis is placed in an anti-gravity position. It would be interesting to see whether patients obtained further relief by bending their knees and keeping their heads off a pillow, hence lessening the tension placed along the tract.

A decrease in lumbar CSF pressure can be expected in 80% of these patients and headaches can be eased by intrathecal injections of saline (Thorsen 1947, Wolff 1963). Blockage of the leak by epidural blood patch, whereby venous blood is injected into the epidural space, is very successful for abolishing the headaches (Ostheimer et al 1974).

Similar mechanisms may occur with misplaced epidural injections or minor tears of the dura mater.

T4 SYNDROME

A collection of symptoms and physical signs worthy of the designation 'syndrome' undoubtedly guides patient management but often points to a lack of exact understanding of cause and pathology in an individual patient. (Phillips & Greive 1986)

This statement was directed towards the thoracic outlet syndrome. It is equally relevant for the T4 syndrome.

The T4 syndrome describes a symptom complex denoted by widespread and vague upper limb and head pain, all of which are apparently eased by manipulation of the T4 vertebral segment or vertebral segments in the vicinity (McGuckin 1986). I believe this syndrome should be debunked on a number of grounds:

1. The offending levels could be above or below this level, ranging below T2 and T7 (Maitland 1986). The T4 joints are not always at fault.

2. To label a pattern of signs and symptoms as the 'T4 syndrome' would deny our clinical reasoning skills, including the ability to differentiate the source of the symptoms manually. T4 suggests a joint

dominance. Adverse neural tension and muscle weakness are common findings.

3. The concept has been discussed for many years, but there is no proof to incriminate the T4 absolutely. Nor is there any particular anatomy specific to the T4, and not elsewhere, that could form the basis of the syndrome.

Over the last few years, many manual therapists have noted that patients with the symptom complex which could be called T4 syndrome, have positive Upper Limb Tension Tests and some have positive Slump Tests. This clinical observation affords an explanation of the symptom distribution and of the apparent epiphenomena of sympathetic involvement. The T4 joints alone surely cannot be responsible for such widespread symptomatology. The T4 to T9 segment of the spinal canal is a narrow zone (Dommisse 1974) where minimal reduction in the size of the canal will result in possible compromise of the neuraxis and the meninges. With injury to surrounding joints, a site of adverse tension may be initiated. As well as local sources of pain from the structures initially injured, other structures such as the thoracic sympathetic trunk and ganglia, dura mater and nerve roots may eventually be irritated. The possibility of involvement of the preganglionic neurones in the cord cannot be excluded.

Treatment

Maitland (1986) described manipulative techniques for specific thoracic spine levels. McGuckin (1986) endorsed this and emphasised the 'Klapps crawling exercises'. An example is shown in Figure 13.5. While the manipulative techniques can have dramatic results, other structures need consideration, especially if the

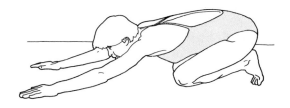

Fig. 13.5 An example of thoracic extension with the arms in tension — a 'Klapp's crawling exercise'

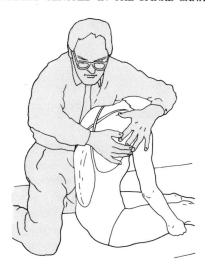

Fig. 13.6 In Slump Longsitting, the costotransverse joints can be mobilised. The technique can be performed as a postero-anterior pressure on the joint or over a rib. In this position, a physiological movement such as rotation could be utilised

disorder has persisted or is recurrent. Mobilisation, as described by Maitland (1986), may be required for the costo-transverse joints. I suggest that both Upper Limb Tension Tests 1 and 2 be utilised and also the Slump Test in sitting and Longsitting, with combinations of thoracic rotation and lateral flexion. They can be used in treatment if needed. A technique where the costo-transverse joint is mobilised in the Slump Longsitting and thoracic rotation position may be utilised (Fig. 13.6). I believe this technique mobilises the sympathetic trunk via the overlying costo-transverse joints.

Another recommended technique uses antero-posterior pressure through the chest wall and is useful for the thoracic spine down to the T6 level. A wedge or towel roll can be placed below the level requiring mobilisation. Mobilisation is then performed through the chest wall or by retraction of the low cervical spine or the upper thoracic areas. This technique can be performed in bilateral ULTT with bilateral SLR if needed.

TRAUMA AND INFLAMMATION OF THE NEURAXIS

I believe that mobilisation of the nervous system has an as yet unidentified role in the physiotherapy management of disorders such as stroke and Guillain Barré. In this section, some observations are made. The main aim is to encourage the neurologically orientated physiotherapist to consider the issues raised in this book and test their relevance to the patients they encounter. I see the role as:

1. Symptomatic treatment for pain from the nervous system, for example the hemiplegic shoulder and Guillain Barré syndrome.
2. Minimising post inflammatory scarring.
3. A possible role in assisting healing, for example by postural alterations to minimise tension.

Cerebrovascular accidents

If there has been bleeding in the brain or brainstem and the neural tissues are attempting to recover function, tension on the nervous system should be minimised to allow the best recovery. Prolonged tension in particular should be avoided. Consider the patient who has recently suffered a stroke and is left with some paralysis. If he/she is put into a low chair, with the legs on a stool, the nervous system will be tensioned. This tension will be increased if the patient falls asleep and his/her head flops forward. If the hypotonic arm were to fall out of a sling or constraint and be dependent, further tension will be placed upon the nervous system already faced with great obstacles to healing.

The concepts of tension raised by this book can be applied to these patients and perhaps used clinically by physiotherapists who are already aware of the benefits of correct positioning. While most physiotherapists are well aware of the consequences of unphysiological compression, perhaps fewer are aware of the possible consequences of prolonged stretch. In this regard, the paralysed patient could suffer adversely if placed in prolonged nervous system stretch positions. Some examples are protraction of the shoulder stretching the suprascapular nerve, tightly tucked in sheets holding the foot in plantarflexion and inversion and Slump sitting.

The painful hemiplegic shoulder often presents an impediment to treatment. Like any shoulder and especially one that has lost associated mus-

cle, the pain could come from the joint, rotator cuff or be referred from the cervical spine. These issues have been reviewed by Van Langenberghe et al (1988). While some have shown that the brachial plexus could be stretched and a source of pain in the hemiplegic shoulder (Kaplan et al 1977, Chino 1981), most authors in Van Langenberghe's review point to the rotator cuff and the shoulder joint. From my observations and experiences with ULTT2, the forced shoulder girdle positions in many hemiplegics would be enough to place a pain provoking tension on the brachial plexus, more so if the elbow is extended. Structural differentiation would be easy, just by investigating whether wrist extension alters the shoulder pain. If symptoms are neurogenic, sources could be hypoxic and stretched peripheral nerve fibres, stretched connective sheaths, referral from nerve roots, dural sleeve or dura mater. With the co-existing brain injury there is the possibility of central pain.

The incidence of peripheral nerve injuries in the adult head injured patient has been studied. Stone & Keenan (1988) investigated 50 head injured patients, none with a premorbid history of peripheral neuropathy. Thirty-four percent of this group had neurophysiological evidence of peripheral nerve injuries. The most common areas were the ulnar nerve in the cubital tunnel and brachial plexus. Most injuries were in the spastic limb and in the neurologically affected limb.

It is easy to assume, in the head injured patient, that the signs and symptoms are from a central source. What might be a rather insignificant musculoskeletal abnormality in the normal may be catastrophic for the handicapped. Such reports provide excellent support for the benefits of early rehabilitation and provide an awareness of the effects of flexor spasticity on the vulnerable ulnar nerve. In this group of patients presented by Stone and Keenan (1988), not one patient complained. This stresses the need for careful and skilled observation of target structures, particularly skin and muscles.

Guillain Barré

Guillain Barré is an acute polyradiculoneuropathy characterised by sudden development of muscular weakness and sensory symptoms. In the acute stage, the disorder is extremely painful. Genis et al (1989) reported that 61% of a group of 26 patients complained of significant pain with pain most frequently affecting the thigh, buttocks, legs, and lumbar spine. Marked adverse neural tension signs in two case studies has been presented (Simeonato et al 1988). I was involved in the Simeonato et al (1988) case studies, where a patient with an acute disorder (just out of intensive care) and a patient about to be discharged were examined. The acute patient lay in an anti-tension position, yet displayed an odd movement pattern if the altered mechanics of the nervous system were considered. For example, while some tension increasing movements (such as shoulder depression) increased pains, in others a decrease in tension increased pains. This was particularly so in the arms. Here, a painful position could be held, but the addition of cervical lateral flexion towards the positioned limb increased pain. Following the hypotheses in this text, I interpreted this as the nervous system hurting while being moved, not while the intraneural pressures were increased. This does fit with Thomas's view (1982) that, in the inflammatory poly-radiculopathies, the nervi nervorum are involved. Pain could well come from the connective tissues of the nervous system as well as the obvious source from the nerve fibres. I felt this patient could benefit from passive movement but that it would have to be movement in a particular way. This was not tension increasing movements such as the SLR, but gentler, through range movements. An example of such a particular movement is shoulder depression and elevation with the limbs out of tension or knee extension in a few degrees of hip flexion or ankle dorsiflexion with the limb out of tension.

The second patient, just about to be discharged, complained of some lumbar pain. His SLRs were restricted and reproduced this pain. He also had a positive Slump Test. Both pains and his movement restrictions improved rapidly after the tension test examination.

Hopefully this text has presented enough material to encourage further examination of impaired neurobiomechanics in these kinds of patients.

REFERENCES

Benoist M, Ficat C, Baraf P et al 1980 Postoperative lumbar epiduro-arachnoiditis: diagnosis and therapeutic aspects. Spine 5: 432–436

Blikra G 1969 Intradural herniated lumbar disc. Journal of Neurosurgery 31: 676–679

Bogduk N 1986 Cervical causes of headache and dizziness. In: Grieve G P (ed.) Modern manual therapy of the vertebral column. Churchill Livingstone, Edinburgh

Bogduk N 1986 The anatomy and pathophysiology of whiplash. Clinical Biomechanics 1: 92–101

Bogduk N 1989 Anatomy of headache. In: Dalton M (ed.) Proceedings of headache and face pain symposium, Manipulative Physiotherapists Association of Australia, Brisbane

Breig A 1978 Adverse mechanical tension in the central nervous system. Almqvist & Wiksell, Stockholm

Chino N 1981 Electrophysiological investigation on shoulder subluxation in hemiplegics. Scandinavian Journal of Rehabilitation Medicine 13: 17–21

Clark K 1969 Significance of the small lumbar spinal canal: cauda equina compression syndromes due to spondylosis: clinical and surgical significance. Journal of Neurosurgery 31: 495–498

Clemens H J, Burrow K 1972 Experimental investigation on injury mechanisms at frontal and rear-front vehicle impacts. In: Proceedings of the Sixteenth Stapp Car Crash conference 76–104

de la Porte C, Siegfried J 1983 Lumbosacral spinal fibrosis (spinal arachnoiditis). Spine 8: 593–603

Dommisse G F 1974 The blood supply of the spinal cord: a critical vascular zone in spinal surgery. The Journal of Bone and Joint Surgery 56B: 225–235

El Mahdi M A, Latif F Y A, Janko M 1981 The spinal nerve root innervation, and a new concept of the clinicopathological interrelations in back pain and sciatica. Neurochirurgia 24: 137–141

Elvey R L 1986 Treatment of arm pain associated with abnormal brachial plexus tension. Australian Journal of Physiotherapy 32: 225–230

Fahni W H 1966 Observations on straight leg raising with special reference to nerve root adhesions. Canadian Journal of Surgery 9: 44–48

Fernandez E, Pallini R 1985 Connective tissue scarring in experimental spinal cord lesions: significance of dural continuity and the role of epidural tissues. Acta Neurochirurgica 76: 145–148

Ford D J, Ali M S 1985 Acute carpal tunnel syndrome. Journal of Bone and Joint Surgery 65B: 758–759

Genis D, Busquets C, Manubens E et al 1989 Epidural morphine analgesia in Guillain Barré syndrome. Journal of Neurology, Neurosurgery and Psychiatry 52: 999–1001

Hoyland J A, Freemont A J, Denton J et al 1988 Retained surgical swab debris in post-laminectomy arachnoiditis and peridural fibrosis. Journal of Bone and Joint Surgery 70B: 659–662

Kaplan P E, Meredith J, Taft G et al 1977 Stroke and brachial plexus injury: a difficult problem. Archives of Physical Medicine and Rehabilitation 58: 415–418

Lee S, Fairholm D 1983 Intradural rupture of lumbar intervertebral disc. The Canadian Journal of Neurological Sciences 10: 192–194

Louis R 1981 Vertebroradicular and vertebromedullar dynamics. Anatomica Clinica 3: 1–11

MacNab I 1971 The whiplash syndrome. Orthopaedic clinics of North America 2: 389–403

Maimaris C, Barnes M R, Allen M J 1988 Whiplash injuries of the neck: a retrospective study. Injury 19: 393–396

Maitland G D 1986 Vertebral manipulation, 5th edn. Butterworths, London

Marinacci A A, Courville C B 1962 Radicular syndromes simulating intra-abdominal surgical conditions. American Surgery 28: 59–63

McGuckin N 1986 The T4 syndrome. In Grieve G P (ed) Modern manual therapy of the vertebral column. Churchill Livingstone, Edinburgh

McKenzie R A 1981 The lumbar spine: mechanical diagnosis and therapy. Spinal Publications, Waikanae

Mikawa Y, Hamagami H, Shikata J et al 1986 An experimental study on prevention of postlaminectomy scar formation by the use of new materials. Spine 11: 843–846

Murphy R W 1977 Nerve roots and spinal nerves in degenerative disc disease. Clinical Orthopaedics and Related Research 129: 46–60

Ommaya A K, Faas F, Yarnell P 1968 Whiplash injury and brain damage. The Journal of the American Medical Association 204: 285–289

Ostheimer G W, Palahniuk R J, Shnider S M 1974 Epidural blood patch for post-lumbar-puncture headache. Anesthesiology 41: 307–308

Pan G, Kulkarni M, MacDougall D J et al 1988 Traumatic epidural haematoma of the cervical spine: diagnosis with magnetic resonance imaging. Journal of Neurosurgery 68: 798–801

Phillips H, Grieve G P 1986 The thoracic outlet syndrome. In: Grieve G P (ed.) Modern manual therapy of the vertebral column. Churchill Livingstone, Edinburgh

Pountain G D, Keegan A L, Jayson M I V 1987 Impaired fibrinolytic activity in defined chronic back pain syndrome. Spine 12: 83–85

Quiles M, Marchisello P J, Tsairis P 1978 Lumbar adhesive arachnoiditis. Spine 3: 45–50

Quintner J L 1989 A study of upper limb pain and paraesthesiae following neck injury in motor vehicle accidents: assessment of the brachial plexus tension test of Elvey. British Journal of Rheumatology 28: 528–533

Ransford A O, Harris B J 1972 Localised arachnoiditis complicating lumbar disc lesions. Journal of Bone and Joint Surgery 54B: 656–665

Richards H J 1954 Causes of coccydynia. Journal of Bone and Joint Surgery 36B: 142–148

Scott B B, Quisling R G, Miller C et al 1976 Spinal epidural haematoma. The Journal of the American Medical Association 235: 513–515

Simionato R, Stiller K, Butler D 1988 Neural tension signs in Guillain Barré syndrome: two case reports. Australian Journal of Physiotherapy 34: 257–259

Smyth M J, Wright V 1958 Sciatica and the intervertebral disc. Journal of Bone and Joint Surgery 40A: 1401–1418

Stoddard A 1969 Manual of osteopathic practice. Hutchinson, London

Stone L, Keenan M E 1988 Peripheral nerve injuries in the adult with traumatic brain injury. Clinical Orthopaedics and Related Research 233: 136–144

Thomas P K 1982 Pain in peripheral neuropathy : clinical and morphological aspects. In: Culp W J, Ochoa J (eds) Abnormal nerves and muscles as impulse generators. Oxford, New York

Thorsen G 1947 Neurological complications after spinal anaesthesia and results from 2493 follow-up cases. Acta Chirurgerie Scandinavica 95 (Suppl 121): 7–272

Triano J J, Luttges M W 1982 Nerve irritation: a possible model of sciatic neuritis. Spine 7: 129–136

Van Langenberghe H V K, Partridge C J, Edwards M S et al 1988 Shoulder pain in hemiplegia: a literature review. Physiotherapy Practice 4: 155–162

Vandam L D, Dripps R D 1956 Long-term follow-up of patients who received 10,098 spinal anaesthetics: syndrome of decreased intracranial pressure (headache and occular and auditory difficulties). The Journal of the American Medical Association 161: 586–591

Wittebol M C, van Veelen C W M 1984 Spontaneous spinal epidural haematoma. Clinics in Neurology and Neurosurgery 86: 265–270

Wolff H G 1963 Headache and other head pain, 2nd ed. Oxford, New York

14. Selected case studies

This chapter presents a selection of various disorders from case notes. The five patient histories I have selected are discussed in a different manner to bring out aspects of assessment, treatment and prognosis.

An unusual and vague foot pain. The emphasis here is on the clinical reasoning processes, including techniques to identify the origin of symptoms.

An example of extraneural pathology. A day by day treatment description is made emphasising the use of pathological knowledge in the treatment decision.

The 'pain everywhere' kind — where to start? Aspects of analysis of the multiple pain area patient, making features fit and selecting the initial treatment are discussed.

A straight forward tennis elbow? Clinical reasoning is illustrated in the process of identifying the adverse tension component, prognosis making and treatment selection.

A quick mention of a fingertip pain. The use of the symptom aggravating position in treatment and some thoughts about the possible effects of treatment are included.

AN UNUSUAL AND VAGUE FOOT PAIN

Subjective examination

A healthy looking 26-year-old woman presented for treatment with a vague right foot pain. At first she indicated that she did not really want to come for treatment as previous electrotherapy treatment had been unsuccessful, but her doctor had insisted. She could not identify any specific area of pain and referred to it as a 'dull ache, a heaviness, a feeling of swelling'. These symptoms began three years previously when, she thought, an incident whilst water-skiing may have initiated the problem. She could not recall any particular injury mechanism, and could not be sure about the history. She denied any spinal pain and said that apart from the foot the rest of the leg felt exactly the same as the opposite leg. Exercise such as a game of netball seemed to help the foot a little. Other than walking a long distance and a painful restriction in squatting, she could not describe any particular aggravating activity. She was not greatly concerned about the foot as it did not limit her in any way though she did feel it was stiffening up a little. There were no indications from precautionary questioning of any possible sinister pathology, and she had been referred after a thorough examination from her doctor.

Initial thoughts

'This is a little odd' was my first thought. At this stage the features did not seem congruent. There did not seem to be any reason for the continuation of an ankle problem from apparently minimal trauma in a young healthy person. My initial hypothesis was that although there would be some signs in the foot joints and associated muscles (the painful squat was the clue), there had to be other structures involved. The vague symptoms, chronicity, complaints of heaviness, and feelings of swelling prompted this reasoning. As well as the foot, on my first examination I knew the lumbar spine and the nervous system would require examination (and the knee if time permitted). I reasoned that tension tests would have to be performed with the foot in a variety of positions, although I knew dorsiflexion was painful in the squatting position. Yet, this was not necessarily solely a mechanical problem of the nervous system since the knee flexion involved in squatting relieves tension in the tibial and peroneal tracts.

Physical examination

There was nothing remarkable on observing the patient's posture, although her lumbar erector spinae looked a little tight, associated with an increased lumbar lordosis. I also noted a flat, almost lordotic thoracic spine. Again, on questioning, she denied any spinal symptoms. Her foot posture was fine, although there was minimal swelling around the malleoli and on the dorsum of the foot. I also thought her right calf bulk was slightly decreased.

From the information gained, I wanted to examine two functional positions — walking and squatting. On fast walking she limped a little, though without pain. I thought the dorsiflexion on push-off was probably pain-inhibited and that I would probably prove this when dorsiflexion of her ankle was physically examined. The squat position reproduced pain around the talocrural joint, both anterior and posterior, and was clearly limited by the restricted dorsiflexion in the foot. I noted the range (buttocks to heels minus 12 inches), and felt that there was no sensitising manoeuvre I could add to the squat; for my own learning experience, however, I did ask her to squat with her head flexed and compare this to squatting with the head extended. The foot pain was the same. I hypothesised that the limitation was a combined talocrural (from the area of pain) and soleus limitation and I made a mental note to carefully test these structures.

The other relevant physical signs are discussed below.

• Lumbar extension was limited to about 10° and the movement caused pain locally in the lumbar region. There was a slight thoracic list to the right on extension. If corrected, the pain and restriction on lumbar extension was worse. Spinal flexion and lateral flexions were limited to what I thought to be three quarters of normal range. In sitting, rotations of the thoracic spine were about 60° and reproduced a 'crampy feeling' on the contralateral ribs.

• The complete foot pain could be reproduced by a right SLR of 50° without including any foot movements. In this position, the pain was increased by hip adduction.

• Dorsiflexion of the right ankle was painful and reproduced the 'squat pain'. I held dorsiflexion to the point of pain reproduction and added the SLR. Although the range of SLR was more restricted with dorsiflexion, the pain only worsened a little. This confirmed my hypothesis that I was probably dealing with two or more sources of symptoms. SLR/DF increased foot symptoms more than DF/SLR. With the right SLR there was some posterior knee pain not present during SLR of the left leg. This pain was worse when DF/SLR was tested.

• Right ankle plantarflexion reproduced the same foot pains as ankle dorsiflexion. This symptom response was worsened by the addition of SLR.

• The trunk and neck flexion components of the Slump test were clear, but with right knee extension to 60° (no DF) her foot pains were reproduced. Release of neck flexion completely eased her foot symptoms and she could extend her knee another 10° before the pains were further reproduced.

• I palpated her lumbar spine. The L2 spinal segment on the right was difficult to palpate due to spasm. At L4/5, both the left and right sides felt thick and rubbery, not a 'joint feel' (see Ch. 4). I also palpated around the T6 level. At this level and for a couple of levels below, pressures centrally, laterally on the zygapophyseal joints and over the costo transverse joints, especially on the right, revealed stiffness and reproduced some local pain.

• On neurological examination, sensation was normal, however, there was a generalised weakness of the muscles around the right ankle compared to the left. I did note that her balance, whilst standing on the right foot, was impaired compared to standing on the left foot.

• There was a general increased sensitivity to palpation of her peroneal and tibial nerves in her foot and posterior knee compared to the left side.

Thoughts following the physical examination

The features of this disorder were now making more sense. However, there were some unexpected physical findings. Some lumbar signs were expected, although not the findings from palpation of the L2 segment. I also thought it odd that she did not complain of any lumbar pains. Overall, the pattern of signs and symptoms indicated a strong neural tension involvement with the primary source of adverse tension being in the spine. The evidence suggesting this was the positive Slump Test, the palpation findings and SLR/DF worse than DF/SLR (see Ch. 2). It also seemed logical that, if ankle plantarflexion and ankle dorsiflexion brought on the same pains, there had to be an upper leg or spinal component that was extraneural and common to both nerves, such as the piriformis muscle.

I thought perhaps the patient sustained an old ankle injury which was being maintained by some spinal injury. Perhaps the lumbar sympathetic trunk was in some way involved and irritated at L2. Other thoughts about the possible symptom sources included the dura mater, nerve root, local foot neural structures, the ankle joint and tendons crossing the ankle. Examination would eventually have to include all structures between the foot and the spine.

I considered the relevant features related to prognosis. With a three year history of unchanging, non-specific pain with widespread and relevant contributing signs, I thought that prolonged treatment would be necessary. My aim was to ease about 60% of her symptoms in approximately 6 weeks. Yet, the disorder had never been treated manually before, it was non-irritable, and there was a recognisable pattern to the signs and symptoms. Although there was a significant adverse neural tension component to the

disorder, conduction was not measurably altered. On reconsideration, I adjusted my hoped for improvement to at least 75%.

These findings needed explaining to her. She needed to understand why, when presenting with a foot pain, I had palpated her thoracic spine.

Treatment

Treatment 1. The initial technique selected was rotation of L2,3 (right side up, pelvis to the left). I wanted to implicate or clear this segment as part of the disorder. While coaxing the movement, the joint gave a loud 'clunk'. The technique was then continued as a grade IV. Significant findings on reassessment were:

SLR improved
Foot signs and squat ISQ
DF/SLR improved
PFI/SLR worse
L2 palp. improved
L4/5 palp. worse

It was rather odd that a rotation of L2 should change the DF/SLR and make the PFI/SLR worse. It did, however, form a link between the L4,5 joints and the PFI/SLR test. I mobilised the lower lumbar joints in the same manner. There was no clunk, as in the technique for the higher joint, but the PFI/SLR improved. Other improvements were maintained. Encouraged by the response to treatment of the interfacing structures, I gently manipulated the T5,6 area. On reassessment, all signs had improved except the foot signs and the squat. I explained to her that I could not be sure of the response after treatment, but I was very pleased by the reactions to treatment.

Treatment 2 (four days later). I could see she was a bit angry as soon as I saw her in the waiting room. 'You've brought back my RSI,' she said, referring to repetition strain injury. 'What RSI?' I said. 'You didn't tell me about any arm pains.' 'Both arms are now aching,' she said, 'and I hadn't had it since my new job, and all my arm pains have come back since the last treatment.'

After my initial and natural despair, I thought that this actually made more sense of some of the features — more than after the last visit. The thoracic spine could perhaps be a source of the arm symptoms. It made the thoracic posture and the positive Slump Test more appropriate to her disorder. She said that she had not wanted to tell me about her repetition strain injuries last time. I realised that I would have to be particularly careful how I communicated with her. On physical examination findings were as follows:

- ULTT1 and 2 (radial and median) were positive for arm symptoms.
- ULTT1 reproduced a mid thoracic pain.
- Thoracic spine palpation of T4,5 was very stiff with local pain.
- Lumbar joint and tension signs related to the SLR were improved.
- Foot signs had not changed.

As a treatment, I manipulated the T4,5 level. On reassessment, there was a significant improvement in the ULTTs. There was some improvement also in the Slump and the SLRs. I also mobilised the T5,6 and the L2 to L4 levels, at a grade IV+. I also spent some time reassuring her and telling her that I understood her symptoms and how they could spread as they did.

Treatment 3 (4 days later). She was much happier than on the previous occasions and thought she was getting somewhere. All symptoms had eased, 'overall 30% better,' and the arm symptoms had nearly completely abated. There was a commensurate improvement in her signs, although her foot dorsiflexion, plantar flexion and the squat were only marginally better.

I thought of two broad directions to follow. I would continue to mobilise the relevant joints, and additionally assess the effect of nervous system mobilisation. I was also keen to assess the effect of local treatment of the foot. After all, that is what she came in for.

The last treatment was repeated, and in addition, I performed a technique on the foot. Rather than add a plantar flexion or dorsiflexion mobilisation, I preferred an accessory technique, one that would affect the joint but have a minimal effect on the adverse tension components. After examination, an anteroposterior pressure on the talus was found to be the most relevant sign, and I mobilised this well into resistance and local pain. On reassessment, ankle signs, including the squat, were improved. The SLR, both PFI/SLR and DF/SLR, were also improved. The extent of improvement, especially on the tension signs, surprised me.

Treatment 4 (3 days later). Subjective and physical improvements were maintained. The ULTT's were normal. The same treatment was repeated.

Treatment 5. All signs improved, '50% better'. The patient commented, 'I wasn't aware of how much this was limiting me in the past, I not only move better, I feel better in myself.'

The treatment was repeated, except for the thoracic spine which no longer required mobilising. With the response from treating the interfacing structures now known, I began to directly mobilise the nervous system. The techniques chosen were IN: SLR 60 reproducing foot pain, DID: Hip adduction $2 \times III$; and IN: DF, DID: SLR $2 \times IV$ (see Ch. 9 for notes on recording). Note that one SLR technique was performed by taking up the distal component first (dorsiflexion) and the second by taking up the hip flexion first. The through range technique (grade III) was performed because a detectable resistance and foot pain existed throughout the range of adduction.

On reassessment, this treatment provided an excellent response. After the nervous system mobilisation, the Slump Test and joint signs remaining in her lumbar spine and foot were improved.

I treated this woman once weekly for another 8 weeks, continuing to mobilise and manipulate her joints as required and progressing the nervous system mobilisation. This progression included adding the Slump Test as a treatment technique. Hunting for the foot pain necessitated that the SLR and the Slump be performed in combined spinal movements. I became more vigorous with tension techniques and the patient was conscientious with a home programme involving SLRs on the wall and Slump in longsitting, with the foot in both dorsiflexion and plantarflexion (see Ch. 11). One technique I found helpful with her (and subsequently with other patients) was an anteroposterior pressure on the talus while in Slump

Longsitting. Treatment also included balance work on a wobble board and self mobilisation of the ankle and spine. The patient continued netball and took up swimming. Her spinal posture improved. She said that she was '80% back to normal' and was prepared to continue to work on her ankle. Since her tension signs and spinal signs were clear, I felt this was appropriate to discharge her with the invitation to contact me if the disorder worsened or persisted.

AN EXAMPLE OF EXTRANEURAL PATHOLOGY

This patient's history was presented at a symposium by a fellow physiotherapist well versed in mobilisation of the nervous system.

Subjective examination

A 54 year old woman had a catheter inserted into her right brachial artery, as part of a series of tests for kidney function. Immediately after, she reported pins and needles in the inner aspect of her arm and down into her thumb, index finger and thenar eminence. Severe, constant pain in the same area began 2 days later. A mass of bruising, firm to palpate, extended from her axilla to her mid forearm.

She reported that any arm movement increased the pain and that the pain was not allowing her to sleep. The referral for physiotherapy was 12 days post catheterisation. At this time her symptoms were stable.

The physical examination on the first day of treatment was, by necessity, very limited due to pain and an apparently irritable disorder. All arm movements were stiff and painful. Cervical spine movement was close to full range. There were no neurological signs of altered conduction on manual testing, although muscle power could not be adequately examined due to pain. ULTT1 reproduced her pins and needles and hand pain with shoulder abduction to 80° and slight elbow extension. In this position, a small amount of cervical lateral flexion towards the left increased all symptoms.

Treatment

Treatment 1. The initial treatment was carefully performed with the patient's arm cradled in glenohumeral abduction of 80°, with elbow extension as the technique. Two sessions of 20 seconds duration, just short of increasing the symptoms (IN: gh ab 80, DID: ee II–2 × 20secs). The alternative position for performing an ULTT1 was used because more support could be given to the arm (refer to Fig. 8.2).

Treatment 2 (1 day later). The patient said she had no pain on the afternoon after treatment, although the same pains began again the next day. Paraesthesia had not altered. On examination, the painfree range of elbow extension in glenohumeral abduction of 80° was improved. The treatment selected was elbow extension, 2 sessions of 20 seconds duration at a grade III. While this technique was performed into resistance, great care was taken not to aggravate the symptoms (IN: gh ab 80, DID: ee III 2 × 20).

Treatment 3 (1 day later). The patient reported no pain since the previous treatment and although the tingling was still present, it was a little decreased. She was still not using her arm. On examination of ULTT1, at glenohumeral abduction of 80°, elbow extension was painless, although with wrist extension her pains could be provoked. If wrist extension was examined in 100° of abduction, the symptoms came on earlier in range. The treatment was wrist extension 2 × IV + performed in glenohumeral abduction of 80°, elbow extension and supination.

Treatment 4 (2 days later). The patient reported she had been free of symptoms since the previous treatment, although while walking her dog the previous night, it pulled on the leash and all of her symptoms had returned including some paraesthesia. On a re-examination of the neurological status, no measurable conduction deficit existed. The treatment techniques were repeated.

Treatment 5 (2 days later). She reported no pain since the previous treatment, although a persistent pins and needles remained. Wrist extension in the full ULTT1 position reproduced the symptoms. Unilateral passive accessory movements on the right C5,6 zygapophyseal joint reproduced a stiffness and local pain that was not present on the left side or higher and lower in the cervical spine. There was a positive ULTT2 (median), although the ULTT1 was the more symptomatic test. ULTT3 was negative. The stiff zygapophyseal joint was mobilised. On assessment of the ULTT1, the wrist could be taken further into extension before the pain came on. The same tension treatment as at the last session was performed.

Treatment 6 (+ 7 days). The patient reported there had been no pain, just occasional minimal paraesthesia in the thumb. The same treatment was performed and she was given a self mobilising exercise (see Ch. 11). Her cervical spine had normal movements on overpressures and palpation. The patient was discharged and advised to contact the physiotherapist if any symptoms reoccurred. At a 3 month telephone checkup, she reported that there had been no symptoms and no limitations placed by her arm.

Discussion

In the lower part of the arm, the brachial artery runs alongside the median nerve. In the case study, uncontrolled bleeding appears to have surrounded the nerve and also tracked up and down the arm in fascial and muscle planes. Lundborg & Dahlin (1989) referred to this situation where the nerve bed appears occluded with blood thus limiting the normal excursion of the nerve as the 'stuck nerve'.

After damage to a blood vessel, especially an artery, damage to a nerve is possible. Two mechanisms could be implicated in this case study. Firstly, if the blood vessel is a crucial feeder vessel, neuroischaemic damage may occur. More likely, however, the pressures around the nerve have been altered by the physical presence of blood. Alterations of blood flow to axons may have occurred and a process of nerve hypoxia and intrafascicular oedema proceeded (see Ch. 3). If the situation persists, intraneural fibrosis could ensue, some of which may be irreversible. Co-existing with these events, the epineurium would be irritated and probably involved in the fibrosing

blood and oedema. Dunkerton & Boome (1988) noted in a series of patients with stab wounds affecting brachial plexus signs and symptoms, that 'many patients' had a false aneurysm without a direct nerve injury. Some required urgent surgery and some required later neurolysis.

From the presenting signs and symptoms and the history, it may be hypothesised that this patient's tension test limitation is primarily due to an extraneural pathology. There is no evidence of a conduction deficit, it is of recent origin, there is no direct trauma to the nervous system, and all movements hurt. It can be hypothesised that the symptoms are likely to come from irritated epineurium. However, nerve fibres could possibly be hypoxic and discharging ectopically, especially given the extent of the bleed and the symptoms of paraesthesia. It is notable during treatment that changes in pain were not necessarily accompanied by changes in paraesthesia. Perhaps the symptoms have come from different sources: pain from the connective tissues and paraesthesia from the nerve fibres. Other innervated tissues, such as the blood vessels, fascia and muscles may also contribute to the symptomatology.

Clinical reasoning processes associated with treatment must relate to the high likelihood that the disorder, at this stage, is primarily related to an extraneural pathology and that movement of the nerve in relation to the surrounding structures is necessary. To use Lundborg & Dahlin's terminology, it must be 'unstuck'. The response to treatment, via gentle through range movements, is further proof of the site of the disorder. The attention given to the cervical spine provides a good example of thinking along the tract. The stiffness in the C5,6 joint could have been there prior to the injury but it may have been initiated by the injury. A more complex presentation would have been evident if the joint began to refer pain into the arm. The reasons for performing a technique employing more tension (Treatment 3) were the symptoms of tingling (perhaps from an intraneural source). There is also the possibility of an intraneural oedema after this period of time. Of course symptoms would have to be reproduced by such a technique.

Some physiotherapists may consider that 2 sessions of 20 seconds of actual manual treatment is not giving the patient value for money. The physiotherapist treating this patient wanted to find the origin of the symptoms and to evaluate the new concept of nervous system mobilisation, without complicating the management by using other modalities. Some physiotherapists may like to add in other modalities such as electrotherapy. However, this physiotherapist learnt an enormous amount about this disorder without applying a basket of treatments. The result has justified the treatment selection.

As well as a good public relations exercise, check-ups after treatment are a good learning exercise. A telephone call is often all that is necessary.

THE 'PAIN EVERYWHERE' KIND — WHERE TO START?

Subjective examination

A 45 year old woman fell onto her outstretched hands and sustained bilateral Colles' fractures 12 months prior to seeking treatment. The fractures were reduced and placed in a plaster of Paris cast for 6 weeks. There were no wrist or arm problems prior to the accident, although she had complained of some neck aches and pains: 'the kind that everyone gets'. Four months of physiotherapy to her hands had given her some relief and could ease her symptoms. However, she dropped things, her hands were swollen and were puffy and red. The right hand was worse than the left. She complained of spinal symptoms, headaches, and right leg pain as shown on the body chart (Fig. 14.1), all of which she said began after the fractures. Other than her general practitioner and the previous physiotherapist, no-one believed that her symptoms were genuine. Since the accident happened at work, she was on worker's compensation. Nobody had examined her spine.

During my examination, she seemed quite genuine and angry about the persistence of symptoms. She thought she would just have to put up with them. I thought it rather odd that she was still having wrist problems. She was otherwise healthy, and had received excellent physiotherapy to her wrists. My hypothesis was,

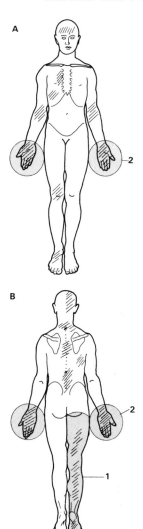

Fig. 14.1 Body chart showing the distribution of symptoms. The headaches were occasional, the chest pains were referred to as 'stabs'. The patient's whole leg (1) felt dead and 'wooden'. Both hands (2) were red, puffy and were constantly painful. She felt that her spinal pains were related and were worse when her hands were aggravated and swollen.

although there had to be local structural changes in wrist joints and muscles, there would be something maintaining the symptoms and that this could be spinal. There was a tension point pattern to the spinal symptoms suggesting a strong neural tension component. I accepted all her complaints and went on to see what physical findings there were that could match them.

Physical examination

Her wrists had about half the usual range of movement. Her elbows had full range of movement. Her grip was weak, the right more than the left. I wondered whether this could be a pain inhibited weakness, but otherwise there were no detectable changes in conduction. Her neck movements were limited to about half to two thirds normal range by stiffness and pain in the ipsilateral suprascapular fossa area, right worse than left. I had a quick look at her thoracic rotations. These were grossly restricted to about 10% and reproduced the same neck pains as elicited by neck rotation. Lumbar flexion caused central lumbar pain and midthoracic pain when her hands reached patella level. The addition of cervical flexion made these symptoms worse. Lumbar extension reproduced neck pain, even when the neck was carefully supported.

A recognisable pattern of symptom presentation was now becoming obvious and I felt reassured that her symptoms were valid. On examination of her nervous system, the right SLR at 20° caused back pain and a pulling sensation in her neck. Similar pains were produced by the left SLR at 40°. I did not need to add any sensitising movements because the neck pain had already been reproduced and I was a little unsure of how irritable the disorder was. On tension testing, if wrist extension was held on pain, this could be worsened by the addition of elbow extension and further worsened if the shoulder was taken into abduction. There were also limitations to all of the base ULTTs.

The initial treatment

With such widespread, marked and potentially confusing signs and symptoms, it can be difficult to know where to start. There are some factors related to the assessment that must be taken into account when deciding the treatment:

• The spine, neuraxis and meninges, i.e., the spinal canal component to the adverse tension, must be addressed.
• Attention will have to be directed to joints, nerves and later, muscles.
• Techniques will need to be taken into some resistance to alter pathomechanics.

• The disorder is potentially irritable.
• With such a lengthy duration of symptoms and spread of symptoms and signs, the prognosis is only fair.
• Treatment may be prolonged and will require the patient to do plenty of self mobilisation.

There were three alternative suggestions for the starting treatment.

• With the knowledge that the wrist had been mobilised quite vigorously in the past, this could be treated firmly, and an ULTT manoeuvre added. For example, the wrist could be held in a position of symptom reproduction, elbow extension added and then a glenohumeral movement such as abduction or depression used as the technique. The cervical spine, wrist, and the tension tests, including the SLR, need reassessment.
• Any spinal joints could be mobilised and perhaps manipulated. One should be prepared for changes in any of the signs and symptoms with treatment to one area.
• If mobilisation of the nervous system was decided on, techniques such as the SLR, or ULTT on the left (less painful) arm could be attempted. For example, IN: Hip flexion DID: Knee extension, or IN: SLR 20 degrees DID: Hip Adduction.

My treatment selection with this patient was to attend to the interfacing structures first. There were plenty of comparable signs in the joints and muscles and no overt conduction changes. I mobilised relevant joints in her lumbar and thoracic spine.

I treated this woman for 3 months, twice per week. Her spinal movements and tension signs improved markedly and to a much lesser extent, her hands improved as well. One of the first symptoms to change was the feeling of swelling in her hands. Although I achieved only a small increase in wrist ranges of movement, her functional ability improved greatly. Progression was not straightforward. There were some periods of up to a fortnight where she was worse, although at each time I could point to an improvement in physical signs. I think it takes time for structures to get used to different relations with the adjacent structure, and this was a helpful idea to give her to work through the difficult periods. I was also aware that I had to treat all relevant structures. A typical treatment session could involve mobilisation of the lumbar cervical and thoracic spine, trapezius and levator scapulae stretches, wrist mobilisation and mobilisation of the SLRs and ULTTs. This would take half to three quarters of an hour.

Overall, she thought she was 60% back to normal. I was happy with that and left her with mobilising exercises and the knowledge that she could contact me or her doctor if there were any exacerbations. She required three treatments to loosen up a stiff neck three months later. I would not be surprised if she requires further treatment in the future.

Thoughts on the 'pain everywhere' type

All physiotherapists have stories about patients who, on being asked where the problem is, describe vast and often apparently unrelated areas of their body and give descriptive and sometimes colourful explanations of their symptoms. The patient has often tried various remedies and a variety of practitioners. The patient's descriptions of symptoms often invite disbelief. Thoughts about whether physiotherapy can help and 'where do I start' emerge. Sometimes the doctor referring the patient may not have the answer either, and the patient is referred on to physiotherapy because the doctor does not know what to do with him/her, or because physiotherapy is seen as a last resort.

These patients must be believed, at least initially. With an understanding of the patterns of presentation of adverse tension, bizarre and odd symptoms may be quite feasible. For some of these patients with widespread symptoms it is hoped that the information contained in the first two parts of this book will allow some elucidation. We need to remember always that we are an unknown distance on the way to total understanding of neuro-orthopaedic disorders.

Thoughts should arise with any unfamiliar presentation regarding the possibilities of a sinister process, such as carcinoma or rheumatoid arthritis. This kind of patient must be under medical referral. To go on with an assessment and treatment, there has to be some evidence on physical examination that matches in some way with the complaint, or at least part of the complaint.

A TYPICAL TENNIS ELBOW?

Subjective examination

An extremely cheerful 62-year-old woman presented with an 8-month history of right sided lateral elbow pain or 'tennis elbow', as she said. She could not recall any initiating incident, but thought it may have been due to a lot of knitting during the winter. She could isolate a spot pain just distal to the right lateral epicondyle and an ache in the extensor muscle belly about 5 cm–7 cm distal to the elbow crease. The symptoms were constant. She could recall similar pains in the same elbow 12 years ago. These pains were worse in the morning, and with most activities, especially repetitious movements. She adored knitting but she had to limit this to short sessions of 15 minutes. A number of electrotherapy treatments had not helped her.

Physical examination

The relevant findings were as follows:

• There were limitations of right cervical rotation and extension.
• Unilateral passive accessory movements on the right C5 segment were stiff and produced local pain.
• The spots on the lateral epicondyle of the elbow and in the extensors were painful to palpate. The pain elicited on palpation of the common extensor belly could also be reproduced by palpation of the supinator muscle, full pronation of the forearm and resisted supination.
• Extension/adduction movements of the elbow reproduced the spot pain.
• Static resisted contraction (SRC) of wrist extension reproduced both elbow pains. Only a minimal contraction was possible before pain was produced.
• SRC of extension of the middle finger reproduced both elbow pains, and to a lesser extent, so did a SRC of the index finger extension.

• All base ULTTs had more resistance to movement on the right side than the left side. The ULTT2 radial bias test reproduced a 'familiar' elbow pain, made worse by shoulder abduction and eased by the most gentle release of depression.

• Her trapezius and levator scapulae were tight especially on the right side.

• A neurological examination of muscle strength was difficult due to the pain. On questioning, she said her web space on the right side had 'lost a bit of feeling'. On examination, light touch and vibration sense were decreased compared to the left side. The decrease in vibration sense was noted on the radial styloid and at the base of the first metacarpal.

Thoughts regarding management

This is a rather typical case of chronic tennis elbow. I also find that adverse neural tension is a common finding, especially a positive ULTT2 radial bias test. Often electrotherapy does not help or gives temporary relief only.

I recognised a pattern from the subjective and physical examination and felt sure there was a component of adverse tension in the disorder that would need addressing. This hypothesis was based on the following findings:

• The positive radial nerve bias tension test.
• The evidence of neurological involvement.
• Co-existing cervical signs, perhaps indicative of a double crush type of syndrome.
• SRC of the middle finger was positive. This contracts the extensor carpi radialis brevis muscle which presents a fibrous edge to the posterior interosseus nerve (deep radial nerve) in the radial tunnel in the supinator muscle.
• Contraction and stretch of supinator reproduced symptoms. This possibly suggested some involvement of the posterior interosseus nerve in the radial tunnel.

I also felt the area of symptoms was indicative of nervous system involvement. Entrapment in the radial tunnel is well known but I am of the opinion that the common spot pain on or around the lateral epicondyle is often neurogenic in origin.

Small nerves destined for the epicondylar structures may be caught in scarred muscle or fascia and an abnormal impulse generating site may form. The pain can often be proven as neurogenic in origin by structural differentiation. It is also easy to treat via mobilisation of the nervous system.

I was also aware of joint and muscle signs in the cervical spine and neck that would need addressing.

Making a prognosis

Following the examination, I weighed up my findings to make some sort of prognosis. I thought that she could be helped. My reasoning for this was there had been inadequate treatment in the past. The patient was 'on side' and would assist me in any way possible. There was no history of severe trauma, and she presented with a pattern of lateral elbow pain that I had been able to assist in the past.

On the other hand I had to consider factors that would go against a good prognosis. There was constant chronic pain. It was probable that multiple structures and contributing factors were involved (elbow joint, cervical spine, nervous system). The nervous system component was probably intraneural and intrafascicular given the constant pain, lengthy history and the conduction changes. There was heightened nervous system mechanosensitivity. The nervous system was involved in a number of areas (deep and superficial radial nerves, perhaps nerve root, perhaps some sympathetic maintenance). And there was muscle weakness and disuse.

I took an educated guess and wrote down on my patient's notes that I was hopeful for 60% improvement in 6 weeks. I saw her twice a week.

Treatment

Treatment 1. Mobilisation of the right C5,6 zygapophyseal joints via unilateral posteroanterior pressure. The technique was performed into resistance with reproduction of local pain (2 × IV+). Reassessment showed improvement in all SRCs, ULTT (radial) and range of cervical rotation. This was more of an improvement than I expected. I discussed the possibility of treatment soreness and impressed upon her that I needed to know about any changes on her return.

Treatment 2. (3 days later). I noted the improvement had been maintained. The patient commented that the pain below the elbow had eased somewhat and was now more above the elbow. I felt this made the hypothesis of adverse tension a bit stronger as the common extensor muscles or even the radiohumeral joint was unlikely to behave in this way. Treatment was repeated, plus IN: ULTT2 (rad) DID: GH abduction 2 × IV. All signs improved again.

Treatment 3. (4 days later). No improvement. General elbow soreness for 4 days, settled now to the level of the previous treatment. She also reported she been quite dizzy for 2 days after the treatment. On questioning, she suffered dizziness for 8 years; it had been extensively examined by medical specialists and no reason found for it. However, it was worse during the 4 days that the elbow was aggravated. I realised the error of not enquiring about dizziness earlier, but understood how this error had occurred. My hypothesis was initially strongly elbow and adverse tension. I did not expect such an initial beneficial response from the cervical spine and the necessary change in hypothesis caught me off guard.

On examination, all improvements in physical signs from the previous treatment were maintained, except the SRC of supinator and the wrist extensors. I repeated the cervical mobilisation and then, in an ULTT2 (radial bias) position, mobilised the wrist in extension. All signs improved.

Treatment 4. (3 days later). Improvement maintained. Dizziness had settled. The cervical mobilisation was repeated, plus upper trapezius stretches. Trapezius stretches had a beneficial effect on the relevant physical signs, especially the ULTT, and were notably more painful with the elbow straight. The same ULTT mobilisation, as in the previous treatment, was performed.

Treatment 5. All improved. The cervical joint and muscle treatment was repeated. The tension technique was progressed to IN: ULTT2 (rad) DID: elbow extension 1 × IV+.

Treatment 6. Marked improvement in elbow pains and functional levels. She was able to knit

for several hours but still experienced some pains on lifting. There was still some dizziness, but she felt this was 'back to the normal level'. She thought that overall she was 70% improved. On physical examination:

- SRC wrist — slight pain.
- SRC middle finger — painless.
- ULTT2 (radial bias) — slight pain only.
- Extension/adduction of the elbow produced a sharp pain at the lateral epicondyle.
- Light touch and vibration sensation were improved, but still not normal.

I treated IN: ULTT2 (rad) DID: Elbow extension/adduction 1 × IV+. I felt sure I could treat this strongly and that my combined technique getting at the joint and the nerve component would be beneficial. On examination there was a good improvement in physical signs.

Treatment 7. (14 days later). The patient had been on holidays. She reported she had been particularly sore for 9 days including all pains in her elbow. There was no aggravation of her dizziness. 'This doesn't fit,' I thought, and went back through my treatment to try and work out why. I ascertained that she had not done anything unusual that could have aggravated the elbow. I felt I had misread the irritability of the disorder and should have questioned the patient further when she said she felt 70% improved. I should have asked more questions about what activities she had been doing. If the prognostic factors were weighed up and I considered my initial 60% hoped for, perhaps the last treatment had been a little too vigorous. On examination, I thought the physical signs had maintained their improvement.

For treatment, I performed a similar treatment IN: ULTT2 (rad) DID: elbow extension 2 × IV. I also performed a more joint orientated technique of elbow extension and adduction 1 × IV.

This woman continued to improve a little and was left at about the 70% improvement mark. Her dizziness was no different to her pre treatment level. I felt comfortable about leaving her at that. She was far happier, especially now that she could knit. We discussed some anti-tension position for her to knit in. I told her to avoid low chairs and to take her body out of the knitting position regularly. I advised cervical retraction mobilisation and some hand above head activities. She asked me about Tai Chi activities. I thought they would be marvellous for her.

The role of adverse tension in lateral elbow pain

Tennis elbow provides a superb example of mechanical involvement of the nervous system in a disorder. 'Radial tunnel syndrome' has been described by many authors, among them Roles & Maudsley (1972), Lister et al (1979), Dawson et al (1983) Lundborg (1988), Mackinnon & Dellon (1988), Peimer & Wheeler (1989). They reason that a possible source of failure in treatment for tennis elbow is if the symptoms are neurogenic, and if this component has not addressed surgically. I also feel that branches of the radial nerve, prior to entry into the supinator, may also be responsible.

From my anecdotal clinical experience, I believe adverse neural tension plays a significant role which needs treatment in approximately 75% of lateral elbow pains. Many clinicians now prescribe tennis elbow straps, the rationale being that compression around the common extensor muscle a few centimetres below the epicondyle gives the muscles a false origin, thus taking some pressure off the pathological origin. Note that this could well alter nerve biomechanics. A colleague of mine told me a story of a patient who inadvertently put the strap on above the elbow rather than below and came back for treatment saying that it was a wonderful help for his pain. Elbow joint and muscle could not be altered in this case, but the nerve probably is.

A PASSING MENTION OF FINGER TIP PAIN.

I treated a 60-year-old gentleman for some weeks for knee pain due to osteoarthritis of the knee. There were no tension signs relevant to the knee and he was making good progress with mobilisation of the tibiofemoral joint, heat, and strengthening of his quadriceps and hamstrings. One day just as he was leaving the treatment area, he said, 'You couldn't do anything for the tip of my finger could you?' Before I could tell him how busy I was and that I could perhaps look at it next time, he said, 'I get it when I push a door closed with my outstretched arm. It's just annoying.' I quickly became interested and told him that I would look at it for a couple of minutes. He had no history of trauma and I knew from the knee examination, that there were no systemic or general health concerns. I got him to demonstrate the position and noted that it appeared to be the protraction of the shoulder girdle that hurt the tip of the finger. A quick examination of finger and wrist joint and muscle revealed no abnormality. Light touch and vibration sense were normal. ULTT2 with the shoulder in depression/protraction reproduced the symptoms. I held him in this position and did 3 firm grade IV+ techniques of depression in protraction. On reassessment, he could push on the wall with decreased pain.

At the next treatment, we initially forgot about it since he was in the gymnasium. When I checked my notes and enquired about his finger he said that all symptoms went after that treatment. I wished that osteoarthritic knees could be as easy, but I also thought, '— What did I do?' Had I stretched some scarred epineurium? Had I perhaps freed up a blood vessel caught in some scar around a digital nerve? Perhaps the problem was more proximal in the plexus. What would have happened if the problem had persisted? Would a double crush type symptom have appeared elsewhere? Would it have improved by itself? I rechecked the tension tests related to the knee, convinced myself they were normal and went back to mobilising the tibiofemoral joint.

REFERENCES

Dawson D M, Hallett M, Millender L H 1983 Entrapment neuropathies. Little, Brown, Boston

Dunkerton M C, Boome R S 1988 Stab wounds involving the brachial plexus. Journal of Bone and Joint Surgery 70B: 566–570

Lister G D, Belsole R B, Kleinert H E 1979 The radial tunnel syndrome. Journal of Hand Surgery 4A: 52–60

Lundborg G 1988 Nerve injury and repair. Churchill Livingstone, Edinburgh

Lundborg G, Dahlin L B 1989 Pathophysiology of nerve compression. In: Szabo R M (ed) Nerve compression syndromes. Slack, Thorofare

Mackinnon S E, Dellon A L 1988 Surgery of the peripheral nerve. Thieme, New York

Peimer C A, Wheeler D R 1989 Radial tunnel syndrome/Posterior interosseus nerve compression. In: Szabo R M (ed) Nerve compression syndromes. Slack. Thorofare

Roles N C, Maudsley R 1972 Radial tunnel syndrome: resistant tennis elbow as a nerve entrapment. Journal of Bone and Joint Surgery 54B: 499–508

COURSES

Manipulative physiotherapy/clinical reasoning courses including the concepts and practice of mobilisation of the nervous system are available. They are taught by physiotherapists skilled in the use of the Maitland concept who have also attended advanced courses in mobilisation of the nervous system.

Those interested should get in touch with:

David Butler
P O Box 8143
Adelaide 5000
AUSTRALIA

Mark and Helen Jones
20 Rossall Road
Somerton Park 5044
AUSTRALIA

Bern and Ellen Guth
17248 Rolando Avenue
Castro Valley CA 94596
USA

Hugo Stam
Rheumaklinik
8437 Zurzach
SWITZERLAND

Robin Blake
Harrogate Physiotherapy Practice
37 East Parade
Harrogate HG1 5LQ
UNITED KINGDOM

Peter Wells
The Courses Secretary
The Physiotherapy Centre
37 Harwood Road
London SW6 4QP
UNITED KINGDOM

Index

Abbreviations: ANS autonomic nervous system; CNS central nervous system; CSF cerebrospinal fluid; NS nervous system; PKB Prone Knee Bend; PNF Passive Neck Flexion; PNS peripheral nervous system; RSI repetition strain injury; SLR Straight Leg Raise; ULTT Upper Limb Tension Tests

Achilles tendon rupture, 63
Activity specific mechanosensitivity, 86
Adverse neural tension, 1–86
    anomolies, 69–71
    chronic, 84
    clinical consequences of injury to ANS, 75–86
    clinical neurobiomechanics, 35–52
    defined, 55
    disorders based on the spinal canal, 231–246
        coccydynia and spondylisthesis, 238–239
        epidural haematomas, 238
        headache, 241–242
        loss of spinal tension, 235–236
        nerve root injuries, 231–235
        post lumbar spine surgery, 239–241
        T4 syndrome, 242–243
        trauma and inflammation of the neuraxis, 243–245
        whiplash *see* Whiplash
    disorders centred in limbs, 213–230
        extremities, 213–214
        foot and ankle, 214–218
        hand and wrist, 218–222
        intraneural and neural sites, 166–167
        meralgia paraesthetica, 222–223
        nerve lesion in lower limb muscle, 223–224
        peripheral nerve surgery, 224–226
        RSI *see* Repetition strain injury (RSI)
        thoracic outlet syndrome, 222
    functional anatomy and physiology of NS, 3–30
    pathological processes, 55–71
    syndromes, 81, 83
    temporal factors, 71
AIDS, 105, 109
Ankle *see* Foot and ankle

Arachnoiditis, 64, 239
Arthritis, cervical, 65–66
Autonomic nervous system (ANS), 10
    adaptive mechanisms, 44–45
    biomechanics, 35–52
    postganglionic fibres, 10
    preganglionic fibres, 10
        head and neck, 10
    preganglionic neurones, 45
    and somatic NS, 10
    sympathetic ganglia, 10
    sympathetic trunk, 10
    tests of, 122
Axonal transport systems, 25–26, 79
    antegrade, 25 26, 64
    injuries, 63
    retrograde, 26, 64
Axons, 3, 4, 5–6
    in ANS, 10
    axoplasm, 5, 63–64
    in central nervous system (CNS), 13
    not straight, 14

Birth paralysis, 11
Blood nerve-barriers, 23–25
Bowstring test, 135
Brachial neuritis, 65
Brachial plexus
    as force distribution, 5
    injuries to, 11
    internal and external formations, 110
Brachial Plexus Tension Test *see* Upper Limb Tension Tests (ULTT)
Brachialgic sciatica, 50

Carpal tunnel
    interfacing structures, 58
    pressure gradients, 59–60
    wick catheter experiments, 61–62
Carpal tunnel syndrome, 65, 66, 124

bilateral, 50
chronic, 84
in hand or wrist, 220–221
testing, 122
Case studies, 247–259
    extraneural pathology, 251–253
    finger tip pain, 258
    foot pain, 247–251
    pain everywhere, 253–255
    tennis elbow, 255–258
Cauda equina
    examination, 109
    treatment, 106
Central nervous system (CNS), 10–16
    continuous tissue track with PNS, 3
    junction with PNS, 11
    meninges *see* Meninges
    nerve roots *see* Nerve roots
    neuraxis *see* Neuraxis
Cerebrospinal fluid (CSF)
    in subarachnoid spaces, 15–16
    in subdural spaces, 16
Cerebrovascular accidents, 244
Circulation, 19–25
Clinical correlations, 50
Clinical neurobiomechanics, 35–54
    ANS adaptive mechanisms, 44–45
    concept of tension points, 46–49
    other biomechanical considerations, 49–52
    SLR, 41–43
    spinal canal, neuraxis and meninges, 37–41
    upper limb adaptive mechanisms, 43–44
Clinical reasoning, 91–106
    analysing structures and contributing factors, 96–98
    characteristics of expertise, 95–96
    inquiry strategies, 98–101
    precautions and contraindications, 104–106
    process, 92–95
    structural differentiation, 102–104

Coccydynia and spondylisthesis, 238–239
Colles' fracture, 218–220
Connective tissues
    dural pain, 75–77
    injuries to epineurium, 62
    innervation, 29, 75
    sheath, 7
    see also Meninges
Cord function testing, 122–123
    physical, 123
    subjective, 122–123
Cumulative Trauma Disorder see Repetition strain injury (RSI)
Cuteaneous innervation fields, 112–113

De Quervain's disease, 213, 221–222
    misdiagnosis, 227
Demyelination, 62
Dermatomes, 111
Diabetes, 50, 66, 67, 105, 109
Diagnosis and prognosis see Clinical reasoning
Disc surgery, 65
Dizziness, 105, 109
Dorsal root ganglion (DRG), 61
Double crush syndrome, 65–68, 81
Dura mater, 16, 17, 26–27
    as source of pain, 75–77, 81
Dural headache, 241–242
Dural ligaments, 16–18, 19, 28
'Dural pain', inadequacy of term, 75–77

Electrodiagnosis, 123–125
Elvey's Test see Upper Limb Tension Tests (ULTT)
Endoneurial fluid pressure (EFP), 24
Endoneurium, 6, 7
Epidural haematomas, 238
Epineurium, 8
    fascicular arrangement, 9–10
Examination, 91–180
    application, analysis and further testing, 147–159
    clinical reasoning, 91–106
    nerve conduction, 107–125
    palpation techniques, 172–175
    tension testing of lower limbs and trunk, 127–145
    tension testing of upper limbs, 147–159
    see also Tension testing; Testing
Extension and flexion see Flexion and extension
Extraneural pathology (Case study), 251–153

Failed back syndrome, 65, 240
Fibrosis
    consequence of, 68
    extraneural, 179–180
    friction fibrosis, 60
    intermeningeal, 239

intraneural, 60, 71, 179–80
    and nerve injury, 64–65
    and pressure gradients, 59, 60, 61, 69
    spinal, 239
Fingertip pain (case study), 258
Flexion and extension, 4, 14, 62
    ankle dorsiflexion, 49, 50, 132–133
    cervical, 49, 134–135
    peroneal nerve, 214–216
    spinal canal, 37–41, 51–52
    sural nerve, 218
    tibial nerve, 216–218
Flexion/inversion
    plantar,
        of ankle, 63
        of foot, 52
Foot and ankle
    ankle dorsiflexion, 49, 50, 132–133
    disorders, 214–218
    foot pain (case study), 247–251
    plantar flexion/inversion, 52, 63, 133
Force distribution, 11, 12
    brachial plexus, 5, 14
Frank cord injury, 105
Frozen shoulder, 69

Gravity, effects, 52
Guillain Barré, 244–245

Hamstring
    pain, 140
    tears, 224
Hand and wrist disorders, 218–222
    carpal tunnel syndrome, 220–221
    Colles' fracture, 218–220
    de Quervain's tenosynovitis, 221–222
Headaches
    dural, 241–242
    post lumbar puncture, 242
Hip adduction, 133–134
Hip medial rotation, 134
Hurdler's stretch, in self treatment, 208
Hypoxia, 59, 60

Injuries
    and axoplasmic flow, 63–64
    bullet, 71
    carpal tunnel see Carpal tunnel syndrome
    chronic, 56, 57
    clinical consequences, 75–88
    connective tissues, 62, 68
    denervation supersensitivity, 69
    double crush syndrome, 65–68, 81
    frank cord, 105
    frank trauma, 58
    irreversible, 71
    irritative, 65, 66
    kinds, 57
    mechanical factors, 58, 62–63
    and movement, 80

multiple crush, 66, 81
nerve, 175–180
    classification of, 175–180
    contracture of NS, 68–69
    neural lesions, 65
    peripheral nerve, 176–177
    postural and movement patterns, 84–86
    pre-existing, 56, 69, 83
    predispositions to, 56, 57
    prespondylosis, 69
    repercussions, 57
    reversed crush, 66
    secondary, 57
    sites of, 55–57
    spinal cord, 106
    subclinical entrapment, 56, 57, 69
    sudden more severe, 71
    temporal factors, 71
    triple crush, 66
    vascular factors, 58–62
    whiplash see Whiplash
Interfacing structures, treatment, 193–194
Intervertebral foramen (IVF)
    effects of movement, 39–40
    plugging of, 12
Irritable disorder, treatment, 188–190

Joint-specific treatment, disadvantages of, xiii

Klapp's crawling exercise, 243

Lazarevics test, 130
Leprosy, 105
Leptmeninges see Meninges
Leseague's test, 130, 131
Lhermitte's sign and movement, 85
Limbs
    adverse neural tension disorders, 212–230
    carpal tunnel see Carpal tunnel syndrome
    Colles' fracture, 218
    de Quervain's disease, 213, 221–222
    disorders in extremities, 213–214
    foot and ankle see Foot and ankle
    hamstring tears, 224
    meralgia paraesthetica, 222
    nerve lesion, 223–224
    peripheral nerve surgery, 224–226
    peroneal nerves, 214–216
    sural nerve, 218
    thoracic outlet syndrome, 222
    tibial nerve, 216–218
    see also Repetition strain injury (RSI)

Maitland techniques in examination, 79, 86, 98–101, 108, 187
Martin Gruber anastamosis, 70
Mechanical interface, 35–36
    spinal canal as, 37–40

Meninges, 4, 5, 14–16, 17
  arachnoid mater, 14–15
  and CSF, 15–16
  dural innervation, 26–28
  flexion and extension, 40–41
  innervation, 26–29
  pia mater, 14–15
  spinal canal contents, 15–16
  subarachnoid space, 15–16
  subdural space, 15–16
  see also Dura mater
Meralgia paraesthetica, 222
Mesoneurium, 8
Mobilisation, basic principles,
  187–188
Motor function
  examination, 115–122
  muscle power testing, 117
  muscle testing lower limb, 120–122
  muscle testing upper limb, 117–120
  reflex testing, 115–117
  wasting, 115
Movement and injuries see Injuries
Multiple crush syndromes, 66, 81
Multiple sclerosis, 105, 109
Myelin, 4
  biomechanics of myelin sheath, 6
  in neurones, 5, 6

Nerve conduction examination,
  107–125
  cord function, 122–123
  electrodiagnosis, 123–125
  further testing and analysis, 122
  general points, 107–108
  motor function, 105–122
  subjective neurological, 108–109
Nerve fibres
  autonomic, 7
  motor, 7
  sensory, 7
  see also Axons
Nerve injury, classification, 175–80
Nerve roots, 10–13
  angulated or 'ascending', 12–13
  common causes of injuries, 11
  connective tissues, 10–11
    epidural, 11
    innervation, 29
    not joined to meninges, 11
    peripheral, 11
  and CSF, 12
  radicular pia, 11
  safety mechanisms, 11
  sheath, 11
  susceptible to injury, 10
  vasculature, 21–22
Nerve trunks, 4
  connective tissues, 10
Nervous system (NS)
  adapatations to movement, 36–37
  and AIDS, 105
  basis of symptoms, 19
  clinical consequences of injury,
    75–88

area of symptoms, 80–82
  history, 83–84
  pain, 75–79
  postural and movement patterns,
    84–86
and diabetes, 105
external connections of dura, 16–18
functional anatomy and physiology,
  3–33
impulse conduction, 3, 4
injury, 55–58
innervation, 26–30
interconnectedness of, 3, 55–57, 97
internal attachments of dura, 18
and leprosy, 105
movement and tension, 37
and multiple sclerosis, 105
neurotransmitters, 3
and pain, 75–79
palpation, 172–175
protective tissues, 4
signs and symptoms of injury,
  79–83
spaces and attachments, 16–19
and tumours, 105
vascularisation and tension points,
  47–48
see also Autonomic nervous system;
  Central nervous system;
  Peripheral nervous system
Neuraxis, 4, 5, 13–14, 17
  autonomic fibres, 44
  cerebrovascular accidents, 244
  flexion and extension, 40–41
  Guillain Barré, 244–245
  trauma and inflammation, 243–245
  vasculature, 20–21
Neurobiomechanics
  and neuropathology, 58, 65
  see also Clinical neurobiomechanics
Neuroglia, 4
Neurological signs, and treatment,
  105
Neurones, 5–7
  myelinated and unmyelinated, 5,
    6–7
Node of Ranvier, 5, 6
Normative studies, 49–50

Oedema, 59, 60, 61, 62
  and plaster of Paris, 69
Overuse injury see Repetition strain
  injury (RSI)

Pain
  'dural' inadequate term, 75–77
  hamstring, 140
  lateral elbow, neuro-orthopaedic
    sources of, 97
  lines and clumps, 81–82
  pain dysfunction syndrome, 227
  in peripheral nerve disorders, 77
  peripheral nerve trunk, 77–78
  and PNF, 50
  and SLR, 46–47

sources, 75–79
  see also Injuries; Symptoms
Parathesia and movement, 85
Passive Neck Flexion (PNF), 76,
  105, 128–130
  and movement, 51
  responses to, 50, 76
  test, 40
Pathological processes, 55–71
  factors in adverse tension
    processes, 69–71
  injury to NS, 55–58, 64–69
  minor nerve injury, 69
Pathology
  intraneural and extraneural, 57–58
  see also Injuries
Patients, importance of questioning,
  79, 82
Perineurium, 4, 7–8
Peripheral nervous system (PNS),
  5–10
  attachments, 18–19
  autonomic fibres, 44
  connective tissue, 3, 7, 48, 78
  defined, 5
  endoneurium, 6, 7
  epineurium, 8
    fascicular arrangement, 9–10
  innervation, 29–30
  junction with CNS, 12
  mesoneurium, 8
  more vulnerable than CNS, 4–5
  neurones, 5–7
  and pain, 77–78
  peripheral nerve surgery, 224–226
  vasculature, 22–23
  see also Autonomic nervous system
    (ANS)
Plantar flexion/inversion see Foot and
  ankle
Plaster of Paris and oedema, 69
Post lumbar puncture headache, 242
Post lumbar spine surgery, 238–241
  acute post-surgical patient, 240
  chronic post-surgical patient,
    240–241
Posture
  antalgic tension, 84, 85
  fixed forward head, 85
  movement patterns, 85–86
  poked chin, 84
  postural patterns, 84–85
  in self treatment, 209–210
Prespondylosis, 69
Prone Knee Bend (PKB), 136–139
  biomechanics, 138–139
  in self treatment, 206
  and Slump Test, 137–138

Radial nerve
  and de Quervain's disease, 221–222
  in palpation, 175
  'Saturday night palsy', 57
  vulnerability, 56
Rats tail formation, 69

Renaut bodies, 65
Repetition strain injury (RSI), 47,
    83, 86, 226–228
  aspects of treatment, 228
  and posture, 227–228
  and ULTT, 226–227
Reversed crush syndromes, 66

Saphoneus nerve
  in foot, 214
  tension test, 138
'Saturday night palsy', 57
Schwann cells, 4, 5, 6
  necrosis, 62
Sciatic brachialgia, 50
Self treatment
  assistance in, 204
  combination slumps, 206–208
  hurdler's stretch, 208
  mobilisation, 203–205
  PKB, 206
  posture, 209–210
  prophylaxis, 210
  self mobilisation, 203–205
  SLR, 205–206
  slump positions, 206–208
  ULTT, 208–209
  useful techniques, 205–209
Sensation, 109–115
  and age, 115
  light touch, 110–111
  physical examination of, 109–115
  pinprick, 111–114
  proprioception, 114
  two point discrimination, 115
  vibration, 114
Slump Test
  biomechanics, 144–145
  care required, 104, 105, 141–142
  and kneee extension, 14
  in longsitting, 143
  responses to, 45, 85
  and spinal flexion, 40
  and tension, 47, 51–52
  and traction, 39
Somatic nervous system see
    Autonomic nervous system
    (ANS)
spasticity, 69
Spinal canal, 17
  adverse neural tension disorders,
    231–246
  cervical,
    flexion and extension, 39, 51–52
    meninges in, 38
    neuraxis in, 38
    shape, 38
  flexion and extension, 4, 37–41,
    51–52
    loss of spinal extension, 235–236
    lumbar, 2
  headaches, 241–242
  low lumbar, shape, 38
  as mechanical interface, 37–41
  mid thoracic, shape, 38

nerve root injuries, 231–235
  acute cervical, 231–233
  chronic cervical, 233–235
  loss of spinal extension, 235–236
  and SLR, 232
  thoracic syndromes, 235
  and ULTT, 232
post lumbar spine surgery, 239–241
T4 syndrome, 242–243
trauma and inflammation of
  neuraxis, 243–245
vasculature, 20–21
whiplash see Whiplash
Spinal cord
  of child, 15
  compression post injury, 61
  tethered cord syndrome, 106
Spinal fibrosis, 239
Spinal stenosis, 64
Spinal surgery, 69, 239–241
Spiral bands of Fontana, 6
Stoop test (Dyck), 38–39
Straight Leg Raise (SLR)
  back pain, 75–77
  bilateral, 135
  biomechanics, 136
  crossed, 135
  and diagnosis, 130–136
  and dizziness, 109
  and NS, 35
  and pain, 46–47, 50, 76
  with PFI, 52
  responses to, 45, 50–51, 52, 76, 85
  in self treatment, 205–206
  symptoms evoked by, 45, 76
  and tension, 37, 39, 41–43, 103
Subclinical entrapment, 69
Sural nerve disorders in foot and
    ankle, 174, 218
Sympathetic chain, 44–45
  lumbar, 46
Sympathetic ganglia, 10
Sympathetic trunk, 44–45
  of ANS, 10
Symptoms
  abnormal impulse generating
    mechanisms, 68
  area, 80–82
  basis, 19
  intermittent and constant, 82
  kinds, 82–83
  patterns, 80, 81–82
  shifting, 81
  time of day, 83, 85
  of tumours, 50

T4 syndrome, 242–243
Tennis elbow, 63
  case study, 255–258
Tension
  and compression, 51
  and movement distribution, 50–51
  in neck flexion, 49
Tension points, 46–49
Tension testing, 80

analysis of, 161–165
development, 167–170
essential features of analysis,
    163–165
establishing sites of adverse
    tension, 165–167
lower limbs and trunks, 127–145
  base tension tests, 127–128
  PKB, 136–139
  PNF, 128–130
  SLR, 130–136
  Slump Test, 139–145
recording, 171–172
sites of adverse tension, 165–167
taking tension testing further,
    167–170
upper limbs, 147–180
  see also Upper Limb Tension
    Tests (ULTT)
Testing
  classification of nerve injury,
    175–180
  essentials, 161
  free arm hanging test, 169
  Lazarevics test, 130
  Leseague's test, 130, 131
  palpation of the NS, 172–175
  quick, 170
  and recording, 171–172
  relevance of findings, 161
  stoop test (Dyck), 38–39
Tethered cord syndrome, 106, 109
Thoracic nerve root syndromes, 235
Thoracic outlet syndrome, 222
Tibial nerve disorders in foot and
    ankle, 174, 216–218
Tinel's sign, 10, 122, 173
  and movement, 85
Traction, 39
Treatment, 185–201
  basic principles of mobilisation,
    187–188
  commonly asked questions,
    194–198
  communication, 199–201
  general points, 185–187
  history, 185, 188
  interfacing structures, 193–194
  irritable disorder, 188–190
  non-irritable disorder, 190–193
  pathomechanical dominance,
    190–193
  pathophysiological dominance,
    188–190
  prognosis making, 198–199
  and treatment potential, 183–210
  see also Self treatment
Triple crush syndromes, 66
Tumours
  Pancoast's, 105
  symptoms, 50

Ulnar nerve in palpation, 175
Upper limb adaptive mechanisms,
    43–44

Upper Limb Tension Tests (ULTT)
  and adaptive mechanisms, 44, 45
  biomechanics, 152–153
  care required, 104, 105
  and diagnosis, 147–159
  and reassment, 101
  in self treatment, 208–209
  symptoms evoked, 50
  and tension, 103

Wallerian degeneration, 65
Whiplash
  and adaptive mechanisms, 45
  and ankle dorsiflexion, 50
  associated injuries, 68, 71, 97,
    236–237
  and NS, 236–238
  prognosis, 237–238
  and sympathetic chain, 61

  and tension, 47
  treatment, 237
Wrist and hand disorders, 218–222
  carpal tunnel syndrome, 220–221
  Colles' fracture, 218–220
  de Quervain's tenosynovitis,
    221–222